CLINICAL RADIOLOGY
OF THE
EAR, NOSE AND THROAT

CLINICAL RADIOLOGY OF THE EAR, NOSE AND THROAT

Second Edition

by

ERIC SAMUEL, C.B.E.

B.Sc., M.D., F.R.C.S. (Eng. & Edin.), F.R.C.P.E., F.R.C.R., D.M.R.E.
Forbes Professor of Medical Radiology, University of Edinburgh

and

GLYN A. S. LLOYD

M.A., D.M., F.R.C.R.
Director, Department of Radiology,
Royal National Throat, Nose & Ear Hospital, London

Foreword by

DONALD F. N. HARRISON

M.D., M.S., F.R.C.S.
Professor of Laryngology & Otology, University of London

LONDON
H.K. LEWIS & CO. LTD.
1978

First Published 1952
Second Edition 1978

©

H. K. LEWIS & Co. Ltd.
1978

ISBN 0 7 186 0437 7

PRINTED FOR H. K. LEWIS & CO. LTD.
BY THE WHITEFRIARS PRESS LTD., LONDON AND TONBRIDGE

Foreword

By DONALD HARRISON   *Professor of Laryngology & Otology, University of London*

The Radiologist and his colleagues are without doubt an essential and integral part of every medical team. Naturally, their role will vary with different disciplines but to the Otorhinolaryno-ologist they are absolutely essential to the proper practice of his specialty. In the last decade tremendous advances have been made in the development of radiological equipment and techniques, few specialties have benefited more from these advances than my own and this book is a comprehensive and detailed account of the multitudinous ways in which the experienced radiologist can assist the ENT surgeon. We are most fortunate to have as editors two radiologists who have achieved international recognition for their contributions to ENT Radiology. Each chapter therefore, is a condensation of a wealth of experience illustrated by examples taken from their own unique material. This ensures that this book is up to date and reliable thus filling a gap in both the Radiological and ENT literature. Nothing has been omitted and its assured success must bring credit to both them and their specialty.

Preface

The time lapse since the previous edition has seen many major advances in the diagnosis and treatment of diseases of the ear, nose and throat. The advent of antibiotics has had a major influence on the treatment of infections and the demands for radiological examination are of a different calibre from those requested at the time of the original edition.

Likewise the development of sophisticated tomographic equipment has made the detailed visualisation of the middle and inner ear feasible and more accurate.

Newer techniques of laryngography have now become accepted methods of early diagnosis of lesions of this structure.

The illustrations throughout this book are now printed in the negative mode to conform with current practice.

The authors are deeply indebted to their surgical and medical colleagues for their collaboration and helpfulness through the preparations of the text and their readiness to allow access to their clinical notes – in particular Professor D. Harrison, Mr J. F. Shaw, Mr C. J. Duncan, Dr A. Maran and Mr J. F. Birrell who have provided us with clinical photographs of cases under their care. Our numerous radiological colleagues have also been ready to help in all circumstances – Professor B-S. Jing, Dr S. P. Rawson, Dr S. Goldberg, Dr G. Green, Dr M. B. Denny, Dr G. T. Vaughan, Dr A. Langlands, Dr G. H. M. Landman, Dr N. Lewtas and Dr A. J. A. Wightman have all generously provided illustrative cases.

We are also indebted to Dr A. J. A. Wightman for reading the proofs and to Mrs P. Drake for her care and diligence in the typing and checking of the manuscripts.

The Departments of Medical Photography at the University of Edinburgh and the Royal National Throat, Nose & Ear Hospital have given invaluable assistance in the preparation of illustrations and the publishers have given us great help in the organisation of the text.

We are indebted to publishers Grune & Stratton, W. B. Saunders Co. and Churchill Livingstone for permission to reproduce illustrations used by the author in Seminars in Roentgenology, "Textbook of Radiology" and "Radiology of the Orbit".

September 1977

ERIC SAMUEL
GLYN A. S. LLOYD

Contents

CHAPTER 1

Radiographic examination of the paranasal sinuses

Pathological conditions affecting the paranasal sinuses encroach on the air in the sinuses, consequently they present on the radiograph as alterations in the translucency of the sinus. The extent of this loss of translucency may not be marked and thus a standardised technique producing films of the highest quality is essential for accurate assessment of disease involving the paranasal sinuses.

Furthermore, as many pathological conditions affecting the sinuses produce fluid, every effort must be made to demonstrate it. For this reason examination of the sinuses should be carried out in the erect position, thus allowing the fluid and air to separate into easily recognisable fluid levels (figs. 5, 6).

STANDARD POSITIONS

The radiographic positions for examination of the paranasal sinuses are standardised around three planes; two anatomical, the **coronal** and **sagittal**, and one radiographic, the **"radiographic base line"**. The anatomical planes need no definition; the radiographic base line represents a line drawn from the external canthus of the eye to the midpoint of the external auditory meatus. The radiographic base line should not be confused with the anatomical Reid's base line which is not used in radiography of the paranasal sinuses.

The standard positions used to demonstrate the paranasal sinuses by plain x-ray are:

(a) Occipito-mental (Waters, Law) position
(b) Occipito-frontal (Caldwell) position
(c) Submento-vertical (Hirtz) position
(d) Lateral position
(e) 39° oblique (Rhese, Goalwin) positions

Occipito-mental view. The patient sits facing the film with the radiographic base line tilted to an angle of 45° to the horizontal, the sagittal plane being vertical (fig. 1). The incident beam is horizontal and is centred over a point 1 in (2·5 cm) above the external occipital protuberance. In patients with short, fat, or stiff necks where it is impossible to tilt the radiographic base line to 45°, the head should be tilted as far as possible and the tube angled a corresponding degree towards the feet.

If the mouth is kept open, particularly in edentulous patients, a view of both sphenoid sinuses can be obtained through the open mouth (fig. 2). This open mouth view of the sphenoid sinus may prove an extremely useful supplement to the routine views of the sphenoid sinus.

The correctly positioned radiograph obtained gives a slightly foreshortened view of both antra with the petrous temporal bone lying immediately below the lowest point of the antrum.

If the antrum in the occipito-mental view shows a loss of translucency suggestive of a fluid level, a tilt of

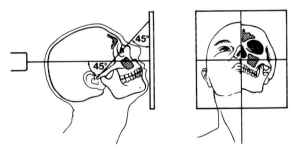

Fig. 1. Occipito-mental view. The radiographic base line is angled at 45° to the film and the incident beam centred on a point 2·5 cm above the external occipital protuberance. The positions of the frontal sinus and antrum are shown diagrammatically.

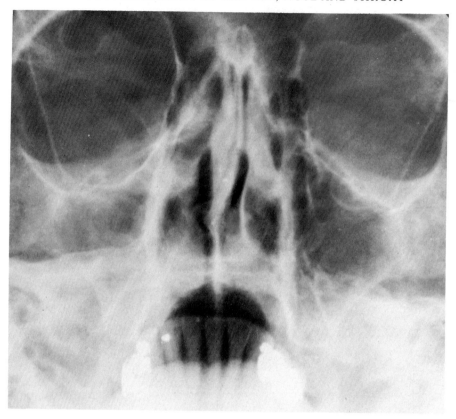

Fig. 2. Occipito-mental view illustrating the commonest error, namely the base line has been insufficiently tilted and consequently the petrous bones obscure the lower half of the antrum.

the sagittal plane to an angle of 30° and further radiography in the occipito-mental position will show movement of any fluid present in the antrum. The head should always be tilted so that the fluid runs into the lateral part of the antrum where the fluid level may be more easily seen. It must also be appreciated that the demonstration of the level is dependent on the incident beam passing tangentially along the line of the fluid level; when there is a marked obliquity a level may be obscured.

Occipito-frontal view (Caldwell). The patient sits facing the film with the radiographic base line tilted to an angle of 10° upwards from the horizontal and with the sagittal plane vertical. The incident beam is horizontal and is centred ½ in (13 mm) below the external occipital protuberance. The same view may be obtained by keeping the radiographic base line horizontal and inclining the incident beam 10° towards the feet (fig. 7).

In this position the frontal sinuses are almost in direct contact with the film, little or no distortion occurs, and geometric blur is minimal and their outlines are shown with great clarity (fig. 8). In this view the antra are overlapped by the petrous bone and the view consequently provides little or no useful information about the antral translucency. However, a tangential view of the lateral wall of the antrum is obtained and erosion of the lateral wall of the antrum by a tumour can be recognised early.

If fluid is suspected in either frontal or ethmoid sinuses the head should be placed in the occipito-frontal position and tilted to 45° on either side of the sagittal plane. Care must be taken that the sagittal plane is not rotated during this tilt and that the head should remain tilted for a sufficient period to allow the fluid to gravitate and attain its own level. In the case of viscid exudates this may take as long as 10 minutes. An occipito-mental or occipito-

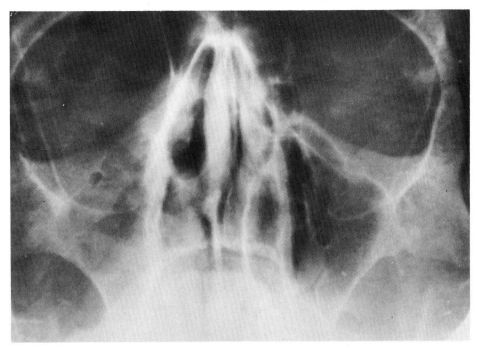

Fig. 3. Same patient as shown in Fig. 2 with the head correctly tilted. The extensive mucosal thickening in the right antrum, largely obscured in Fig. 2, is clearly seen.

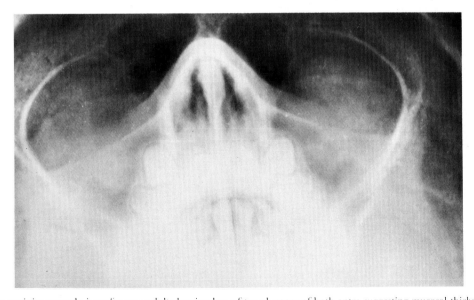

Fig. 4. Erect occipito-mental view of young adult showing loss of translucency of both antra suggesting mucosal thickening. These appearances are produced by over-tilting of the skull, and the foreshortening of the antrum is the key to the cause of the loss of translucency.

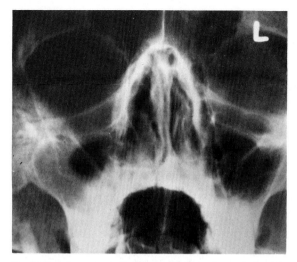

Fig. 5. Occipito-mental view showing thickened mucosa in right antrum and to a lesser extent in left antrum. No fluid level seen.

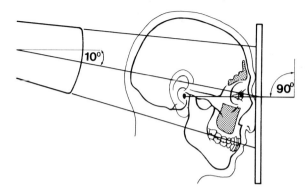

Fig. 7. Occipito-frontal view. The base line may either be horizontal as in this illustration and the tube inclined caudally at 10° (Grainger position), or the base line may be tilted 10° upwards and the incident beam kept horizontal (Caldwell).

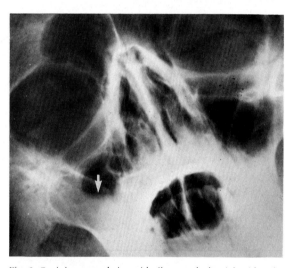

Fig. 6. Occipito-mental view with tilt towards the right side. The fluid level is now readily seen in the right antrum.

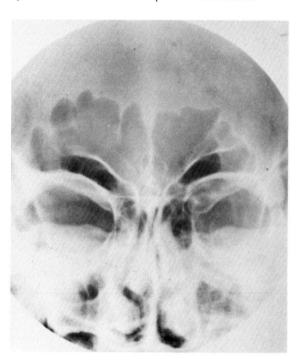

Fig. 8. Occipito-frontal radiograph showing the extremely good visualisation of the frontal sinus. The petrous bones cross the antra.

frontal projection with the patient lying in a horizontal position may improve the demonstration of small quantities of fluid.

Submento-vertical view. The submento-vertical position is primarily utilised to demonstrate the sphenoid sinuses. Fluid levels in the sphenoid sinus and its bony outlines can be demonstrated in this position. For this position the back is arched as far as possible so that the base of the skull is parallel to the film. The incident beam is centred in the midline at a point midway between the angles of the jaw (figs. 9, 10). In elderly patients the submento-vertical position may be easier to achieve if the examination is carried out in the supine position with the head hanging back over the end of the table.

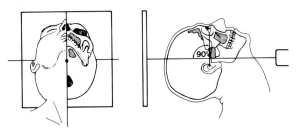

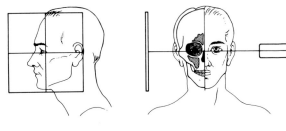

Fig. 9. Line drawing showing position for submento-vertical position. The base line is parallel to the film and the incident beam centred at a point mid-way between the angles of the mandible. If the base line cannot be made parallel to the film the incident beam must be angled cranially to cross the radiographic base line at right angles.

Fig. 11. Line drawing showing patient's position for lateral view of sinuses and, diagrammatically, the position of the antrum and frontal sinus.

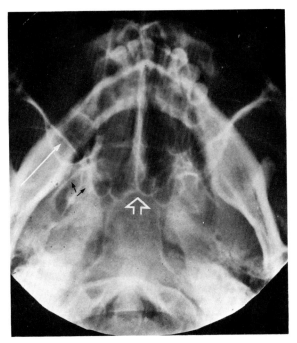

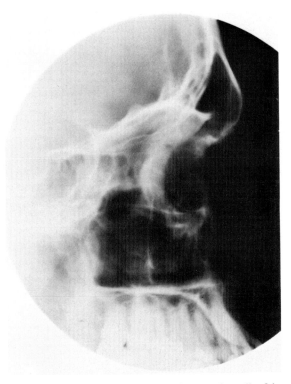

Fig. 10. The radiograph in the submento-vertical position showing the sphenoid sinuses (hollow arrow), the pterygoid plates (black arrows), the posterior orbital wall (white arrow) and the posterior margin of the antrum.

Fig. 12. Lateral radiograph of sinuses. The posterior walls of the sinuses are clearly shown in this view. The zygomatic recess may be seen superimposed on the antrum.

The submento-vertical view is also of considerable assistance in determining the relative thickness of the bony walls of the antrum and the frontal sinuses. A knowledge of the thickness of these walls is of importance as the translucency of a shallow frontal sinus is particularly affected by the thickness of its bony walls.

Lateral view. The lateral projection is difficult to interpret as the overlapping shadows make the appreciation of changes in the antra and frontal sinuses difficult. Nevertheless, the view is indispensible for routine sinus radiography. It is necessary for the assessment of frontal sinus abnormality, to determine whether a loss of trans-

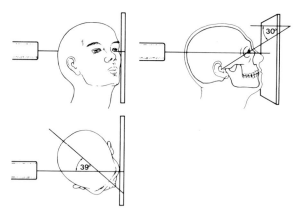

Fig. 13. Line drawing illustrating the position for the oblique view to show the posterior ethmoid cells.

lucence is due to thickening of the anterior bony wall or infection in the sinus. It is frequently the view that best demonstrates fluid levels in the antrum and is essential for the appreciation of sphenoid sinus disease.

The lateral view also gives information on the radiographic appearances of the nasopharynx and soft palate. Soft tissue masses involving the naso-pharynx and palate can be readily seen in this view, and it is the standard projection for detecting enlargement of the adenoid pad. It should be remembered that tumours and masses involving the lateral wall of the nasopharynx may be invisible as they do not give an edge between the mass and the air space. Submento-vertical views may be needed for the visualisation of laterally placed

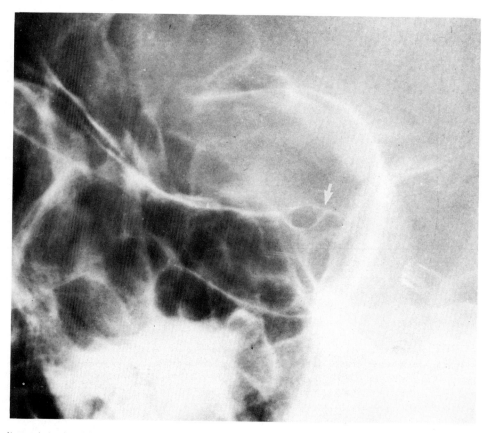

Fig. 14. Radiograph in the oblique position. The optic foramen is seen end-on in the centre of the illustration and the posterior ethmoid cells lie anteriorly.

nasopharyngeal tumours. For the lateral view the patient sits with the sagittal plane parallel to the film and the radiographic base line horizontal. The incident ray is horizontal and the incident beam is centred at the midpoint of the antrum (figs. 11, 12). Lateral projections for the nasopharynx should be taken in a true lateral position, that is a 2 metre focal-film distance with the film against the shoulder, rather than the "turned head" position used in skull radiography.

Oblique view (39° oblique position). This is designed to demonstrate the posterior ethmoid cells and also the optic foramen. To obtain the projection the patient first sits facing the film. The head is rotated so that the sagittal plane is turned through an angle of 39°. The radiographic base line is at an angle of 30° to the horizontal. The incident beam is horizontal and is centred so that the emergent beam passes through the centre of the orbit nearest the film. In this position the supra-orbital ridge, the external orbital margin, and the lateral surface of the nose are all in contact with the film (fig. 13). In the resulting film the posterior ethmoid cells occupy the anterior two-thirds of the medial wall of the orbit and the optic foramen should appear in the upper and posterior quadrant of the orbit (fig. 14).

SPECIALISED METHODS OF RADIOGRAPHIC EXAMINATION

Tomography

Tomography is an essential part of the x-ray investigation of the paranasal sinuses. Abnormalities not readily visualised on plain x-ray may be demonstrated on tomographic section and changes seen on plain x-ray are frequently better delineated in size, extent and relationship to adjoining structures by this means. For complete tomography of the sinuses films are required in three planes: coronal, lateral and axial, and for optimal results specialised tomographic units capable of pleuridirectional or circular movements such as the Polytome (Philips Massiot) should be employed.

Technique. There are three general points of radiographic technique that require emphasis. First, the choice of tomographic movements should be such as to produce a maximum blurring effect and relatively thin tomographic section. With the Polytome the hypocycloidal movement meets

these requirements and is recommended for sinus tomography. Secondly, complete immobility is needed during the examination. With the Polytome apparatus exposures of up to 6 seconds are required and with these long exposures some means of immobilisation of the head is indispensable. The head fixation clamp supplied with the Polytome apparatus, with suction pads for adherence to the table top has proved totally adequate in this respect.

The third important point of radiographic technique concerns the reduction of radiation dosage to the eye during sinus tomography. Chin, Anderson & Gilbertson (1970) have shown that in full hypocycloidal tomography of the temporal bones in the antero-posterior position, the cornea may receive a dose of 10·5 rad, and lens opacities have followed the exposure of the eyeball to a single 15 rad dose in animal experimental work (Upton, Christianberry & Forth, 1953). As exposures only slightly less are also involved in sinus tomography it becomes essential to modify radiographic technique to reduce eye dosage. For this reason all coronal tomography should be performed in the postero-anterior position of the head. This effectively reduces the dose to the front of the eye to less than 5 mrad per exposure. For lateral and axial tomography a lead mask can be employed to protect the eyes without detriment to the x-ray film image.

Coronal tomography. For coronal tomography the patient is placed prone and there are two useful projections which may be employed.

(1) An under-tilted occipito-mental position of the skull in which the orbito-meatal line is angled 30°–35° cranially with a straight tube. This is used primarily to show the maxillary antra and associated orbital abnormalities to best advantage. An important example is a blow-out fracture of the floor of the orbit in which both the herniation of orbital contents and the fragments of displaced and depressed bone from the orbital floor will be best demonstrated in this position, since the central ray is virtually parallel to the roof of the maxillary antrum.

(2) The second projection corresponds to the standard postero-anterior skull view, the nose and forehead being placed in contact with the table top with the orbito-meatal line at right angles to it. This projection is recommended for a general survey of the paranasal sinuses, using a 5 mm separation of the tomographic sections and hypocycloidal

movement of the tube. It demonstrates the ethmoids and sphenoids optimally and provides the best view of the floor of the anterior cranial fossa and the cribriform plate. It has its most important application in the demonstration of expanding processes and bone destruction, either inflammatory or neoplastic in paranasal sinus disease. In the maxillary antra the integrity of the medial wall is particularly well demonstrated and coronal tomography is the optimum method of demonstrating associated masses in the nasal cavity.

Lateral tomography. For lateral tomograms of the paranasal sinuses the patient should be placed in the prone oblique position with the uppermost leg raised and the knee bent. This will help to maintain a true lateral position of the head during examination. The hypocycloidal movement of the tube is the recommended procedure but it may also be useful to employ high kilovoltage zonography with 3 mm of brass filtration in studies of the naso-pharynx and sphenoids. In the maxillary antra lateral tomography is useful to show bone erosion of the anterior and posterior walls, for example the indentation caused by an angiofibroma on the posterior wall of the antrum is best demonstrated by lateral tomography (see Chapter 3). Lateral tomography is also useful preoperatively to estimate the posterior extent of a blow-out fracture. Other applications of lateral tomography include the demonstration of mucoceles of the frontal sinuses invading the orbital roof. It is sometimes possible to demonstrate a thin rim of expanded bone forming the inferior border of the mucocele on these lateral films. In frontal sinus mucoceles it is also important to determine whether or not the posterior wall of the frontal sinus is intact since the sac of the mucocele may be in contact with the dura if erosion of the posterior wall is complete. Lateral tomography is also the optimum way of demonstrating anterior bone erosion in the frontal sinuses in neoplasms or inflammatory disease. The most important application of lateral tomography is, however, in the demonstration of tumours and other expanding lesions in the sphenoid sinus, adjacent ethmoids and in the nasopharynx.

Axial tomography. In the technique evolved for axial tomography (Lloyd, 1971) the Philips Massiot Polytome has been used exclusively. The hypo-cycloidal movement has been found to produce the best results, but other rotational tomographic movements will give adequate results in most

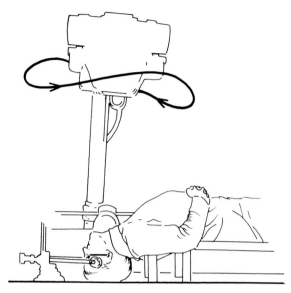

Fig. 15. Position for tomography in half-axial position. The patient lies on a specially designed table placed on the x-ray table and this allows the half-axial position to be more easily achieved.

instances. The position of the patient is illustrated in fig. 15. A light wooden platform is placed on the table top so that the submento-vertical position of the skull can be maintained with the patient horizontal. For axial tomography of the paranasal sinuses a standard submento-vertical projection is adequate, with the orbito-meatal line placed parallel to the film, but to show the optic canal in the axial plane, a more hyperextended position than this is required. This view is needed to show fractures of the sphenoids involving the optic canal and also in neoplasms and mucoceles of the sphenoid when erosion of the medial wall of the canal can be evaluated. The hyperextended position of the head and neck required for this view is physically impossible for most adult patients, but this problem can be overcome by angling the x-ray film in the cassette holder. The attachment for macrotomography on the Polytome apparatus allows angles of inclination of 45° or more. With the patient in the submento-vertical position the film needs to be inclined 25°–30° for the tomo-graphic cut to lie in the plane of the optic canal. The inclined plane method is also very useful in patients who for any reason find it difficult to maintain a full submento-vertical position, as may happen in the elderly or in patients with a dorsal kyphosis; the inclination of the x-ray tube will compensate for any under-tilt of the head.

Axial tomography is the optimum method of demonstrating the ethmoid cells radiologically. It provides a plan view of the whole of the ethmoid labyrinth on a single film (fig. 80). Thus the exact extent of a tumour can be demonstrated; whether it extends across the midline or into the sphenoid sinuses; if the medial orbital wall has been breached and the orbit involved. In malignant disease of the sinuses the presence and degree of orbital involvement is particularly important since this will influence the decision to exenterate the orbit at surgery.

Other expanding processes in the ethmoid cells are well demonstrated by this technique; for example axial tomography is the optimum method of demonstrating an ethmoid mucocele (Lloyd, Bartram & Stanley, 1974). Fractures of the medial wall of the orbit are best shown by this means (fig. 80) and the method is also invaluable for the assessment of fractures involving the optic canals (Lloyd, 1971).

CONTRAST MEDIA

The introduction of radio-opaque media into the paranasal sinuses is seldom used nowadays.

The contrast medium usually employed is Lipiodol or Pantopaque although other preparations such as oily Dionosil have been used. The watery contrast media are of little value.

Barium suspensions have also been instilled into the nose to outline the walls of the nasopharynx.

The oily preparations may be introduced into the paranasal sinuses by one or two methods:

(1) Through a cannula following direct puncture of the antral wall.
(2) By displacement technique (Proetz therapy).

When proof puncture of an antrum is performed further information as to the size and shape of the antral cavity may be obtained by the introduction of Lipiodol through the cannula (see figs. 86, 87).

The value of the time taken for the oil to clear from the sinus as a means of assessing function of the mucosal cilia has been disputed. Some authorities believe that if significant quantities of

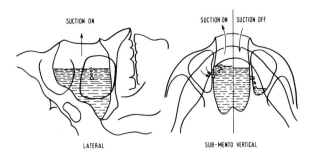

Fig. 16. Line drawing illustrating the underlying principle of Proetz displacement therapy. The negative suction applied to the nose (with a closed nasopharynx by phonating "KK") causes air to flow from the antrum into the nose, thus creating a partial vacuum in the antrum. When suction is released the contrast medium bubbles back into the antrum.

contrast medium remain in the sinuses after 7 days then considerable impairment of ciliary function is present.

Displacement (Proetz technique, Proetz, 1931). This is another means of introducing Lipiodol into the sinuses as it is painless, easily performed and does not involve puncture of any of the paranasal sinuses.

The technique of displacement is as follows. The patient lies in the supine position with the head extended and below the level of the shoulders. Oily contrast medium is slowly dropped into the nose, care being taken not to run any medium into the nasopharynx. The nasopharynx is closed off from the nose by repeating the syllable "K" and negative suction is applied to the nasal cavity (fig. 16). Air is consequently removed from the paranasal sinuses and the Lipiodol runs back into the sinus. The patient is then radiographed in the erect position and routine views of the sinuses are taken.

Although many of the assumptions made with regard to the filling and emptying of Lipiodol from the sinuses are controversial, there is no doubt that this method may be extremely valuable in determining the origin of many aberrant cells and the presence of septa within the antrum (fig. 25).

ULTRASOUND

Ultrasound has considerable limitations in the diagnosis of the paranasal air sinuses as the air content of the sinuses limits the penetration of the ultrasound beam.

Kametan (1966) found that benign tumours and

cysts showed only surface and bottom echoes whilst malignant tumours showed irregular transverse echoes throughout the tumours.

Abdurasulor (1966) found ultrasonics particularly useful in the diagnosis of disease of the maxillary sinus particularly in children.

In practice the most useful function of ultrasound in sinus disease is to distinguish between a cystic mass (mucocele) and a solid tumour arising from the anterior ethmoid cells and frontal sinus.

THERMOGRAPHY

Thermograms of the face will reveal increased infra-red emission with a hot spot over an infected sinus. However, in chronic sinus infections the degree of thermal change may be insufficient to produce significant changes which can be recognised. It has been found that the thermograph has been of no value in determining whether an opaque antrum represents a chronic infective process or a sequela of a previous infection.

COMPUTERISED TOMOGRAPHY
(C.A.T., EMI SCAN)

The EMI Scanner system, which is a computer-aided technique for brain tissue examination, was originally described by Ambrose & Hounsfield in 1972. A detailed description of the apparatus has been given by Hounsfield (1973) and its clinical application in neuroradiology has been described by Ambrose (1973) and by Paxton & Ambrose (1974). In this new imaging system the head is scanned by a collimated beam of x-rays in a series of layers of 13 mm thickness. Each slice of tissue is irradiated from a large number of different but sequential positions of the x-ray source over the circumference of the skull, and the transmission of x-ray photons is recorded for each position of the scan. The measurements obtained are processed by computer and an image of the tissue slice is reconstructed as a series of absorption values. Lesions can then be recognised as alterations in the normal pattern of soft tissue densities. Although originally devised to detect intracranial space-occupying lesions the apparatus may also show soft tissue abnormalities in the paranasal sinuses and orbit.

Neoplasms and other expanding lesions in the sinuses are shown by C.A.T. in plan view as in axial hypocycloidal tomography (see above). The technique is complementary to the latter in that it provides better demonstration of the extent of soft tissue changes in the adjacent pterygoid fossa, orbits and the anterior and middle fossae of the skull. Forssell et al. (1976) have shown the value of this technique for demonstrating anterior soft tissue extension of maxillary tumours. Computerised tomography is also a very useful method of delineating the extent of malignant disease prior to radiotherapy and also monitoring the effects of treatment.

REFERENCES

ABDURASULOR, D. M. (1966) The Use of Ultrasonics in the Diagnosis of Max. Sinus. *Nord. med. Tekh.*, **2**, 30.

AMBROSE, J. (1973) Computerised Trans-axial Scanning (Tomography). *Br.J. Radiol.*, **46**, 1023.

CALDWELL, E. W. (1918). Skiagraphy of the Accessory Nasal Sinuses. *Am.J. Roentg.*, **5**, 569.

CHIN, F. K., ANDERSON, W. B. & GILBERTSON, D. J. (1970) Radiation Dose in Petrous Tomography. *Radiology*, **94**, 623.

FORSSELL, A., LILLIEQUIST, B. & WICKMAN, G. (1976) Computer Tomography of the Paranasal Sinuses. In *VII International Congress of Radiology in O.R.L.*, Copenhagen.

GOALWIN, H. (1926) The Roentgenography of the Orbit and Petrous Pyramid and its Clinical Value. *J. Ophthal. Otol. Lar., Phila.*, **30**, 7.

HIRTZ, E. J. (1922) Le Diagnostic Radiologique des Sinusites. *Bull. Mém. Soc. Radiol. méd. Fr.*, **10**, 22.

HOUNSFIELD, G. N. (1973) Computerised Transverse Axial Scanning (Tomography) I. *Br.J. Radiol.*, **46**, 1016.

KAMETAN, H. (1966) A Study on the Diagnosis of the Max. Diseases by Ultrasound. *J. Rad. Soc. Japan*, **68**, 751.

LAW, F. M. (1931) Interpreting Sinus Roentgenograms. *Ann. Otol. Rhinol. Lar.*, **40**, 82.

LLOYD, G. (1971) Axial Tomography of the Orbits and Paranasal Sinuses. *Br.J. Radiol.*, **48**, 460.

LLOYD, G., BARTRAM, C. I. & STANLEY, P. (1974) Ethmoid Mucoceles. *Br.J. Radiol.*, **47**, 646.

PAXTON, R. & AMBROSE, J. (1974) The EMI Scanner. A Brief Review of the First 650 patients. *Br. J. Radiol.*, **47**, 530.

PROETZ, A. W. (1931) *The Displacement Method of Sinus Diagnosis and Treatment.* St. Louis: Annals Publishing Co.

RHESE (1910) Die Diagnostik der Erkrankungen des Siebleinlabyrinthes und der Keilbeinhohlen durch das Rontgen Verfahren. *Dt. med. Wschr.*, **36**, 1756.

UPTON, A. C., CHRISTIANBERRY, K. W. & FORTH, J. (1953) *Archs Ophthal.*, **49**, 164.

WATERS, C. A. & WALDRON, C. W. (1915) *Am. J. Roentg.*, **2**, 633.

CHAPTER 2

Development and radiological anatomy of the nose and accessory nasal sinuses

The nose and nasal cavity may be subdivided into:

(i) The external nose, and
(ii) The nasal cavity proper.

The external nose is readily available for detailed examination by clinical means and radiological examination is seldom needed. The nasal cavity proper lying enclosed within the framework of facial bones, surrounded by bony walls and filled with air, is more suitable for radiological study.

THE EXTERNAL NOSE

The external nose is a pyramidal-shaped structure with its base directed downwards and supported by the facial bones. It is a cartilaginous structure covered by skin and subcutaneous tissue and lined by mucoperiosteum. The cartilaginous portion of the external nose is composed of numerous small cartilages which largely determine the configuration of the nose. The nasal cartilages which take part in the structure of the external nose comprise:

(a) Two major alar cartilages forming the tip and lateral aspects of the nose;
(b) Two lateral nasal cartilages, and
(c) Minor alar cartilages forming the lateral wall of the nose.

The major and minor alar cartilages are all supported by a midline triangular plate of thin cartilage (mobile nasal septum) which is attached along its inferior surface to the nasal maxillary spine anteriorly, and to the perpendicular process of the ethmoid and vomer, posteriorly. This cartilaginous plate is continuous posteriorly with the bony nasal septum.

The paired nasal bones form the support for the nasal cartilages and show well defined neurovascular markings on their inner surfaces (fig. 17).

THE NASAL CAVITY PROPER

Most of the bones which take part in the formation of the facial skeleton play some part in forming boundaries of the nasal cavity. Superiorly, the nasal

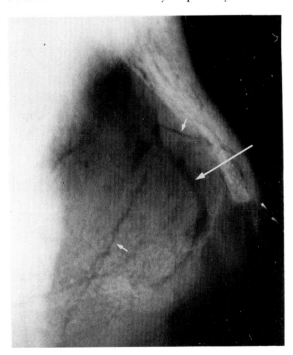

Fig. 17. Dental film showing the neurovascular groove visible on most normal nasal bones, and the grooves formed by the vascular branches.

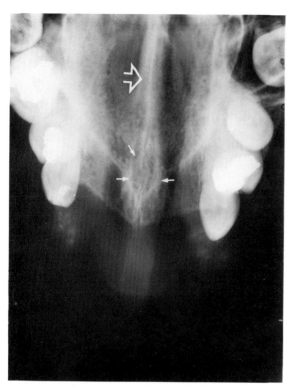

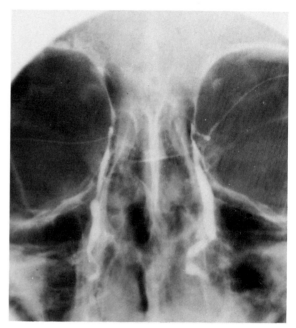

Fig. 19. Dacrocystogram showing filling of the lachrymal sac and the naso-lachrymal duct, extending into the inferior meatus of the nose.

Fig. 18. Occlusal view of palate showing bony septum (hollow arrows), incisive canal (white arrow) and nasolachrymal ducts.

cavity has a narrow roof which is formed by the cribriform plate of the ethmoid bone. Its lateral walls, which slope outwards and downwards, are formed from behind – forward by the orbital plates of the ethmoid and palatine bones and by the lachrymal bones, whilst its extreme anterior margin is formed by the nasal process of the maxilla. The floor of the nasal cavity is formed by the palatal process of the maxilla (fig. 8).

Resting on the horizontal processes of the maxilla is the vomer which forms a thin midline section of the bony floor of the nose and whose vertical portion also forms a considerable portion of the nasal septum proper.

Posteriorly the nasal cavity opens into the nasopharynx by two oval-shaped openings – the posterior nares.

Projecting into the nasal cavity and dividing it into a complex series of channels and depressions designed to enhance its physiological function of moistening and warming inspired air, are the turbinate bones. Subdividing the nasal cavity is the bony nasal septum which is formed by the vertical plate of the ethmoid in its upper two-thirds whilst the lower third is formed by the vomer. The junction of the two bones frequently forms a spur (vomerine spur). Apart from infants and young children, only in exceptional cases does the bony nasal septum occupy a completely midline position. More often, it bulges into one side, the vomerine spur usually projecting into the opposite half of the nasal cavity.

Projecting from the lateral wall of either side of the nose are the three turbinate bones which are arranged in a roughly horizontal plane. The largest is the inferior turbinate which hangs from a thin linear attachment, is curved upon itself, and is seen from the antero-posterior plane as presenting a scroll-like appearance. The projecting inferior turbinate results in the formation of a sulcus beneath the turbinate bone which is known as the inferior meatus. The INFERIOR MEATUS is bounded above and medially by the inferior turbinate, laterally by the lateral wall of the nasal cavity. It is the largest meatus.

The MIDDLE MEATUS lies between the middle and inferior turbinates. The middle turbinate is far less complex in design than the inferior turbinate; its anterior margin is free and extends to a curved free border known as the agger nasi. It arises from the lateral wall of the nose beneath the inferior aspect of the ethmoid labyrinth.

On the lateral wall of the middle meatus lies a curved depression known as the hiatus semilunaris. Into the anterior end of this depression opens the fronto-nasal duct draining the frontal sinus, whilst halfway along its length lies the ostium which drains the maxillary antrum.

Projecting into and forming the roof and lateral aspect of the middle meatus is a curved portion of the ethmoidal bone which contains the main bulk of the ethmoidal cells. This portion of the ethmoidal bone is known as the ethmoidal capsule (bulla ethmoidalis).

The SUPERIOR MEATUS lies above the middle turbinate bone. Into this uppermost part of the nasal cavity open the posterior ethmoid and sphenoid cells. Projecting into the superior meatus is the uncinate process of the ethmoid. The superior turbinate and the superior meatus are small in comparison with the other nasal structures but their importance in the problem of nasal infection is not correspondingly diminished.

The POSTERIOR NARES (choanae) form the openings between the true nasal cavity and the nasopharynx. These apertures are oval in shape and are bounded above by the body of the sphenoid and to a lesser extent by the alar process of the vomer; below by the posterior edge of the hard palate and laterally by the medial plates of the pterygoid processes. They are separated by the posterior free edge of the bony nasal septum.

Radiological features

Only the nasal bones themselves and the nasal process of the frontal bone can be demonstrated radiologically. The radiological differentiation of the constituent cartilages of the nose is not possible. However, the contrast formed between the soft tissues and the contained air makes the demonstration of abnormalities in the nasal cavity proper relatively easy. The nasal bones themselves are symmetrically paired bones on which the anterior ethmoidal nerve and vessels form a groove (the ethmoid sulcus). The bony groove formed by this nerve runs a longitudinal course along the nasal bone and is a well-defined radiological landmark.

Its paired nature enables it to be differentiated from a vertical fracture. When the ethmoidal sulcus is seen to branch, its differentiation from a fracture is simple. A small foramen in the centre of the nasal bone (for the passage of a vein) forms a second constant anatomical marking (fig. 17).

Two suture lines can be seen and must be identified as normal anatomical markings. The single central nasal suture between both nasal bones which can best be seen in the postero-anterior view whilst the lateral suture between the nasal bones and the nasal process of the maxilla is best seen in the lateral views.

Radiological examination of the nasal bones can best be made by placing a dental film in direct contact with the side of the nose and centering the incident beam horizontally through the nose. A cranio-caudal view of the nasal bones is obtained by inserting an occlusal film between the teeth and directing the vertical beam through the nasal bones on to the film. In the dental film the exquisite detail of the nasal bones can be clearly demonstrated whilst the cranio-caudal projection is invaluable in detecting lateral shifts and displacements of fractured nasal bones.

The nasal cavities proper are best demonstrated in the submento-vertical and occipito-frontal projection. Postero-anterior tomograms are, however, the only real means of obtaining full radiological views of the nasal fossae and the detailed anatomy can be clearly followed (fig. 123). In the postero-anterior tomograms the detail of the ethmoid labyrinth, the turbinates and the ethmoidal capsule can readily be made out. The bony edge of the anterior nares can be seen overlying the true outline of the nasal cavity proper. Postero-anterior tomograms are superior to conventional projections and help considerably in demonstrating the bony details of the nasal cavities (fig. 52).

The inferior turbinates vary considerably in size but the scroll-like appearance of the bony structure can generally be clearly seen. Considerable variation in the size of the inferior turbinates occurs in normal individuals. The development of the inferior turbinates is seldom symmetrical and they may be congenitally absent.

The middle turbinates are less easily recognised and overlapping shadows of the ethmoid capsule may obscure these structures. The ethmoidal capsule is recognised from the honeycombed appearance produced by the contained ethmoidal air cells.

Many of the ethmoidal cells may migrate during development from the ethmoidal capsule into the surrounding bones. The inferior turbinate frequently contains ethmoidal cells whilst aberrant ethmoidal cells (agger cells) frequently migrate into the orbital plate of the maxilla, producing a double radiographic appearance of the roof of the maxillary antrum. This appearance may be confused with a septate antrum.

The higher level of the floor of the nasal cavity in relation to that of the antrum can be appreciated and the relationship of the antral wall to the nasal cavity can be seen in the postero-anterior projection.

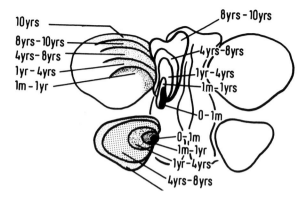

Fig. 20. Line drawing (after Caffey) showing the relative sizes of the frontal sinuses and antra at various ages during their development.

PARANASAL SINUSES

The paranasal sinuses whose function is not understood, are a series of air-containing cavities lying in the bony framework surrounding the nasal cavity. They are composed of two paired frontal sinuses lying in the frontal bone, two maxillary antra lying mainly in the body of the maxillary bone but part of whose walls are formed by other facial bones, and ethmoidal cells sub-divided into anterior, middle and posterior groups lying within the ethmoidal labyrinth. The fourth sinuses, the sphenoid sinuses, are paired and are totally contained in the body of the sphenoid bone.

Development. The sinuses begin to develop during the fourth month of intra-uterine life as an invagination of nasal mucous membrane into the surrounding capsule and further increase at the expense of the surrounding bones.

The maxillary antra are the first of the paranasal sinuses to appear (fig. 20). They begin to develop in the region of the frontal recess of the middle meatus of the nasal cavity, during the fourth to fifth months of foetal life (Schaeffer, 1920). At birth they form small ovoid cavities measuring 8 × 4 × 6 mm, lying close to the nasal wall with their greatest diameter transversely. Thereafter their expansion coincides with the growth of the facial bones. At the age of one year, the outer wall of the maxillary antrum is still medial to the infra-orbital foramen. By the age of two the outer wall of the antrum has extended laterally as far as the level of the infra-orbital foramen. Davies (1938) states that the maxillary sinuses increase their diameter by an

average of 2 mm per year vertically and laterally, and 3 mm antero-posteriorly between the age of three to nine years. Development proceeds until the antrum reaches its full adult size in its transverse diameter at approximately eight years (Schaeffer, 1920; Onodi, 1911) (fig. 20). Thereafter the antrum enlarges in its antero-posterior and vertical diameters as the permanent teeth erupt and the alveolar recess of the maxilla only finally develops with the complete eruption of the permanent

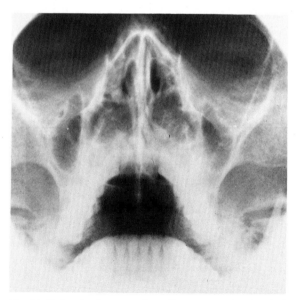

Fig. 21. Under-development of maxillary antrum showing thick lateral wall with infra-orbital foramen lying medially in its embryonic position.

dentition. The infra-orbital foramen and canal initially lie in the middle of the maxilla but as the antrum grows in size, they are displaced upwards until they come to lie in the roof of the antrum (fig. 21).

In the infant and adolescent the tooth buds of the permanent teeth cast shadows which obscure the lower and inner parts of the antra and render the radiological interpretation of pathological changes in the antra difficult. In the immediate postnatal period, however, there are other factors which cause haziness of the antra. Wasson (1933) found that in the newborn the maxillary antra and ethmoids were filled with a jelly-like material, and concluded that in spite of the appreciable size of the antra and ethmoids at birth aeration of these sinuses in the newborn infant takes place relatively slowly. Loss of radiographic translucence in the antra in the neonate should therefore be interpreted with caution.

The adult maxillary antrum is a large pyramidal-shaped cavity which lies in the body of the maxilla. Viewed in the postero-anterior plane, the antra are pyramidal in shape with their apices directed downwards. In the lateral view they are quadrilateral with rounded corners. In the submento-vertical view, they are pyramidal with the apices directed backwards.

The anatomical boundaries are, superiorly the bony floor of the orbit, from which on its medial aspect it may be separated by ethmoidal cells interposed between the roof of the antrum and the floor of the orbit. Running across the roof of the antrum is a bony ridge which is formed by the infra-orbital canal and carries the infra-orbital nerve and vessels.

The floor of the antrum is usually formed by that portion of the alveolar process of the maxilla containing the molar and premolar teeth.

The medial wall of the maxillary antrum is formed by the lateral wall of the nasal cavity. The main portion of the nasal wall of the antrum is formed by the maxilla but to a lesser extent from before – backwards the lachrymal bone, the vertical plate of the ethmoid, and the maxillary process of the inferior turbinates all take part. Inferiorly the vertical process of the palate contributes to the formation of the medial wall.

Anteriorly, the antrum is bounded by the facial aspect of the maxilla whilst its posterior wall is also formed by the maxilla which separates the antrum from the pterygo-maxillary fossa. The ostium of the antrum is placed on the medial wall about halfway between the roof and the floor. The situation of the ostium in relation to the most dependent part of the antrum implies a positive drainage system. This is brought about by the ciliary action of the lining mucosa.

The antra are the most symmetrical of the accessory nasal sinuses although complete symmetry is rare. The most common variation is in the level of the antral floor both with regard to the teeth and the extent of the alveolar sulcus. The teeth are separated from the antral cavity by a solid layer of bone over the apices of the teeth but in a well pneumatised antrum this may be reduced to a thin bony layer. Rarely, there may be only antral mucosa between the sinus and the apices of the teeth and in these cases the antra may be infected from an infected tooth. Likewise during a complicated dental extraction, a fragment of tooth root may be easily displaced into the antrum.

On the lateral wall of the antrum the grooves caused by the branches of the anterior and posterior branches of superior dental vessels and nerves may suggest a fracture. These grooves are remarkably constant in position, occurring approximately halfway down the lateral wall of the antrum. The paired appearance should suggest the anatomical nature of the marking (fig. 22). As the

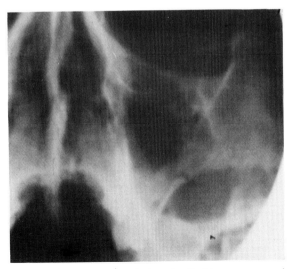

Fig. 22. The bony groove on the lateral wall of the antrum caused by the superior dental vessels and nerves. This must be differentiated from a fracture.

course of the superior dental canals are in an oblique direction extending downwards and outwards they are most easily visible in the occipito-mental projection. When the incident ray extends along the vessel, these neurovascular markings appear as defects in the lateral wall and they appear as a "C" type marking extending into the maxillary antrum. They are particularly well seen in postero-anterior tomograms (Chiang & Innes, 1973).

The alveolar recess projects into the alveolar process of the maxilla and varies considerably in development. In infancy the alveolar recess is absent, being occupied by the permanent tooth buds and complete development does not occur until the permanent dentition has fully erupted. In edentulous patients the absorption of the alveolar process may occur to such a degree that the antrum is separated only by the thinnest layer of bone from the oral cavity. The prolonged wearing of dentures hastens this process.

The zygomatic recess is an extension of the sinus into the zygomatic bone. In the lateral film it appears as a clear central area with a well defined cortex. It is especially well seen in occlusal films of the upper jaw when it may be mistaken for a dental cyst.

Tuberosity recess. The maxillary antrum may extend into and completely pneumatise the maxillary tuberosity, and unless a careful examination is undertaken such a recess may be mistaken for a bony cyst.

Anatomical variations

The antra are the most symmetrical of all the paranasal sinuses. Variations in size of the antra may occur and the commonest defect is a failure of pneumatisation of the alveolar recess. This is the last portion of the antral cavity to develop and its development is dependent on the growth of the tooth buds which normally occupy it until permanent dentition is erupted. If this is incomplete the floor of the antrum may lie at the same level as the floor of the nose, and unless careful radiological study of the antrum is made this change may be mistaken in later life for new bone formation in the antral floor. Bone thickening due to an early Paget's and other bone diseases, has to be differentiated from the thick floor which is the sequel of failure of pneumatisation of the alveolar

recess of the antrum. Diagnosis can be made by the fact that the bone detail on the radiograph is normal in texture in the cases of developmental failure (fig. 21).

Over-pneumatisation of the zygomatic recess of the antrum may give appearances in the lateral films suggestive of cyst formation but the occipito-mental view and the angular appearance of the walls confirms the true nature of the "cyst".

Sub-division of the antral cavities may occur by the formation of septa. These may be bony or membranous and may be partial or complete (figs. 23, 24 and 25). It is important to recognise the presence of such a septum as in the presence of infection the surgeon may inadvertently perforate the unaffected portion of the sinus whereas the other part may be filled with pus. In true septate antra the septum is seen as a thin line crossing the antrum, usually in an oblique direction antero-posteriorly. The lower border of the middle turbinate bone which in the lateral view is seen crossing the antrum, from behind, in an upward and forwards direction, must not be mistaken for a septum. In a true septate antrum two ostia, one for each chamber, are always present. One ostium may open in its normal position, the second ostium opening into the ethmoidal infundibulum (Glass, 1952). In cases of doubt the introduction of Lipiodol through one of these ostia will clarify the position. Not infrequently a posterior ethmoid cell grows downwards into the

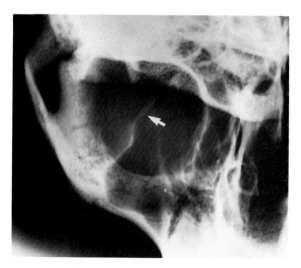

Fig. 23. Radiograph of dried skull specimen showing a bony septum in antral wall.

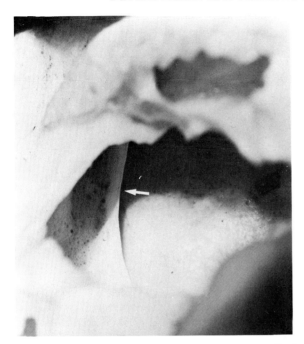

Fig. 24. Anatomical dissection after removal of medial wall of antrum, showing bony septum on lateral wall (see fig. 23).

body of the maxilla and encroaches in varying degrees on the cavity of the antrum. Usually, these maxillo-ethmoidal cells occupy the supero-medial part of the antrum but rarely they may be much

larger and occupy as much as half of the entire vertical extent of the antrum. The relative position of these cells in the occipito-mental view can be seen clearly when they have been outlined with Lipiodol. They may simulate a septate antrum radiographically but anatomically they communicate with the superior meatus, whereas both the ostia from a septate antrum open into the middle meatus. These aberrant cells may become infected without involvement of the antrum and may then appear as opacities in the normal translucent antrum or in cases where the antrum is opaque and the uninvolved ethmoidal cell clear, it may appear as a translucency (fig. 26). Well pneumatised lateral recesses of the sphenoid sinuses are projected over the antra in the occipito-mental view and must not be confused with such aberrant ethmoidal cells.

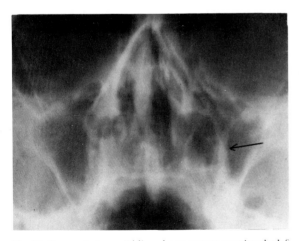

Fig. 25. Septate Antrum. Oblique bony septum crossing the left antrum. Ethmoidal cells projecting into the medial wall of the antrum may closely simulate a septate antrum. The lower part of the linea innominata may also cross the sinus, mimicking a septum.

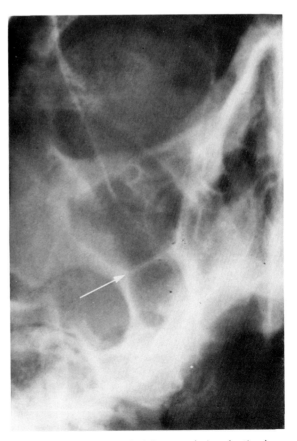

Fig. 26. Septate antrum. Occipito-mental view showing bony septum completely traversing the right antrum.

FRONTAL SINUSES

According to Van Alyea (1941) the frontal sinuses with rare exceptions develop from one or other of two main areas:

(a) The *recessus frontalis* in the ascending ramus of the middle meatus.
(b) The *infundibulum ethmoidale* located in the descending ramus of the middle meatus. (The infundibulum ethmoidale is a crescentic depression or groove in the lateral nasal wall between the uncinate process and the ethmoidal bullae).

These structures – recessus frontalis and infundibulum ethmoidale – develop in the lateral nasal wall at a comparatively early age. In the first few weeks of intra-uterine life the lateral nasal wall is smooth and no irregularity interrupts its even contours. Furrows gradually appear which give origin to the meati and the ridges separating them become rudimentary turbinates.

The cell which gives rise to the frontal sinus is lined with mucous membrane and surrounded by a thin layer of compact bone; it grows upwards simultaneously with the absorption of the cancellous bone substance. By the end of the first year it is still ethmoidal in topography but during the second year of life pneumatisation has reached the frontal bone, and by the third year the apex of the sinus is well above the level of the nasion.

The frontal sinuses are rudimentary at birth and can seldom be demonstrated radiographically until they have extended into the vertical portion of the frontal bone, a process which varies considerably but which seldom occurs to any degree before the age of two years.

The development of the frontal sinus occurs *pari-passu* with the development of the frontal bone. The latter is ossified from two separate nuclei separated by the frontal suture. Union of two centres with disappearance of the suture commences at the age of two and the suture is almost completely obliterated by eight years. By this time the frontal sinuses generally measure less than 1 cm in height and slightly less in their transverse diameter; they reach adult size at puberty. When the two frontal bones remain unfused and the suture persists (metopic suture) pneumatisation of the frontal sinuses is invariably retarded or they may fail to develop and be completely absent.

In childhood the x-ray appearances of the frontal sinus may be confusing. In infants the frontal sinus tends to be rather cloudy and ill-defined, due to the fact that the developing sinus is closer to the posterior than the anterior wall of the frontal bone, with the result that the relatively thick anterior wall gives a diminished translucency to the sinus. The sinus outlines are hazy because their development is incomplete, and the sharply defined outlines of the adult frontal sinus are not seen until the enveloping compact bony layer is formed. This applies equally to all sinuses during development and should be borne in mind when estimating infection of the paranasal sinuses in children.

The fully developed frontal sinuses are two irregular air-filled cavities which lie between the inner and outer tables of the frontal bone. They are composed of a central cavity forming the main body of the sinus, and two extensions; a vertical extension upwards into the vertical portion of the frontal bone, and a horizontal (supra-orbital) component which extends backwards in the orbital plate of the frontal bone (fig. 8). One or either extension may be developed at the expense of the other and one or both may be absent (fig. 27).

The frontal sinuses are seldom symmetrical. One sinus may extend beyond the midline encroaching on the opposite frontal sinus. The central subdividing septum in such cases is deflected, usually in its posterior aspect, its anterior edge being frequently in the midline. Along the roof and anterior wall of the sinuses there are numerous bony ridges which in the postero-anterior radiograph appear to project downwards into the sinus. Arising from these bony ridges are membranous septa which hang into the frontal sinus and may partly or completely subdivide the sinus. Partial subdivision of the sinus is common, complete subdivision on the other hand is rare. The importance of these septa lies in the fact that a complete septum may form a limiting barrier to infection. Partial septa, on the other hand, have no such limiting effect on infective processes.

The posterior wall of the frontal sinus is thin and is fairly constant in thickness. The anterior wall, however, varies considerably and additionally thick bone which is often present over the medial portion gives it a less translucent appearance on the radiograph.

A congenital absence of one of the frontal sinuses is fairly common (fig. 27). More rarely both are

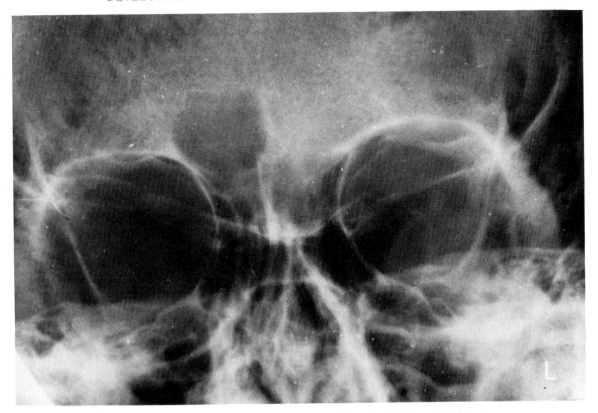

Fig. 27. Congenital absence of left frontal sinus. These appearances must not be confused with opacity of the sinus.

absent, a feature usually associated with a persistent metopic suture. The degree of development of the frontal air sinus appears to be related to the development of the supra-orbital ridges. Well-marked supra-orbital ridges are almost invariably associated with well-pneumatised frontal sinuses. Pathological overgrowth of the supra-orbital ridges such as occurs in acromegaly is associated with a marked enlargement of the frontal sinuses, forming one of the classical radiological signs of acromegaly (fig. 28).

The development of the frontal sinuses is dependent on constitutional, hormonal and racial factors and the radiological features are characteristic for each individual. The frontal sinuses increase in size with ageing and both the vertical and antero-posterior diameter increase in size. The enlargement of the antero-posterior diameter is largely at the expense of the outer table of the skull. The shape of the frontal sinuses is

specific for the individual and for this reason Schuller (1943) and Culbert & Law (1927) have suggested that an investigation of the frontal sinuses in the postero-anterior position would be of considerable medico-legal value in establishing identity.

The radiological features of the frontal sinuses are best studied in the occipito-frontal, lateral and submento-vertical views. These films are mutually complementary and as with the study of the other paranasal sinuses, examination in the occipito-frontal plane alone fails to provide information as regards the thickness of the bony walls and also of the depth of the frontal sinus. Unless these factors are known an interpretation as to the cause of diminished translucency may be completely fallacious.

The frontal sinus communicates with the middle meatus by the fronto-nasal duct. This varies greatly in diameter, length and direction. It is often very

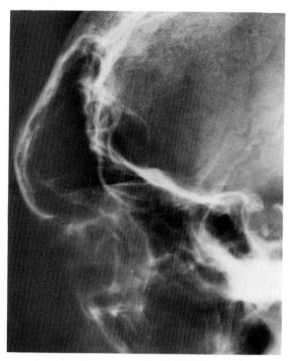

Fig. 28. Acromegaly showing gross enlargement of the frontal sinus. Minimal enlargement of the sella turcica is present.

tortuous, being frequently encroached upon by the fronto-ethmoidal cells. Sometimes the duct opens into an ethmoidal cell instead of directly into the nose. Occasionally the duct is absent and the frontal sinus opens directly into the middle meatus. Owing to the fact that both open into the middle meatus, secretions from the frontal sinuses readily find their way into the anterior cells. Almost invariably, infection of the frontal sinuses is accompanied by some degree of opacity of the anterior ethmoidal cells on the same side. This does not apply to the posterior-ethmoidal cells which open into the superior meatus.

Again, in the majority of cases the fronto-nasal duct opens into the hiatus semi-lunaris of the middle meatus, hence secretion from the frontal sinus is able to pass into the maxillary antrum through its ostium which lies at a lower level in the hiatus semi-lunaris. Unlike the antrum, the ostium of the frontal sinus lies at its lowermost point; it is easily blocked by swollen mucosa, polypi and also by injury to the surrounding bone. This is one of the reasons why mucoceles are more commonly

found in the frontal sinuses than in any of the other paranasal sinuses.

SPHENOID SINUSES

The sphenoid sinus develops as a constriction of the nasal cavity which enlarges into the body of the sphenoid bone. Radiologically, the sphenoid sinus is seldom visible until the age of three years. In the adult the degree of pneumatisation of the sinus varies considerably. The average antero-posterior diameter of the sphenoid sinus involves the anterior two-thirds of the sphenoid bone. On occasions, complete failure of pneumatisation may occur. In such cases ethmoidal cells may grow into the sphenoid bone. Frequently the whole bone is completely pneumatised, the clinoid processes, especially the posterior clinoids, being involved in the pneumatisation. More infrequently the pneumatisation of the sphenoid bone (fig. 24) may involve the pterygoid processes, the greater wings of the sphenoid and, exceptionally, the basilar process of the occipital bone. The sphenoid sinuses may also extend into and occupy the ethmoidal field. Pneumatisation of the greater wings of the sphenoid bone was found in 19·5% of patients and of the basilar portion of the occipital bone in 38·1%. The sinus extended into the pterygoid process unilaterally in 25·7% and bilaterally in only 3%. Pneumatisation in the region of the optic canal was seen in 18·4% of patients but was extensive in only 3% (Peele & Lejeune, 1942) (fig. 30).

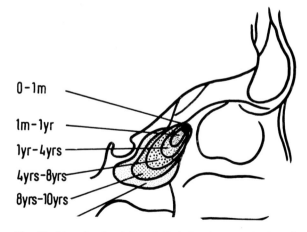

Fig. 29. Line drawing (after Caffey) showing growth size of sphenoid sinus from the neonatal period to adult life.

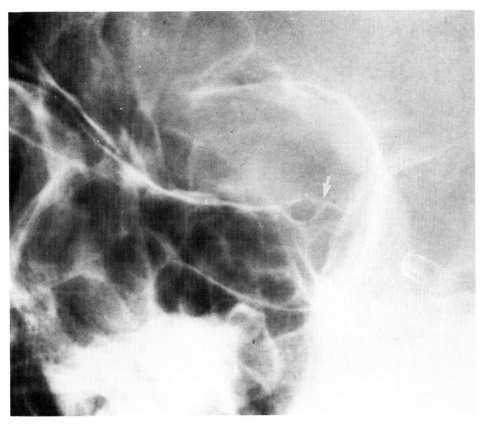

Fig. 30. Double optic foramen. Pneumatised anterior clinoid process simulating a second foramen behind the true optic foramen which lies anteriorly.

Van Alyea (1941) in an anatomical study of the sphenoid sinuses, found that the sinus varied most in its antero-posterior direction. Of 100 specimens the antero-posterior measurement varied from 4 to 44 mm with an average diameter of 23·2 mm.

The sphenoid septum dividing the right from the left sphenoid sinus tends to be in the midline anteriorly whilst posteriorly it deviates to one side or the other. The average width was 25–34 mm with an average height of 19 mm. Accessory inter-sinus septa are seen in 25% of patients and are most commonly seen in the posterior, lateral and postero-lateral regions (Peele & Lejeune, 1942). The position of the intersinus septum has an important bearing on the surgical approach to trans-sphenoidal hypophysectomy and Yttrium implants and preoperative tomographic demonstration of this septum is vital.

The relationship of the sphenoid sinus to the sella turcica is intimate. Whilst normally the posterior border occurs near that of the sella, in some cases the sphenoid sinus extends into the posterior clinoid process. In the oblique view when the anterior clinoid process is pneumatised, lying lateral to the optic foramen it may be erroneously diagnosed as a double or bifid optic foramen (fig. 30). Ossification of the ligament extending from the anterior to the middle clinoid process results in the appearance of another foramen, the clino-carotid, in this region. This foramen is most clearly seen in the lateral view and appears superimposed on the upper end of the superior orbital fissure in the oblique view (Etter, 1952).

All tumours of the pituitary fossa to a certain extent affect the roof of the sphenoid sinus. The factors which determine the spread of a pituitary

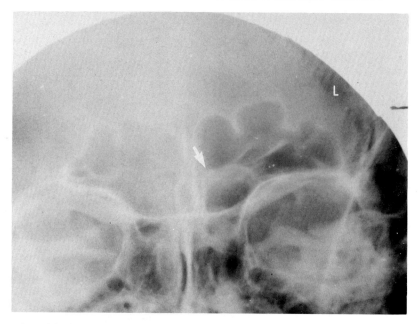

Fig. 31. Frontal agger ethmoidal cell. Occipito-mental view demonstrating an agger ethmoidal cell projecting into the floor of the left frontal sinus. The left frontal sinus shows normal translucency, the right is opaque.

tumour to the sphenoid sinus are probably to a large extent mechanical. Radiologically, the earliest signs are dependent on the rate of growth of the tumour. A rapidly growing tumour decalcifies the roof of the sinus, giving the floor of the sella a decalcified appearance when compared with the anterior and posterior walls. In such cases the significance of this change may be overlooked if only the lateral view is examined. Lateral tomograms will frequently reveal changes in one side of the sella which are completely unsuspected in conventional views. Later the tumour may break through the roof into the body of the sphenoid. In such cases the tumour mass may be visualised within the air-filled sphenoid sinus.

If the tumour is more slow in its growth the floor is pushed downwards retaining its wall and giving the well-known double contour of the sella turcica.

The radiological assessment of the degree of pneumatisation of the sphenoid sinus is of great importance in the surgical approach to tumours of the pituitary. In cases where the tumour has enlarged downwards into a well-developed sphenoid sinus, trans-sphenoid approach is probably the best surgical approach to the tumour (Nager, 1940).

The importance of the trans-sphenoidal approach to pituitary ablation in the treatment of advanced malignancy has focused closer attention on the radiological anatomy of the sphenoid sinus and an examination of the sinuses to exclude infection is essential before undertaking any trans-sphenoid surgery.

Ethmoid cells

The ethmoidal cells form a paired group of cells occupying the lateral masses of the ethmoid bones and placed between the orbits. The ethmoidal cells vary in number from a few large cells to 18 or 20 smaller cells. The development of the ethmoidal cells is proportional to the development of the other paranasal sinuses.

Davies (1938) states that the pneumatisation of the ethmoidal mass is complete at birth and afterwards the cells increase not only in size but by expansion and by invasion into the bony regions around. The extension and increase in size of the ethmoidal cells closely follows the development of the ethmoidal capsule.

Anatomically the ethmoid cells can be divided into anterior, middle and posterior ethmoidal cells.

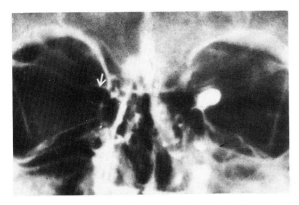

Fig. 32. Agger ethmoidal cell extending into the left anterior clinoid process. On the left side the cell has been filled with contrast medium (Proetz displacement method). On the right side the cell is air-filled. Fragments of contrast medium can be seen in other ethmoidal cells.

Radiologically these cells can be classified into anterior and posterior groups.

The anterior ethmoidal cells vary from 2 to 8 in number (Schaeffer, 1940) in the anterior part of the nasal fossae. They can be classified according to the anatomical sites of drainage.

(a) Frontal ethmoidal cells (figs. 31, 32).
(b) Infundibular anterior ethmoidal cells.
(c) The hilar anterior ethmoidal cells.

The posterior ethmoidal cells vary from one to eight in number. They are located posteriorly to the anterior ethmoid and communicate with the superior meatus.

The ethmoid cells may migrate during development beyond the confines of the ethmoidal capsule, such cells being called agger ethmoidal cells. Agger cells frequently occur in the frontal bone, the sphenoid bone, the palatine and in the nasal bones. Pneumatisation of the ethmoidal concha may result in the development of the conchal cells.

Agger cells in the sphenoid (fig. 33) maxilla or frontal bones may grow to such degree as to be considerably larger than the sinus itself, and radiologically they may be mistaken for the sinus proper. Under-development of a sinus is frequently associated with the corresponding development of an agger ethmoid cell on the affected side. This feature is most frequently seen in the frontal sinus where a congenital absence of a frontal sinus and its

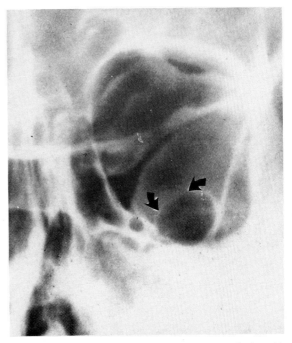

Fig. 33. Agger ethmoidal cell lying in greater wing of sphenoid. The rounded agger cell lying in the greater wing of the left sphenoid bone appears as a translucent defect with a well marked bony wall.

replacement by an agger ethmoid cell is not infrequent. In such cases often it may not be possible radiologically to distinguish between an agger ethmoidal cell and an under-developed frontal sinus.

The agger cells in the middle concha may enlarge to such a degree as to cause obstruction of the middle meatus, whilst enlargement of the agger nasi ethmoid cell may obstruct the lower end of the fronto-nasal duct.

DEVELOPMENTAL VARIATIONS

Variations in development of the paranasal sinuses may be the result of endocrine disturbances as well as of local changes. The maxillary antrum and the ethmoids are less affected than frontal and sphenoidal sinuses. Over-development of the frontal sinuses is particularly seen in acromegaly whilst under-development is a feature of hypo-thyroidism (Cretinism).

Excessive pneumatisation

Acromegaly. An increased pneumatisation of the frontal sinuses associated with over-development of the supra-orbital ridges is usually a prominent feature. Over-development usually affects both the vertical and the supra-orbital extensions of the frontal sinuses.

Cerebral conditions. Agenesis of a cerebral hemisphere or cerebral hemi-atrophy following a birth injury may result in an over-pneumatisation of the nasal sinuses. The frontal sinus and the petrous bone may show over-pneumatisation on the affected side (Dyke, Davidoff & Masson, 1922). The maxillay antra, ethmoid and sphenoid sinuses seldom show any appreciable over-pneumatisation but the sphenoid and frontal sinuses may show this change in the presence of a meningioma (see Chapter 4.

Microcephaly. A relative over-development of the maxillary antra may occur in microcephaly. The frontal sinuses are generally under-developed and may be congenitally absent. The mastoid cells may also show over-pneumatisation.

Defective pneumatisation

General failure of pneumatisation of the paranasal sinuses is usually part of a generalised disease whilst local aplasia is usually the result of local lesions.

Congenital absence of the frontal sinuses is said to occur in 5% of the population (Welin, 1952). The metopic suture subdivides the developing halves of the frontal bone and its persistence is often associated with the absence of the frontal sinuses.

Under-development of one half of the cranial vault as a result of premature fusion of the cranial sutures (cranio-stenosis) is associated with under-development of the frontal sinus on the affected side. This is in direct contrast to hemi-atrophy of the skull secondary to cerebral agenesis when over-pneumatisation of the sinuses on the affected side is a prominent feature and is a valuable sign in the radiological differentiation of the causes of an asymmetrical cranial vault.

Ninety-three per cent of mongols (Down's syndrome) examined by Spitzer & Robinson (1953) showed absence of the frontal sinuses. Cretinism may be associated with a generalised under-development of the paranasal sinuses. Absence of pneumatisation of the maxillay antrum may be seen in sickle-cell anaemia and thalassaemia.

REFERENCES

CHUANG, V. P. & VINES, F. S. (1973) Roentgenology of the Posterior Superior Alveolar Foramina and Canals. *Am. J. Roentg.*, **118**, 426.

CULBERT, W. L. & LAW, F. M. (1927) Identification by Comparison of Roentgenograms of Nasal Sinuses and Accessory Mastoid Processes. *J. Am. med. Ass.*, **88**, 1634.

DAVIES, B. A. (1938) The Paranasal Sinuses in Childhood. *Proc. R. Soc. Med.*, **31**, 1411.

DYKE, C. G., DAVIDOFF, L. M. & MASSON, C. B. (1933) Cerebral Hemiatrophy with Homolateral Hypertrophy of the Skull and Sinuses. *S. G. O.*, **57**, 588.

ETTER, L. E. (1952) Detailed Roentgen Anatomy of the Orbits. *Radiology*, **52**, 489.

GLASS, M. (1952) Duplication of the Maxillary Antrum. Symptomatology, Diagnosis and Treatment. *S. Afr. med. J.*, **26/45**, 895.

NAGER, F. R. (1940) The Paranasal Approach to Intrasellar Tumour. *J. Lar. Otol.*, **55**, 361.

ONODI, A. (1911) *The Accessory Sinuses of the Nose in Children.* Trans. C. Prausnitz. London: John Bale.

PEELE, J. C. & LEJEUNE, F. E. (1942) Roentgenography of Sphenoid Sinus. *Laryngoscope*, **52**, 522.

SCHAEFFER, J. P. (1920) *The Nose, Paranasal Sinuses, Nasolacrimal Passageways and Olfactory Organ in Man.* Philadelphia: Blakiston.

SCHAEFFER, J. P. (1940) *The Head and Neck in Roentgen Diagnosis.* London: Baillière.

SCHÜLLER, A. (1943) A Note on the Identification of Skulls by x-ray Pictures of the Frontal Sinuses. *Med. J. Aust.*, **30**, 554.

SPITZER, R. & ROBINSON, M. I. (1953) Radiological Changes in Teeth and Skull of Mental Defectives. *Br. J. Radiol.*, **27**, 117.

VAN ALYEA, O. E. (1941) Sphenoid Sinus. *Archs Otol.*, **34**, 225.

WASSON, W. W. (1933) Changes in the Nasal Accessory Sinuses after Birth. *Archs Otol.*, **17**, 197.

WELIN, S. (1952) In *Roentgen-Diagnostics*, Vol. II. Ed. Schinz, Baensch, Friedl and Uehlinger. New York: Grune & Stratton. p. 1778.

CHAPTER 3

Pathological changes affecting the nasal cavities

CONGENITAL LESIONS

Choanal atresia

Congenital occlusion of the posterior nares is one of the rare causes of nasal obstruction in infants and young children. Stewart (1931) only found 6 cases in the records of the Edinburgh Royal Infirmary between 1907–26. In the Massachusetts General Hospital during the period 1903–37 there were only 10 cases of choanal atresia. Of these 10 cases, 4 had right-sided, 3 left-sided and 3 bilateral atresia. In 1939 from the Mayo Clinic, Pastore and Williams recorded a total of 12 cases, 4 of which were bilateral and 8 unilateral. Choanal atresia may present as a respiratory emergency in the neonate presenting with asphyxial attacks and feeding difficulties (Medory & Beckman, 1951). Unilateral choanal atresia may go unrecognised until adolescence or even to adult life.

Choanal atresia may be unilateral or bilateral, complete or incomplete, and it may be of membranous or bony structure. The membranous variety probably represents the persistence of the bucco-pharyngeal membrane which is attached to the extreme posterior margin of the choana (Boyd, 1945). The vast majority of congenital atresias are bony (90% according to Lebensohn, 1923) and the thickness of the bony septum may vary from 1–12 mm. Even in cases of bony atresia the bony septum is difficult to see on the radiograph without the use of contrast media. Associated with the choanal atresia there may be facial asymmetry and a high arched palate. The nose is also generally abnormal and Asherson (1930) reported a case showing separation of the nasal cartilages.

Radiological appearances. Radiologically, the following features can be detected in the routine views:

(a) There may be *diminished translucency of the affected half of the nasal cavity*. This can be best seen in the postero-anterior view. Tomographs in the postero-anterior plane also clearly demonstrate that this difference is due to a maldevelopment of the whole of the affected half of the nose (figs. 34, 35).

(b) In the lateral view the *bony obstructing septum may be seen*.

(c) *Paradoxical expiratory ballooning of hypopharynx*. Fluoroscopic examination will show a paradoxical expiratory ballooning of the hypopharynx and its collapse in inspiration (Whitehouse & Holt, 1952).

(d) *The extent and degree of stenosis can be best estimated by instilling oily contrast medium into the nasal cavities* and radiographing the patient in the submento-vertical or lateral positions (Pesti, 1939). An oily contrast medium is introduced through a fine polythene catheter and films taken in the postero-anterior and lateral position using a horizontal ray for the latter view. The contrast material is seen to pool in the posterior part of the nares (figs. 36, 37).

Differential diagnosis. Choanal atresia in the neonate has to be differentiated from post-nasal obstruction due to adenoids or congenital post-nasal polypi. In the older child the causes of intra-nasal occlusion such as due to polypi, bony tumours or new growths, and cicatricial stenosis of the nasopharynx (post-tonsillectomy, syphilitic, diphtheritic or caustic burns) have to be con-

25

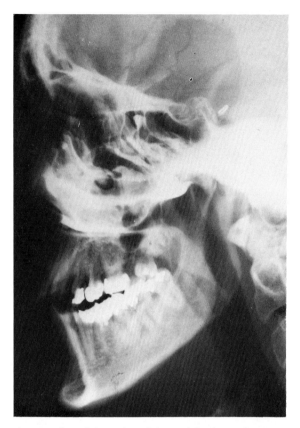

Fig. 34. Unilateral choanal atresia in an adult. The nasal cavity on the affected side is under-developed and the oily medium is at the obstructed choana. Some medium has extended upwards into the spheno-ethmoidal recess.

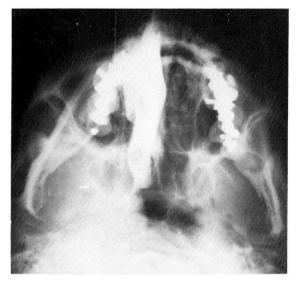

Fig. 35. Choanal atresia. Submento-vertical view of case shown in fig. 34.

sidered, the atresia in this age group being unilateral.

Variations in the size of the anterior nares correspond to the general configuration of the facial bones. The nasal septum almost inavariably shows a deviation to one side or another, except in the newborn or very young. Likewise, there is an almost constant asymmetry of the turbinate bones.

Congenital absence of turbinates

Congenital absence of one or all of the turbinates may occur but radiological investigation of this abnormality is seldom requested as direct inspection is a far more accurate means of investigation.

FOREIGN BODIES

Radiology is an invaluable adjunct in the diagnosis of foreign bodies lodged in the nasal cavities. In infants and small children a persistent or unilateral sanguinous or mucopurulent discharge should always suggest the possibility of an intranasal foreign body. Only intranasal foreign bodies which contain radio-opaque nuclei can be demonstrated, but soft tissue films will often enable foreign bodies of comparatively low radio-opacity to be demonstrated. It must be remembered, however, that a negative radiographic examination does not exclude the presence of an intranasal foreign body, and the plastic toys and buttons which are so frequently the cause of intranasal foreign bodies do not cast a significant radio-opaque shadow.

Foreign bodies either of the radio-opaque or non-opaque type if lodged in the nasal cavity for any length of time frequently form a nucleus for the development of a rhinolith.

Polsen (1943) has defined a *rhinolith* as the result of a complete or partial encrustation of an intra-nasal foreign body with lime salts. The foreign body nucleus is generally of extrinsic but may be of intrinsic origin. The commonest foreign bodies include fruit stones (especially cherry stones), buttons, or fragments of paper. The endogenous

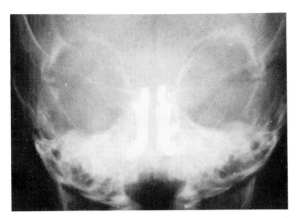

Fig. 36. Choanal atresia in the newborn. Occipito-frontal view of newborn infant after the instillation of lipiodol outlining the nasal fossa but showing complete obstruction posteriorly. (Courtesy of Dr. S. P. Rawson.)

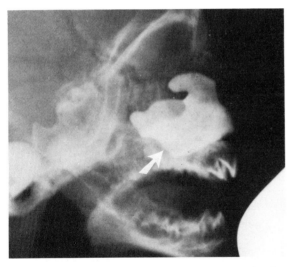

Fig. 37. Choanal atresia. Lateral view of same case showing obstruction posteriorly. (Courtesy of Dr. S. P. Rawson.)

foreign bodies are generally fragments of dried clot, misplaced teeth, sequestra or even inspissated nasal secretions. The coating is formed by calcium phosphate and carbonate, which in turn is derived from inflammatory products.

Nasopharyngeal rhinoliths are extremely uncommon but several cases have been recorded. Rhinoliths are more frequently found in females. No satisfactory explanation for this has been advanced. The age incidence is extensive and they have occurred in patients between the ages of 3 and 76 years. The maximum incidence is in the third decade with only a slightly lower frequency in the adjoining decades. The danger period for the entry of nasal foreign bodies is believed to be in the first decade of life but it has not been possible to determine from clinical evidence the time interval necessary for the development of the rhinolith.

Rhinoliths are generally found in the lower half of the nose situated about midway between the anterior and posterior nares. They are usually situated on the floor of the nose in the inferior meatus or between the inferior turbinate bones and the nasal septum. Bross (1917) found that the vast majority (80%) occupy the inferior meatus.

Rhinoliths have been subdivided into true and false depending on the presence or otherwise of a nucleus. Polsen (1943) considers that an aetiological classification depending on the endogenous or exogenous nature of the nucleus would be more appropriate.

The origin of the calcium salt forming the stone is a source of controversy. Tears have been shown to contain calcium and have been regarded as the source of calcium, whilst other authors believe that it is derived from nasal mucus. The principal source of calcium, however, would appear to be the nasal secretions.

The vast majority of rhinoliths produce clinical symptoms. In only four of a series of cases reviewed by Polsen (1943) were rhinoliths accidentally discovered. In the vast majority unilateral nasal discharge, often purulent and sometimes sanguinous, was present. Subjective or objective unilateral nasal obstruction was discovered in most of the cases. Epistaxis may also occur and in large rhinoliths visible swelling of the nose may be present.

Antral rhinoliths which are excessively rare (only six cases being reported in the literature) are formed by the same processes as nasal rhinoliths developing around foreign bodies located in the antrum.

Lord (1944) records an example of antral rhinolith occurring in a male aged 50 years where the foreign body nucleus consisted of pieces of paper. There was no preoperative radiograph taken but in Zuckerkandle's case (1892) the antrum was expanded, bulging into the nose and along the alveolar margin. Antral rhinoliths are associated with infection and the changes produced by this may obscure the underlying rhinolith.

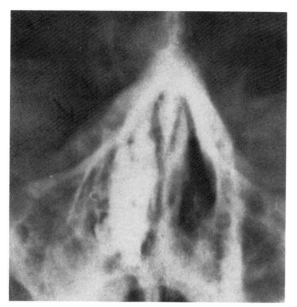

Fig. 38. Large rhinolith lying in the nostril of a male aged 72 years. Nasal obstruction has been present for many years and more recently a bloodstained discharge had been noted. There was actual bulging of the nose on the affected side. Piecemeal removal completely relieved the symptoms.

The first radiological diagnosis of a rhinolith was made by MacIntyre (1900) only four years after Roentgen's discovery of x-rays.

Radiological appearances

(1) *A densely calcified mass lying in the nasal cavity* usually in the sites already mentioned (fig. 38). The calcified mass has a coraline appearance with the central nucleus appearing as a mass of greater or lesser density depending on the nature of the foreign body. Metallic foreign bodies are seldom encrusted to such a degree as to obscure them. Polsen (1943) in a review of rhinoliths emphasised the value of the probe as a method of diagnosis. It is, however, extremely likely that with this method, small rhinoliths will be overlooked. By proper technique radiography will demonstrate the vast majority of rhinoliths, and is a far more satisfactory method of confirming their presence. Radiography will further demonstrate the extent of damage and compression of the bony nasal cavity and septum produced by the stone. Rhinoliths may considerably displace and even perforate the nasal septum and larger ones may considerably expand the nasal cavity (Samuel, 1943).

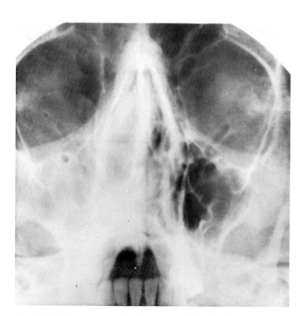

Fig. 39. Rhinitis caseosa. Occipito-mental view showing an opaque right antrum and an opaque right half of nasal cavity.

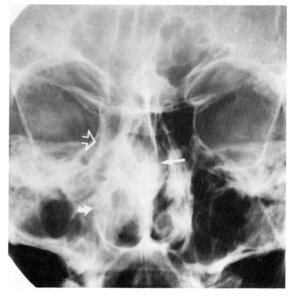

Fig. 40. Rhinitis caseosa. Occipito-frontal view showing thinning and expansion of the walls of the right nasal cavity associated with the large caseous mass.

(2) *Destruction of the nasal bones* is uncommon unless osteomyelitis supervenes. Bony changes are unusual as the diagnosis is generally made long before these changes have occurred, but pressure atrophy of the walls of the nasal cavity may occur with large rhinoliths. Other foreign bodies may enter the nasal cavities by direct penetration through the skin. Foreign bodies, particularly fragments of glass from shattered windscreens in motor accidents, may penetrate into the nose or the anterior ethmoid cells and even into the frontal sinus (figs. 143, 144).

Misplaced teeth occasionally present as foreign bodies in the floor of the nose and give rise to symptoms. The misplaced tooth is usually surrounded by periodontal membrane even when there is no obvious bony cover present.

Rhinitis Caseosa

The nasal cavity becomes filled with a cheese-like mass which may cause widening of the nasal bones (figs. 39, 40).

INFLAMMATORY LESIONS

Inflammatory lesions involving the soft tissues and cartilages of the nose seldom call for radiological examination. Acute inflammatory lesions involving the nose do not give any diagnostic appearances. On the other hand chronic granulomatous lesions may involve the nasal bones, nasal septum and adjacent sinuses. Friedman (1971) classifies nasal granulomatous lesions into specific and non-specific inflammatory processes. The former include syphilis, tuberculosis, sarcoid, leprosy, scleroma, the mycoses and parasitic granulomas (leishmaniasis). Non-specific granulomas include the conditions known as lethal midline granuloma and Wegener's granulomatosis. The disease was first described by McBride (1886) and in 1933 Stewart published a detailed account of the clinical and histological features of the localised disease. In 1939 Wegener described three cases of another necrotising granuloma which also affected the nose but was associated with more widespread lesions in lung and kidney.

Midline lethal granuloma

This is a slowly progressive destructive ulceration of the tissues of the nose and sinuses. Soft tissue, bone and cartilage are eventually destroyed by a chronic inflammatory process leading to severe mutilation (Harrison, 1974). This author considers that this condition is a neoplasm attenuated by the individual's immunological defences and he records instances in which the lesion changed histologically into a proven malignant lymphoma. Radiologically the disease is characterised by massive destruction of the bones of the nasal cavity, palate and adjacent sinuses, with a clear-cut demarcation, a midline distribution and an absence of any significant bone reaction (figs. 41, 42).

Wegener's granulomatosis

This is a systemic disease in which a necrotising granuloma of the nose is associated with lesions in the lungs and kidneys and a vasculitis similar to polyarteritis nodosa. Loss of translucence in the sinuses, especially the maxillary antra, is the earliest radiological change followed by bone destruction in the sinus walls, palate and nasal septum. The

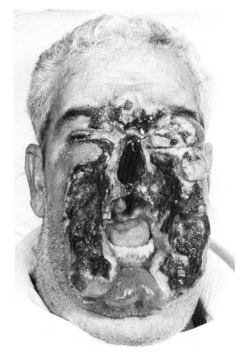

Fig. 41. Midline (lethal) granuloma showing extensive destruction of the soft tissues and bones of the face which has a progressive relentless course. (Courtesy of Professor Harrison.)

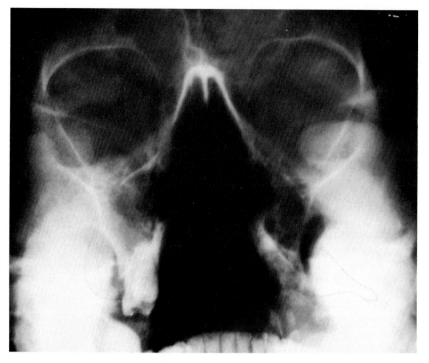

Fig. 42. Occipito-mental view of case shown in fig. 41 showing extensive bony destruction with little or no bony reaction. (By permission of W. B. Saunders Company, Philadelphia from Radiology of the Orbit by G. Lloyd.)

orbit may also be involved by extension from the antrum or ethmoid cells. Massive bone destruction, as in malignant midline granuloma does not as a rule occur. Characteristic changes are frequently found in the chest consisting of multiple areas of infarction appearing as irregular and ill-defined shadows on the radiograph but sometimes as well-rounded opacities. Not infrequently central cavitation is present in these lesions.

SPECIFIC INFLAMMATORY LESIONS

Tuberculosis

Inflammatory lesions such as tuberculosis of the nose are relatively uncommon in civilised communities but still occur with some frequency amongst the primitive people.

Lupus vulgaris. Tuberculous involvement of the nasal bones generally follows a spread of the infection from a lupus vulgaris of the face. Radiographic examination is generally requested for the assessment of the degree of bony damage rather than for diagnosis. The radiological features in such cases are similar to those of tuberculosis in other bones. The lesion is primarily destructive with little reactive change. Sequestration is, however, commoner than in other bone sites as secondary infection is often superadded, and for the same reason bone sclerosis not infrequently occurs.

Tuberculous osteo-periostitis. Tuberculous osteo-periostitis of the nasal bone generally takes one of two forms (Chavanne, 1941). One occurs in young persons and, if untreated, rapidly spreads with a fatal termination; the second type is met with in older persons and is more localised, having a more favourable prognosis. The lesion is primarily destructive. Fistulae may develop and the advent of secondary infection may result in considerable new bone formation.

Syphilis

Other more rare inflammatory conditions are due to a spirochaetal infection of the nasal bones, *e.g.*

syphilis or yaws when the primary lesion is generally a destructive one and the presence of reactive changes with bone sclerosis is unusual. At a later stage, or when secondary infection is super-added, sclerosis may occur to a marked degree. The bone destruction is usually marked, and as a result of the collapse of the nasal bones the typical saddle nose of the congenital or tertiary stage of syphilis appears.

Other more rare lesions involving the nasal bone are **goundou** (a tropical disease of doubtful aetiology) and **leprosy**. In the former condition there is an extensive destruction of the soft tissues of the nose, the nasal cartilages and the nasal bone proper. An extensive infiltration and destruction involving the walls of the nasal cavities themselves also occurs. A curious feature is the absence of any reactive change along the edges of the areas of destruction. Leprosy also frequently affects the nose. In a discussion of lesions of the upper respiratory system due to leprosy, Pinkerton (1938) found that the nasal cartilages were frequently destroyed but the nasal bone was seldom involved. Destruction of the nasal septum results in the "saddle nose" similar to that seen in congenital syphilis.

oedematous swelling caused by allergy. Hyper-trophy of the posterior end of the turbinates as a cause of nasal obstruction may be more difficult to detect clinically although posterior naso-pharyngeal examination will usually suffice. Lateral and submento-vertical views of the nasal sinuses will often show the soft tissue swelling caused by the enlarged turbinate.

Polypi

Polypoid conditions of the turbinate bone may appear as soft tissue shadows projecting into the nasal cavity. In advanced conditions they may completely obscure the air space, and in long-standing cases may give rise to expansion of the nasal cavity with pressure atrophy of the nasal bones and septum (fig. 43). In generalised poly-posis of the nose, the air spaces between the turbinates are lost, and the whole nasal cavity appears to have a ground glass appearance.

Polypi may project into the nasopharynx (antro-choanal polypi). These are best seen in the lateral view and in the open-mouth view when they appear as smooth well-defined soft tissue shadows projecting into the nasopharynx (fig. 70).

NON-INFLAMMATORY LESIONS

Hypertrophy of the turbinate bones

This can usually be recognised on clinical examination but radiologically can be seen in occipito-frontal view when the enlarged hyper-trophied turbinate bones can be seen projecting into the nasal cavity. The nasal septum may be dis-placed by the enlarged turbinate and the air space on the affected side of the nose may be obliterated. Eagle (1942) found that in cases of spheno-palatine ganglion neuralgia over 80% are due to reflex irrita-tion resulting from a trigger focus in the nose caused by contact between some of the intranasal structures. He found that bony spurs and adhesions between the nasal septum and the turbinates (generally the middle turbinates) which often formed such trigger points, could be visualised on the radiographs. Serial films may be necessary to confirm that the hypertrophy is a constant feature and not a transitory enlargement due to

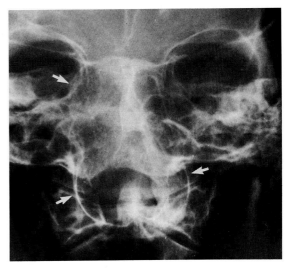

Fig. 43. Nasal polypi – showing ground glass appearance of the right side of the nasal cavity and expansion of the nasal bridge and the marked pressure atrophy of the nasal bones that may occur within polypi of long standing.

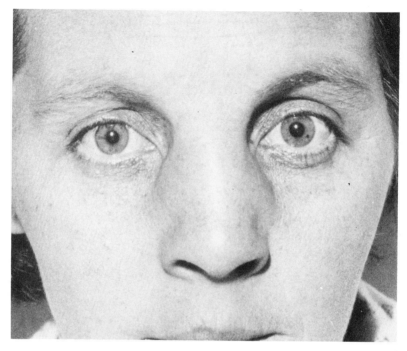

Fig. 44. Sarcoid. Showing broadening of the nasal bridge with soft tissue swelling.

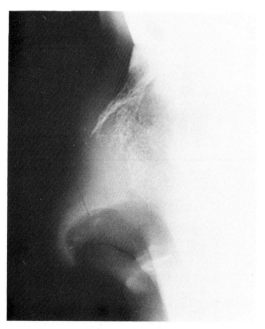

Fig. 45. Radiograph of same case showing irregular destruction and cystic changes in nasal bone. (Courtesy of Mr. C. J. Duncan, F.R.C.S.)

Sarcoid

Black (1973) has reviewed both the clinical and radiological features of nasal involvement in Sarcoid. Isolated involvement of the nasal bones is rare and diagnosis is seldom made until the skin and mucous membranes are involved. Radiological examination of the chest is valuable, as sarcoid changes in the lung field give a clue to the diagnosis. Cystic changes in the nasal bones similar to those found in the hands in sarcoidosis have been recorded (Curtis, 1964) (figs. 44, 45).

Examination and biopsy of the nasal mucosa may enable the diagnosis to be made by the recognition of the typical granuloma, long before there is any bone involvement (Poe, 1948).

PRIMARY TUMOURS

Benign tumours

These may arise from skin or cartilage. Those arising from the skin of the nose are only of radiological interest in regard to the degree of pressure changes on the nasal bones.

Dermoid cysts. Inclusion cysts (dermoids) occur at planes of congenital fusion and frequently present for radiological diagnosis. Lipiodol may be injected into the cyst and enables the extent of the cyst to be visualised pre-operatively (Juers, 1941). These cysts in most cases appear to originate in the upper part of the nose (Luongo, 1933). Crawford & Webster (1952) reviewed the features of five cases of dermoid cysts of the nose and added a further 14. Their radiological findings were:

(a) *Cavitation of the nasal bones* with little or no reactive change as the result of direct pressure on the nasal bones. In rare instances some reactive sclerosis of the nasal bones occurs (Brunner & Harned, 1942). Low-grade infective changes may, however, play some part in the production of this sclerosis. Dermoid cysts may penetrate into the frontal bone producing pressure atrophy.

(b) *Displacement of the nasal bones.* Dermoid cysts occurring in the upper part of the nose may burrow between the nasal bones and cause considerable widening of the nose with diastasis of the nasal sutures.

Encephalo-meningoceles. Encephalo-meningoceles for convenience will be considered with benign tumours and may be grouped according to their anatomical site as occipital, sincipital and basal. The sincipital and basal encephalo-meningoceles are the only varieties of interest to the otolaryngologist. Von Meyer (1890) classified *sincipital cerebral hernia* as follows:

(1) Naso-frontal, in which the herniating cerebral or meningeal tissues pass between the nasal and frontal bone, giving rise to a midline protuberance at the nasal root.

(2) Naso-ethmoid in which the defect lies between the nasal, ethmoid and frontal bones, the swelling presenting at the junction of the cartilaginous and bony part of the nose.

(3) Naso-orbital in which there is a defect in the suture line between the frontal, lachrymal and ethmoid bones, with herniation into the orbit, causing protuberance of the tissues at the inner canthus of the eye.

Radiologically sincipital encephaloceles give rise to a smooth well circumscribed dehiscence in the bone at the site of herniation.

The basal cerebral hernias are those which occur

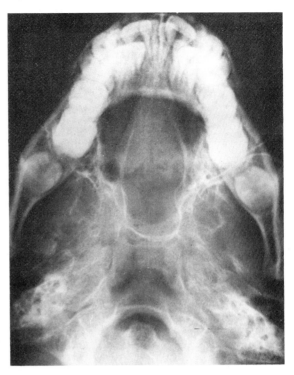

Fig. 46. Midline defect – submento-vertical view of a spheno-ethmoidal meningocele showing hypertelorism, widening of the nasal bridges and loss of bony structures near the nasal bones.

through the cribriform plate and through the sphenoid bone, herniation appearing in the nasal cavity, nasopharynx, epipharynx, sphenoid sinus, posterior orbit or pterygo-palatine fossa. The different varieties of basal encephaloceles may be described as:

(a) Transphenoidal
(b) Transethmoidal
(c) Spheno-ethmoidal (figs. 46, 47)
(d) Spheno-orbital

Transphenoidal. A defect exists in the sphenoid bone and the encephalocele usually extends into the epipharynx but may extend only into the sphenoid sinus.

Transethmoidal. This defect occurs anteriorly through the lamina cribrosa with the hernia appearing in the anterior nasal cavity.

Spheno-ethmoidal. The defect extends through the sphenoid and ethmoid bones with herniation usually appearing in the posterior nasal cavity.

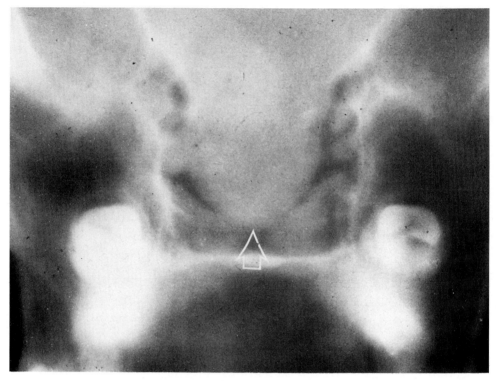

Fig. 47. Axial tomograph of case shown in fig. 46 showing the bone outlines of the defect around the spheno-ethmoidal meningocele.

Spheno-orbital. This type of encephalocele involves the posterior orbit and superior orbital fissure, and is commonly associated with neurofibromatosis.

Pollock, Newton & Hoyt (1968) have described the clinical and radiological features of eight patients with basal encephaloceles; five transphenoidal and three transethmoidal. Two important clinical findings suggest a basal encephalocele:

(a) a facial abnormality with hypertelorism, and
(b) a midline soft tissue mass in the nose or epipharyngeal space.

In the transphenoidal variety a defect in the base of the skull can be shown on plain axial views, but in a transethmoidal encephalocele tomography is necessary to demonstrate the bone defect. Pollock *et al.* (1968) found that both carotid arteriography and pneumo-encephalography were helpful in showing the extent of the cerebral herniations.

Neurofibroma and fibroma. Neurofibroma is an extremely rare tumour found in the nasal cavities (Revesz, 1948). Unless special stains for neurological tissue are made, the neurofibroma may be mistaken for a simple fibroma. Radiologically, the features are those of a soft tissue swelling usually involving the inferior meatus of the nasal cavity. There is no invasion of bone to be seen but pressure atrophy and enlargement of the affected side of the nose may occur (see also Nasopharyngeal Fibroma, Chapter 16, figs. 48, 49).

Papilloma and angioma. These tumours are small and although they frequently cause clinical symptoms, notably epistaxis, they do not give radiological signs.

The development of the technique of selective catheterisation of the external carotid artery and its internal maxillary branches has given a new scope to the diagnosis of epistaxis. In intractable cases embolisation of the bleeding branch (usually a branch of the spheno-palatine artery) has controlled a severe epistaxis. Great care, however, is needed in the selective embolisation as the

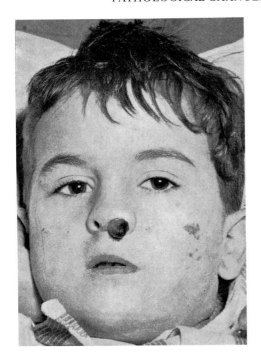

Fig. 48. Angiofibroma of nose presenting through nostril. A six-year-old child whose mother had noticed a bloodstained discharge from the left nostril. Biopsy showed a fibroma with large vascular spaces.

possibility of untoward cerebral embolisation must be guarded against (Sokoloff *et al.*, 1974).

MALIGNANT TUMOURS

Primary tumours. The vast majority of malignant tumours of the nasal cavity are carcinomas, either of the squamous cell variety or, more rarely, adenocarcinoma. Squamous cell carcinomas are especially prone to be superimposed on chronic lesions such as lupus vulgaris. The nasal cavity is more often involved secondarily by an extension of malignant tumours from the paranasal sinuses. The symptoms consequent on such an extension may be the presenting signs of such a tumour and epistaxis and nasal obstruction point to the involvement of the nasal cavity. Radiologically, such lesions can be recognised by the destruction of bony septum and of the walls of the nasal cavities.

Less commonly malignant tumours are melanomas, and Grace (1947) found 66 cases of malignant melanoma recorded. Stewart (1951) found that 4% of all malignant tumours of the nose are melanomas. Wilkinson's case (1912) of melanotic sarcoma is probably a variant of

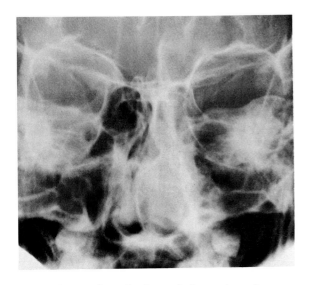

Fig. 49. Fibroma of nose showing marked expansion and pressure atrophy of walls of nasal cavities. (Case shown in fig. 48.)

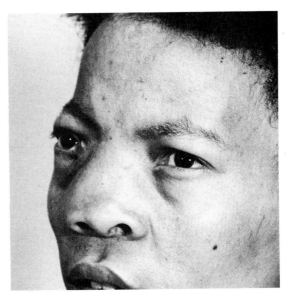

Fig. 50. A young coloured female who complained of nasal obstruction and painless swelling of the nose. Histological section of the tumour, which was easily removed, showed an olfactory neuroblastoma. (Courtesy of Dr. Sam Goldberg.)

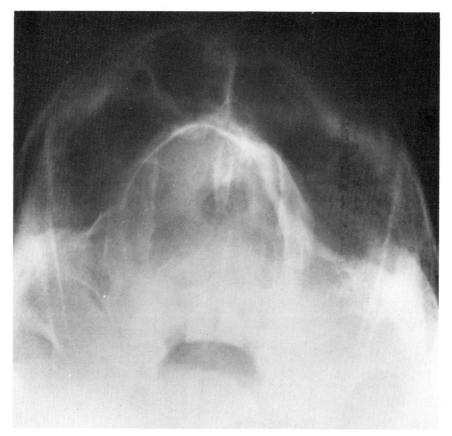

Fig. 51. Occipito-mental view showing marked thinning of the nasal bones and nasal septum together with a soft tissue swelling filling the nose. Radiograph of patient shown in fig. 50.

melanoma. In the absence of pigmentation, and many of these tumours are non-pigmented, there may be no distinguishing features from a carcinoma. Radiologically melanomas show less tendency to bone involvement than carcinoma. In Stewart's series (1951), 7 out of 13 cases showed no evidence of bone involvement.

Secondary tumours. Secondary involvement of the nasal cavity by direct spread from growths arising in the adjoining structures (usually the antrum or ethmoids) is a more frequent occurrence than truly metastatic growths occurring in the nose from distant primary growths.

Radiological appearances

(i) *Destruction of the lateral nasal wall* may be the only sign that the opacity of the nasal cavity is due to malignant disease. In estimating destruction of the lateral nasal wall, great care must be taken as, in many normal subjects, this wall is not demonstrated on the radiograph (Pancoast, Pendergress & Schaeffer, 1940). This apparent absence of the nasal wall may be due to a variety of factors, such as thinness of the bony wall together with an unusual degree of obliquity of the lateral nasal wall.

(ii) *Soft tissue mass.* The soft tissue mass in the nasal cavity may also be visualised. Extension of growths arising from the skin of the nose, *e.g.* basal cell tumours or epitheliomas, into the nasal cavity almost invariably occurs if the growth is of long standing (figs. 53, 54).

Olfactory neuroblastoma (esthesioneuro-epithelioma). The esthesioneuro-epithelioma is an infrequent malignant neoplasm arising from the

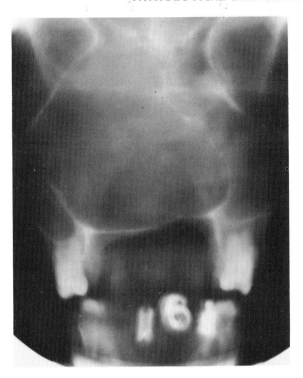

Fig. 52. Postero-anterior tomograph showing the thinned and expanded bone. (Courtesy of Dr. Sam Goldberg) (see figs. 50, 51).

olfactory apparatus, composed of undifferentiated neuro-ectodermal tissue. The neoplasm is slightly more common in males and in a survey of 68 cases compiled by Becker & Jacox (1964), the age incidence ranged from 8 to 79 years, the tumour developing in most patients between 10 and 40 years. The tumour arises most commonly from the middle turbinates and the region of the ethmoid sinuses. The most common presenting symptoms are nasal obstruction, headache and epistaxis. Less common symptoms are proptosis and anosmia. The tumour grows slowly and at times extends locally to destroy the surrounding bone involving the sinuses, orbits and brain (figs. 50, 51, 52).

NASAL FRACTURES

The nasal bones are among the commonest bones to be fractured. Fractures of the nose are frequently associated with other fractures involving the facial bones. Becker (1948) found that 8% of nasal fractures were associated with other fractures of the facial bones. Fractures of the nasal bones may be classified as follows:

(a) Greenstick fractures
(b) Linear fractures
(c) Lateral fractures
(d) Frontal fractures – partial or complete
(e) Lateral frontal fractures
(f) Fractures from below.

Greenstick fractures. The clinical symptoms of this fracture are mild and the radiograph is essentially negative. It is especially liable to occur in children. The bone is impacted at its attachment to the maxilla. The break is generally not associated with any displacement.

Linear fractures. These are simple fractures without displacement or comminution. They constitute 20% of fractures due to a slight blow or fall. The associated oedema generally gives rise to an erroneous diagnosis of a depressed fracture. Radiographs in the lateral position or in occipito-mental position generally demonstrate the fracture (fig. 55).

Lateral fractures. This is the commonest type of fracture and in a consecutive series of 100 nasal fractures it accounted for 37% of the fractures. In this type of fracture there is a depression of the nasal bone under the ascending ramus of the superior maxilla. In the majority of cases the nasal

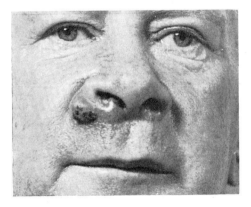

Fig. 53. Carcinoma of the nostril. A male aged 45 years who complained of bloodstained nasal discharge and a persistent "sore" on the lateral aspect of the nose. The clinical photograph shows a raised ulcerating mass present on the right side of the nostril. The clinical impression favoured a basal-celled carcinoma but the histological section showed a squamous-celled carcinoma.

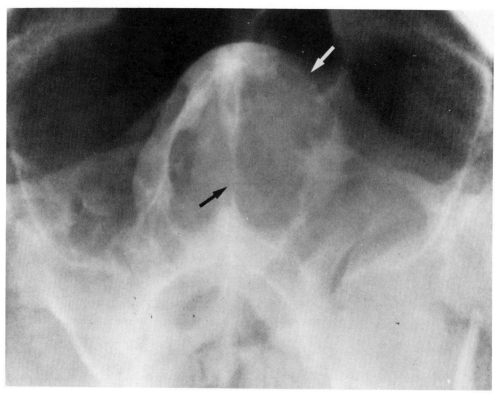

Fig. 54. Carcinoma of nose, showing extensive bone destruction of septum and lateral wall and extension into left maxillary antrum. Histological section showed a papillary mucous adenocarcinoma.

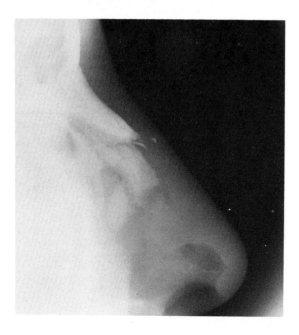

bone overrides the maxilla on the opposite side. There is separation of the nasal bones. The clinical diagnosis in this type of fracture is obvious and radiography is mainly needed to assess displacement (fig. 56).

Frontal fractures. This follows a blow delivered on the nose. In Becker's series it constituted 14% of cases. The fracture generally occurs midway through the nasal bones and is associated with depression and locking under the naso-frontal processes of the maxillary bones. In the severe type of frontal fracture the septum is crushed so that the mucosa and cartilages are telescoped into one another (fig. 57, p. 40).

Lateral frontal fractures. This group forms 10% of all types of nasal fractures. It really represents a

Fig. 55. Linear fracture of nasal bone with comminution and downward displacement of the fractured fragments. In the lateral view no estimate of the extent of lateral displacement can be seen.

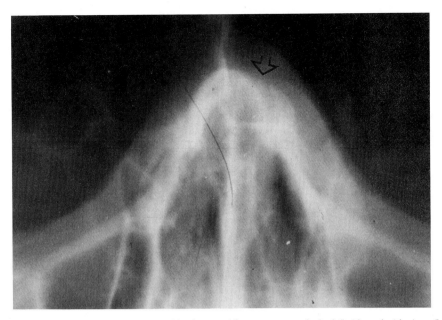

Fig. 56. Occipito-mental view showing displacement of the fractured fragments towards the left side and widening of the nasal bones.

combination of lateral and frontal fractures. The nasal bone on the side of the blow is found in one or two positions, the commonest being a slight overriding of the opposite nasal bone. The opposite nasal bone is depressed and locked under the maxilla so that a space is palpable between the two nasal bones. Small chip fractures of the lower ends of the nasal bones are also present.

Fractures from below. This is a rare type of nasal fracture and only occurred in two cases of 100 consecutive nasal fractures. The nasal bones override the maxillary bones with a resultant widening of the space between the nasal bones.

REFERENCES

ASHERSON, N. (1930) Bilateral Congenital Occlusion of the Posterior Choanae Due to a Membraneous Diaphragm. *J. Lar. Otol.*, **45**, 344.

BECKER, O. J. (1948) Nasal Fractures – Analysis of 100 Cases. *Archs Otol.*, **48**, 344.

BECKER, M. H. & JACOX, H. W. (1964) Olfactory Esthesio-neuroepithelioma: Experiences in Management of Rare Intranasal Malignant Neoplasm. *Radiology*, **82**, 77.

BLACK, J. I. M. (1973) Sarcoidosis of the Nose. *Proc. R. Soc. Med.*, **66**, 669.

BOYD, M. E. (1945) Congenital Atresia of the Posterior Nares. *Archs Otol.*, **41**, 261.

BROSS, K. (1917) Nail Nucleus. (Cited by Key-Aberg).

BRUNNER, H. & HARNED, J. W. (1942) Dermoid Cysts of the Dorsum of the Nose. *Archs Otol.*, **36**, 86.

CHAVANNE, F. (1941) *Oto-rhino-lar. int.*, **25**, 5.

CRAWFORD, J. R. & WEBSTER, J. P. (1952) Congenital Dermoid Cyst of Nose. *Plastic reconstr. Surg.*, **9**, 235.

CURTIS, G. T. (1964) Sarcoidosis of the Nasal Bones. *Br. J. Radiol.*, **37**, 433.

EAGLE, W. W. (1942) Sphenopalatine Ganglion Neuralgia. *Archs Otol.*, **35**, 66.

FRIEDMAN, I. (1971) Changing Pattern of Granulomas of Upper Respiratory Tract. *J. Lar. Otol.*, **85**, 631.

GRACE, C. C. (1947) Malignant Melanoma of the Nasal Mucosa. *Archs Otol.*, **46**, 195.

HARRISON, D. F. N. (1974) Non-healing Granulomata of the Upper Respiratory Tract. *Br. med. J.*, **iv**, 205.

JUERS, A. L. (1941) Dermoid Cyst of the Nasal Septum. *Archs Otol.*, **33**, 851.

KEY-ABERG, H. (1921/22) La Rhinolithase. Monographie et Étude de Cas. *Acta otolaryng.*, **3**, 449.

LEBENSOHN, J. E. (1923) Congenital Atresia of the Postnasal Orifices. *Ann. Otol. Rhin. Lar.*, **32**, 1128.

LORD, O. C. (1944) Antral Rhinoliths. *J. Lar. Otol.*, **59**, 218.

LUONGO, R. A. (1933) Dermoid Cyst of the Nasal Dorsum. *Archs Otol.*, **17**, 755.

McBRIDE, P. (1886) *J. Lar. Otol.*, **12**, 64. (Quoted by McCart, H.)

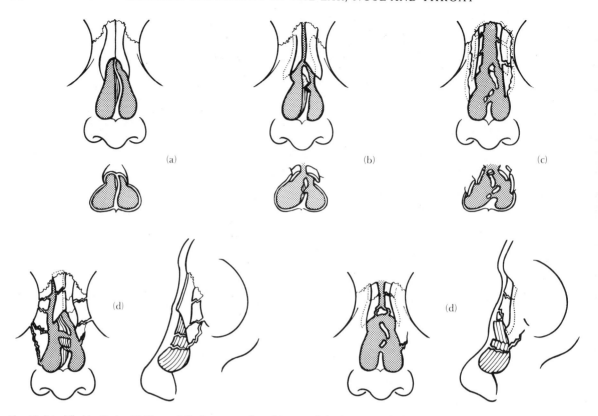

Fig. 57. (Modified by Becker.) (a) Lateral displacement of nasal bone and displacement of septum. (b) Lateral force showing overriding of nasal bone by maxilla and separation of nasal bones with deviation or fracture of the septum. (c) Comminution of the nasal bones with further force. (d) Flattening and commununtion of nasal bones with flattening of naso-frontal angle.

McCART, H. (1950) Malignant Granuloma of the Nose. *Can. med. Ass. J.,* **63**, 357.

MACINTYRE, J. (1900) Early Radiology in Nasal Disease. *J. Lar. Rhin. Otol.,* **15**, 357.

MEDORY, H. & BECKMAN, I. H. (1951) Asphyxial Attacks in a Newborn Infant Due to Congenital Occlusion of Post Nares. *Pediatrics,* **8**, 678.

PANCOAST, H. K., PENDERGRASS, E. P. & SCHAEFFER, J. P. (1940) *The Head and Neck in Roentgen Diagnosis.* Springfield: C. C. Thomas.

PASTORE, P. N. & WILLIAMS, H. L. (1939) Congenital Occlusion of the Nasal Choanae. *Proc. Mayo Clin.,* **14**, 625.

PESTI, L. (1939) Über das Rontgenbild und ein operatives Heilverfahren des Membranßsen Choanalverschlusses. *Mschr. Ohrenheilk. Lar. Rhinol.,* **73**, 245.

PINKERTON, F. J. (1938) Leprosy of Upper Respiratory Tract. *J. Am. med. Ass.,* **111**, 1437.

POE, D. L. (1948) New Diagnostic Procedure for Boeck's Sarcoid. *Archs Otol.,* **47**, 818.

POLLOCK, J. A., NEWTON, T. N. & HOYT, D. F. (1968) Trans-sphenoidal and Transethmoidal Encephaloceles. *Radiology,* **90**, 443.

POLSEN, C. J. (1943) On Rhinoliths. *J. Lar. Otol.,* **58**, 79.

REVESZ, G. (1948) Neurinoma in the Nasal Cavity. *J. Lar. Otol.,* **62**, 241.

SAMUEL, E. (1943) Rhinoliths. *Br. J. Radiol.,* **16**, 186.

SOKOLOFF, J., WICKHORN, I., McDONALD, D., BRAHME, F., GOERGEN, T. G. & GOLDBERG, L. S. (1974) Percutaneous Embolisation in Intra-stable Epistaxis. *Radiology,* **111**, 285.

STEWART, J. P. (1931) Congenital Atresia of the Posterior Nares. *Archs. Otol.,* **13**, 570.

STEWART, J. P. (1933) Progressive Lethal Granulomatous Ulceration of the Nose. *J. Lar. Otol.,* **48**, 657.

STEWART, T. S. (1951) Nasal Malignant Melanoma. *J. Lar. Otol.,* **65**, 560.

VON MEYER, E. (1890) *Virschows Arch. path. Anat. Physiol.,* **120**, 309.

WEGENER, P. (1939) *Beitr. path. Anat.,* **102**, 36.

WHITEHOUSE, W. M. & HOLT, J. F. (1952) Paradoxical Expiratory Ballooning of the Hypopharynx in Siblings with Bilateral Choanal Atresia. *Radiology, 59,* 216.

WILKINSON, G. (1912) A Case of Melanotic Sarcoma of the Nose. *J. Lar. Otol., 27,* 1.

ZUCKERKANDLE, E. (1892) *Normale und Pathologische ihrer der Nasenhohle und Pneumatischen Anhange,* Vol. 2. Wien & Leipzig: Braumuller. p. 158.

CHAPTER 4

Inflammatory and allergic states affecting the paranasal sinuses

Aetiology

The various factors concerned in mucosal changes in the paranasal sinuses may be classified as follows:

(1) Disturbances of function due to anatomical anomalies.
(2) Due to external agents, *e.g.* toxic smokes and gases.
(3) Due to infection elsewhere in the body.
(4) Bacterial infection.
(5) Allergic disease and vasomotor conditions.
(6) A combination of any of the above.

Mechanical disabilities, *e.g.* a deflected nasal septum, or a frontonasal duct obstructed by an aberrant ethmoid cell or bony injury may interfere with the drainage of a sinus. Failure of normal drainage of a sinus predisposes to infection.

The repeated spraying of the nasal passages by pus from a pulmonary infection, *e.g.* a lung abscess or bronchiectasis, may give rise to sinusitis but aspiration of infected material into the bronchial tree from a sinus is much commoner. Noxious fumes and gases may result in a sinusitis from chemical irritation of the mucosa.

Other physical conditions such as alterations in the atmospheric pressure may result in changes in the mucous membrane lining of the paranasal sinuses; this condition of aero-sinusitis (baro-trauma), is not uncommon under unpressurised flying conditions and it is described more fully in Chapter 6. All the diverse aetiological factors forming this group result in a swelling and oedema of the mucosal lining of one or all of the paranasal sinuses, and the changes occurring in the mucosa result in very similar radiological appearances.

There is a general thickening of the mucosa which may be of such a degree as to completely obliterate the cavity of the sinus. A considerable exudation of mucus also occurs. Radiologically, the changes produced by these factors may be indistinguisable from those produced by acute bacterial infection.

With infection the organism usually comes from the nasal cavities but in the case of the maxillary antrum it may originate from the mouth. The buccal source of infection is usually a dental abscess. Generalised systemic disease, *e.g.* exanthemas and indeed any febrile illness, may predispose to sinus infection. Cullom (1941) showed that in routine radiographs of the paranasal sinuses of patients with otitis media and mastoiditis following scarlet fever, concomitant involvement of the paranasal sinuses was present in 91% of cases.

The organisms responsible for sinus suppuration can be divided into two groups:

(a) Those of nasal or mucosal origin such as pneumococci, streptococci, staphylococci and the haemophilus bacillus. These organisms are mainly aerobic and the pus is not foetid. The streptococci are mainly of the haemolytic variety.
(b) Those of dental origin which are mainly anaerobic and produce foetid pus. In a considerable proportion of cases infection of the sinus from a dental source is consequent on some dental treatment.

More rarely, other organisms such as the bacillus tuberculosis or fungal infections may cause an antral infection (Adams, 1944). Radiologically, the appearances are those of an antral infection and there are no distinguishing features. There is no bone destruction to be seen associated with the mucosal thickening.

Primary infection of the paranasal sinuses with actinomycosis is excessively rare (Hersh, 1945). The radiological features show mucosal thickening but there is no evidence to indicate the nature of the infecting organism.

Mycotic infections also include aspergillosis which gives rise to non-specific granulations or a fungal ball mycetoma in the sinuses. Candidiasis and mucormycosis also occur. An example of the former infection has been recorded by Osborne (1963) who described involvement of the frontal sinus and upper part of the orbit by a fibrotic mass with opacity of the frontal sinus, ethmoids and antrum and disappearance of the infero-medial orbital margin.

Mucormycosis is a rare fungal infection most commonly seen in diabetics. The maxillary antrum is usually involved (Friedman, 1971) and often the orbit. Lungs may also be affected and the nasal sinuses are believed to be the port of entry for the organism.

Allergic and vasomotor changes

According to Hansel (1936) allergic reaction is an over-response of the body to foreign protein which has penetrated the tissues and is manifested by changes which vary from a negligible reaction to severe inflammation. It is now generally recognised that a large proportion of cases of sinus disease which were previously thought to be due to infection are in fact the result of allergy. Allergic sinusitis is met with as a component part of hay fever, asthma, vasomotor rhinitis or may occur as a separate isolated entity.

Asthma. An evaluation of the changes that occur in the paranasal sinuses in asthma is of importance as the changes may represent the cause or effect. Russell (1939) believes that many cases of asthma begin in childhood as a result of infection of the paranasal sinuses and that the mucosa is in a state of hypersensitivity from the damage due to the previous infection. Reporting on 50 cases he found that the essential change in sinus mucosa is oedema extending to polypoid formation; pus is infrequent. Other authors (Harrington, 1938; Agar &

Cazort, 1939) feel that the changes in the paranasal sinus in asthma are not primary.

Vasomotor rhinitis. This is a condition closely allied to hay fever. The symptoms are often identical but there is no seasonal incidence; the attacks occurring throughout the year. Wilson (1946) has emphasised that sufferers from this condition show certain stigmata of general vasomotor imbalance throughout the body. Easily recognisable clinical features are the poor circulation in the extremities, the cold blue appearance of the skin and the exaggerated response of the extremities to thermal stimuli.

Protracted exposure to inhaled allergens produces a chronically swollen mucosa in the sinuses which is extremely susceptible to secondary bacterial invasion. This susceptibility to infection is probably the result of disruption of the normal drainage secondary to the allergic changes.

With allergic sinusitis the mucosa of the sinuses is swollen, pale and oedematous. Localised polypoid thickening of the mucosa may occur. Nasal or choanal polypi may be present, and antral polypi when present are almost invariably associated with nasal polypi. Most observers are agreed that polypi have an allergic basis. Microscopically, eosinophils are present in polyps and plasma cells in various stages of development can be found (Lucas, 1952). If, on the other hand, allergic sinusitis becomes secondarily infected the mucosa becomes swollen, reddened and later may become atrophic.

In addition to the changes occurring in the mucosa the underlying mucoperiosteum of the bony sinus wall may be affected. In the acute stage a hyperaemic state of the mucoperiosteum may produce slight decalcification of the bony walls of the sinus.

With chronic bacterial infection, however, the bony walls may become sclerosed and dense (sclerosing osteitis), a feature which may assist in differentiating allergic from bacterial sinusitis.

In other instances, the changes may produce a transient or permanent block of the ostium of the sinus. In such cases the secretions of the antrum, mucus or pus, become retained and an empyema of the sinus may develop. If air remains in the sinus it may be possible to demonstrate a fluid level in the erect position. In other cases the fluid contents may completely fill the sinus producing a homogeneous opacity.

Chronic sinus infection may arise either as a

sequel of acute infection or it may be chronic from its inception. Under these conditions the mucous membrane becomes infiltrated with plasma cells and thickened with an increase in its connective tissue. It may be associated with pus or mucopus in the purulent stage. In chronic sinus infection, the ciliated mucosa of the lining mucosa is generally destroyed and replaced by squamous epithelium, a metaplasia which under certain conditions may be the precursor of a malignant change.

If the ostium of the sinus becomes permanently blocked and the infection subsides the retained secretion may distend the walls of the sinus, forming a mucocele, which most frequently occurs in the frontal sinus.

It is seldom possible on radiological evidence alone to distinguish between bacterial and allergic sinusitis. In some cases radiological signs may be present which may point the diagnosis in one direction.

Radiological appearances which may help in differentiation are:

(i) The visualisation of a polyp is a certain indication of allergy according to Kern & Schenck (1933), although it does not exclude superimposed infection.

(ii) In bacterial infection the thickened mucosal outline is usually parallel to the bony walls of the sinus whereas in allergy it has a crenated border with the bulges of the mucosa directed towards the lumen of the antrum. Marked variation of the appearances from day to day indicates allergic mucosal thickening.

(iii) Additional evidence of the allergic nature of the mucosal thickening may be obtained from an examination of the turbinate bones in the occipito-frontal view. With normal sized turbinate bones allergic thickening of the mucosa of a sinus is unlikely as in the vast majority of cases the mucosa of the turbinate bones is involved in the allergic process and turbinates are swollen.

However, the radiologist because of his inability to distinguish between the two conditions should be careful not to diagnose a "chronic inflammatory hyperplasia of the mucosa" which may be found to have completely disappeared after one week's interval.

Pathological changes in the mucosa of the paranasal sinuses may be roughly grouped into:

(i) Acute, and
(ii) Chronic thickening of the lining membrane.

Whether the activating agent in a case of sinus disease be bacterial or allergic, the only sign which the radiograph shows is a greater or lesser degree of thickening of the lining membrane indicated by a loss of translucency and with or without the presence of fluid.

Radiological interpretation

Normal appearances. In a healthy sinus the mucosa is invisible on the radiograph and the bony walls are clear-cut and distinct. As alteration in translucency forms one of the basic changes seen in sinus disease, appreciation of the variations which may occur normally is of utmost importance. The walls of the sinuses vary considerably in thickness in different individuals, and the wall may also vary in thickness in different parts of the same sinus. Such variations in bony thickness are most frequently seen in the anterior wall of a frontal sinus causing a loss in translucency, but the outline of the normal adult sinus always remains clear-cut and well-defined. In children the bony outlines of the sinus are somewhat less well-defined. This is due to the constant change occurring in the wall of the sinus as a result of the continuing expansion associated with growth. As soon as the process of pneumatisation ceases the sinus outline assumes a hard, clear-cut appearance.

The sinuses are trans-radiant in proportion to their air content and the relative thickness of their bony walls; a normal but small sinus with thick bony walls will therefore be radiographically less translucent than a large well developed sinus with thin walls.

As the individual sinuses differ much in size, in different and even the same individuals, it requires considerable experience to be able to determine whether a sinus of a certain size and air content is or is not normally trans-radiant. Comparison of one sinus with its fellow of the opposite side is a frequent cause of error, as they may be unequally developed or both be equally diseased.

Acute sinus diseases. When a sinus is subjected to disease whether infective or allergic in origin, the primary radiological change is that (i) *the sinus becomes more opaque than normal* owing to swelling of the lining mucosa. This may or may not be

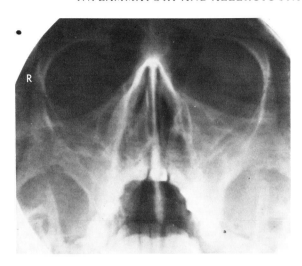

Fig. 58. Complete opacity of antrum. These appearances may occur when the air space in the antrum is obliterated by mucosal thickening with or without fluid being present.

associated with an outpouring of fluid. In the acute stage the bony walls of the sinuses are generally unaffected. The swelling of the mucosa is first seen as a hazy line around the periphery of the sinus. In bacterial infections this rim follows the outline and is parallel to the walls of the sinus. In allergy the oedematous mucosa is apt to vary in thickness with convex bulges into the cavity of the sinus. These features can be readily appreciated by examining the outlines of the air space in the sinus; with bacterial infection the outlines are smooth and approximate to the shape of the bony walls; with allergic states the outlines are wavy.

At a later stage, which both in allergy and virulent bacterial infections may occur within the space of a few hours, the whole sinus becomes (ii) *homogeneously cloudy,* of the transparency of milky water, the bony walls standing out clearly and unaltered in density.

This loss of translucency of a sinus may be mimicked by swelling of the overlying soft tissues of the skin due to trauma, haematoma, infection, *e.g.* cellulitis, but such superimposed shadows are easily

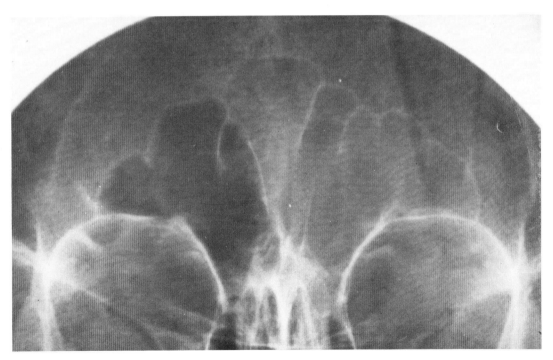

Fig. 59. Acute frontal sinusitis showing complete obliteration of the air space within the sinus with a uniform haziness of the sinus. Radiologically when the sinus is completely opaque it is not possible to exclude the presence of fluid.

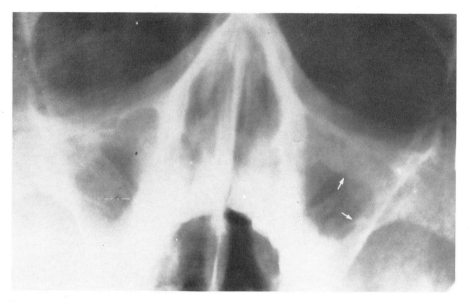

Fig. 60. Mucosal thickening in both antra of bacterial origin. The outlines of the mucosa run parallel to the bony walls in contrast to the wavy outline of the mucosa in allergic sinusitis. The convexity of the mucosa is directed toward the central cavity.

distinguishable by the fact that they extend beyond the confines of the sinus, recognised by careful examination of the sinus in different projections.

Chronic sinus disease. Chronic disease occurs as a sequel to an acute infection or it may result from a low-grade infection and be chronic from its inception. Again, it may be caused by repeated allergic attacks or it may be a combination of allergy and infection; a long-standing allergic condition such as vasomotor rhinitis predisposes to a superimposed infection.

The differentiation of chronic allergic from chronic infective sinusitis may not be possible except that polypi are thought by most observers to be the result of allergy. Also in *chronic infective sinusitis* the sinus walls may undergo a sclerosing osteitis, whereas in *chronic allergy* the sinus walls if at all changed are generally rarefied. In the majority of cases, however, there is little possibility of differentiation between chronic sinus changes due to allergy and those due to infection on purely radiological grounds. Moreover, this is a matter of little practical importance as the rhinologist by his clinical examination can more readily differentiate the two conditions.

Fluid in sinuses. Whilst the demonstration of fluid in a sinus is relatively easy it is impossible on radiological grounds to make any comment on the nature of the fluid. The important point is that if fluid is present, provided that the sinus is not completely filled it can be recognised by radiographing the sinus in the erect position when the air and fluid separate to form a fluid level. As in all air-containing cavities fluid has a horizontal upper air interface which remains horizontal whichever way the cavity is tilted, but is lost if the patient is placed in the recumbent position. The reliability of the radiological detection of fluid has been studied by Chidekel *et al.* (1970) and 86% of those judged as only showing mucosal thickening, 61% showed fluid on proof puncture. The thicker the mucosa the greater the possibility of fluid being present. Equally a normally trans-radiant sinus does not necessarily exclude fluid and in Vuorinen, Kauppila & Pulkkinen's series (1962), 6% of radiologically normal sinuses showed fluid on proof puncture.

The demonstration of a horizontal shadow in the erect position alone is insufficient for the diagnosis of a "fluid level". Retention of this horizontal shadow when the head is tilted to the right or left is essential for accurate diagnosis. Sometimes a thick, viscid fluid may take several minutes to assume the horizontal when the head is tilted so that in doubtful cases time should be allowed for this to

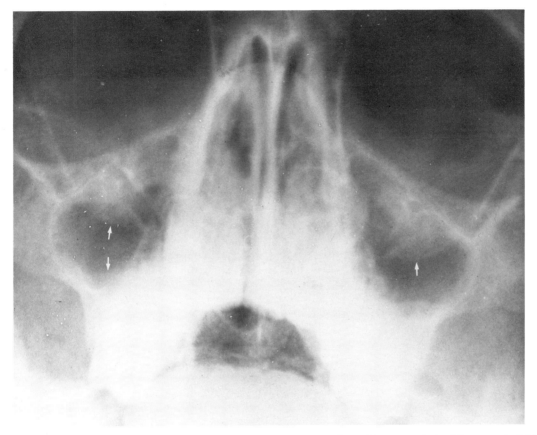

Fig. 61. Allergic sinusitis with polypoid thickening of the mucosa. The irregular swelling of the mucosa in the right antrum is visible. In the left antrum the cavity of the antrum is almost obliterated, appearing as a crescent.

occur. Apart from tilting, confirmation of the fluid nature of the sinus contents can be obtained by radiographs taken in the prone position when the fluid level disappears. When the head is tilted the tilt should be such that the fluid runs to the shallower part of the sinus. In this manner smaller quantities of fluid may not be overlooked.

Complications of sinus disease

Polypi are hyperplastic swellings of the mucous membrane. Histologically the dominant feature is oedematous tissue with relatively little cell content and covered by normal epithelium. The vast majority of polypi are thought to be allergic in origin (Hansel, 1936).

Most polypi originate in the nasal mucous membrane and, less frequently, in the mucosa of the sinuses. Polypi may grow and completely occlude the nasal cavity and in other instances may prolapse through the posterior choana into the nasopharynx (choanal polyp). A choanal polyp may have its origin in the antral mucosa (antro-choanal polyp).

Nasal polypi are seldom individually recognised by radiology but the normal markings of the nasal cavity may be obliterated and the whole nasal cavity has a ground glass appearance. The normal outlines of the turbinates are lost in this opacity. In long standing disease the nasal polypi may enlarge to such a degree as to produce expansion and bone atrophy of the walls of the nasal cavity (fig. 69). This expansion may result in a clinically obvious broadening of the nose (Laff, 1939). This may be

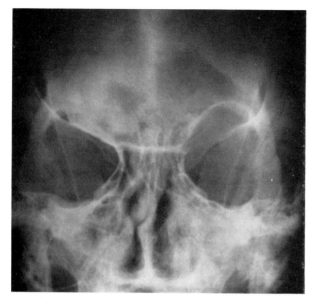 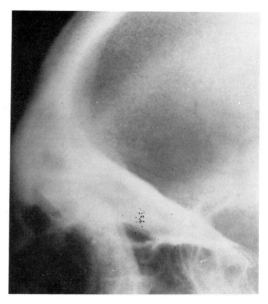

Fig. 62. Female age 72 years. Chronic infection of right frontal sinus for years, presented with proptosis of right eye and a clinical diagnosis of orbital cellulitis. (a) shows the occipito-frontal projection and (b) the lateral view showing extensive new bone formation and sclerosis.

accompanied by a bilateral expansion of the ethmoid cells in some patients, causing displacement of the eyeball and hypertelorism. In a series reported by Lloyd (1975) some degree of ethmoid

expansion was observed in 14% of patients with confirmed nasal polyposis and the change was most commonly found in the young adult patient. The ethmoid expansion affects the whole of the labyrinth, the general form of which is to a large extent retained except for some exaggerated splaying of the cells inferiorly. Although the change

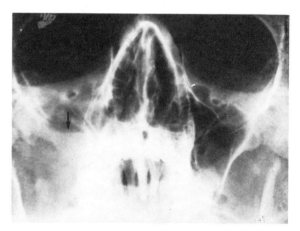

Fig. 63. Tomographic view of same case as Fig. 62 showing the gross thickening of the bony walls and almost complete obliteration of the sinus cavity.

Fig. 64. Occipito-mental view demonstrating fluid level and mucosal thickening in right antrum.

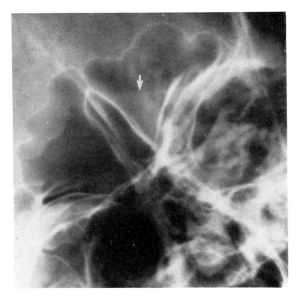

Fig. 65. Fluid level in left frontal sinus. The erect occipito-frontal view clearly reveals the fluid level.

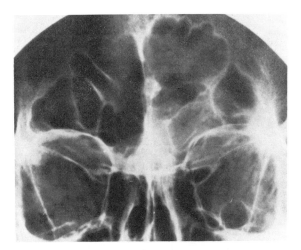

Fig. 66. Erect occipito-frontal view showing mucosal thickening but no fluid level can be seen.

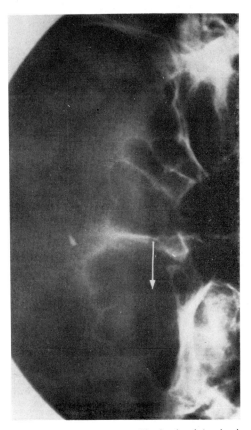

Fig. 67. Occipito-frontal view with the head in the lateral position shows the fluid level clearly (same case as shown in Fig. 66).

is generalised it may show some asymmetry between the two sides.

Choanal polypi are more readily seen when they project into the air-filled nasopharynx, appearing as a soft tissue shadow with a well defined smooth outline (figs. 70, 71). They can be easily seen in the lateral view of the nasopharynx or through the open mouth in the occipito-mental view. Usually the nasal cavity and the maxillary antrum on the side of the choanal polyp are both opaque.

Polypi in the maxillary antra can sometimes be demonstrated as rounded smooth shadows but if they are associated with changes in the remainder of the antral mucosa or if they are multiple the whole antrum may be completely opaque. Polypi may undergo cystic degeneration and under these conditions when the head is tilted their shape may alter slightly. Polypi arising from the floor of the antrum appear as half moon shadows with a convex upper border which in the prone position appear as rounded shadows.

Isolated soft tissue shadows arising from the floor or lateral wall of the maxillary antrum present a problem in differential diagnosis. Such shadows (Ibsen, 1945) may be caused by:

(a) Surface exudate,
(b) Localised acute sinusitis,

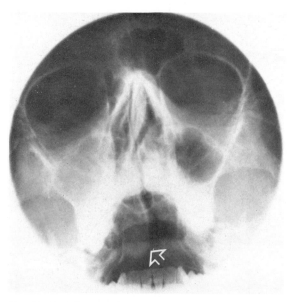

Fig. 68. Occipito-mental view of sinuses showing an opaque right antrum and an antro-choanal polyp seen through the open mouth extending backwards into the nasopharynx.

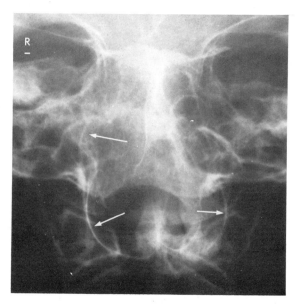

Fig. 69. Bone atrophy with polyps. The nasal cavity is expanded and the nasal bones thinned.

(c) Mucocele,
(d) Solitary mucous polyp,
(e) Retention cysts,
(f) Dental cysts,
(g) Overlap shadows.

Of 35 cases showing such opacities 18 disappeared spontaneously (Ibsen, 1945) and the radiological finding of such a shadow should not be considered as an indication for surgery.

Differentiation of overlap shadows, fluid and cysts of dental origin can be made by tilt views with special dental films but the differentiation of localised mucosal thickening, solitary polypi and retention cysts (non-secreting cysts) may not be possible on radiological grounds.

Mucoceles

Mucoceles of the paranasal sinuses consist of dilated mucus containing sacs lined by sinus epithelium and are due to continuing fluid secretion into an obstructed sinus or air cell. They may result from infection, trauma, tumour formation such as an osteoma or cystic degeneration of the mucosa (Palubinskas & Davies, 1959). In some cases there is histological evidence of an increase in the number of secretory cells in the lining epithelium and in these patients hypersecretion of mucus is a causative factor. When infected, a mucocele becomes a pyocele (empyema) but these two conditions are radiologically indistinguishable.

Mucoceles most commonly occur in the frontal sinus but may also arise in the ethmoid cells, and rarely in the sphenoids and maxillary antra.

Frontal sinus mucoceles. In cases of proptosis, mucoceles are the most common cause to show changes in the radiograph (Zizmor & Noyek, 1968). In most cases the expansion of the frontal sinus displaces the eye forwards and to one side, usually laterally or inferiorly. Expansion of the sinus is palpable in some patients and often the clinical diagnosis is more obvious than the radiological (fig. 78). Radiological signs consist of an expansion of the sinus, which characteristically causes loss of the scalloped margin of the normal sinus wall. In some patients the sinus is more opaque than normal due to fluid accumulation within its cavity, but in others it may appear more radiolucent if the bone loss is such as to counteract the increased density caused by the fluid content of the sinus. Expansion of the sinus may cause a displacement, disappearance or

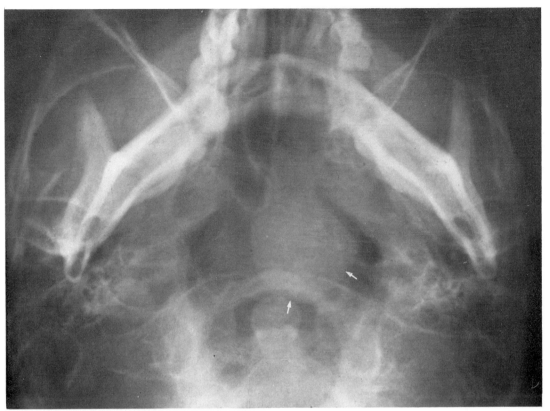

Fig. 70. Antro-choanal polyp. Submento-vertical view showing soft tissue mass projecting into post-nasal space from the right posterior nares.

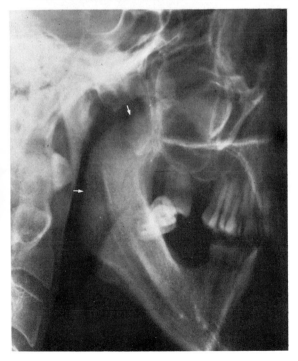

(Figs. 70 and 71 reproduced by permission from Seminars in Roentgenology, April, 1968.)

Fig. 71. Lateral view of case shown in Fig. 70. The shadow of the soft tissue lies over the soft tissue of the palate.

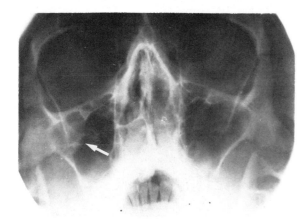

Fig. 72. Polyp on lateral wall of right antrum. Some mucosal thickening is present over the floor of both antra.

"buckling" of the supra-orbital ridge (figs. 75, 76). This is an important observation since in minor degrees of expansion it may be the only positive radiological sign (fig. 77). Lateral tomograms are the

most useful in frontal sinus mucoceles; the thin shell of bone expanding downwards into the orbit may be demonstrated and also the degree of expansion upwards and posteriorly into the anterior fossa (Potter, 1972). The rim of bone expanding into the orbit may be discontinuous and infected mucoceles or pyoceles may rupture outside the peri-orbita and track backwards to the superior orbital fissure, causing ocular motor nerve palsies in addition to exophthalmos.

Ethmoid mucoceles. Under this heading are included expansions arising from the anterior or middle group of ethmoid cells, *i.e.* those cells which drain into the middle meatus. Expansions of the posterior group are considered with sphenoid mucoceles (see p. 54). Mucoceles arising from the frontal sinuses as described above are not as a rule difficult to recognise radiologically, but mucoceles arising from the ethmoid cells may be surprisingly difficult to detect on standard sinus views. They are usually more obvious clinically than radiologically. Twelve patients with ethmoid mucoceles have recently been described (Lloyd, Bartram &

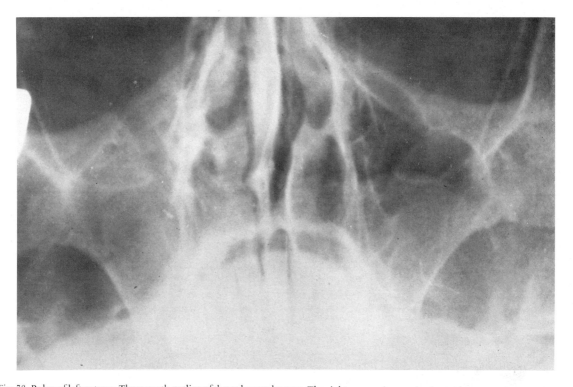

Fig. 73. Polyp of left antrum. The smooth outline of the polyp can be seen. The right antrum is completely opaque.

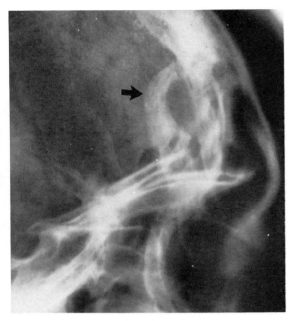

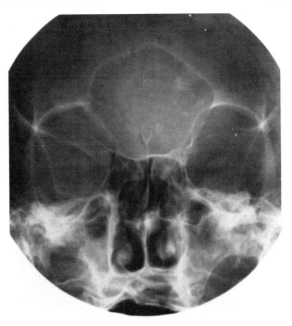

Fig. 74. Thickening and reaction of bone to polyp and infection. Lateral view of frontal sinuses showing the thickened posterior wall of the frontal sinus.

Fig. 76. Frontal mucocele eroding through anterior bony wall of sinus. The clear-cut outline of the frontal sinus is seen together with the erosion of the bony floor.

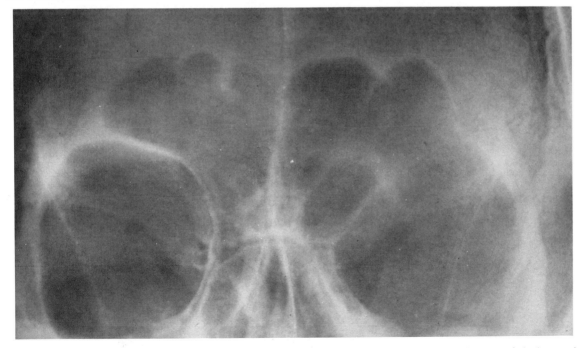

Fig. 75. Mucocele of left frontal sinus. The floor of the left frontal sinus is eroded by pressure atrophy and there is a relative increase in translucency as a consequence of bone loss compared with the right frontal sinus which shows loss of translucency due to mucosal thickening.

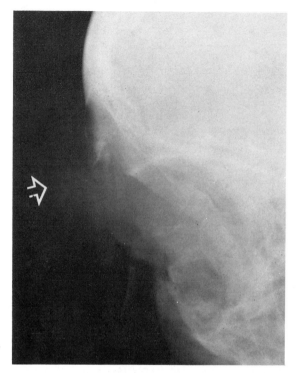

Fig. 77. Lateral view of same case showing loss of bony wall and soft tissue mass.

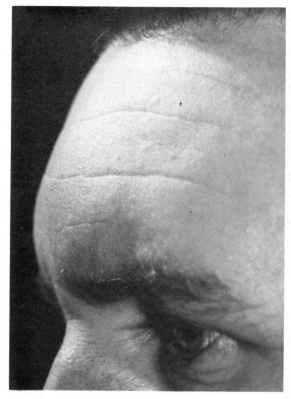

Fig. 78. Clinical photograph of patient. The soft tissue swelling over the left forehead can be seen.

Stanley, 1974). All presented clinically with a palpable mass at the medial canthus; other important clinical features were the presence of proptosis and in some patients epiphora, when the expansion impinged on the lachrymal sec. Loss of translucence in the ethmoid cells was the change most often observed on plain x-ray but was entirely non-specific. Other patients showed loss of the vertical line forming the anterior component of the medial orbital wall (figs. 79, 80), and in some a bony rim may be demonstrated within the orbit due to the ethmoid expansion. Two other signs may be observed; destruction of the ethmoid septa on the affected side, and expansion of the mucocele into the frontal sinus. The two special techniques, which may be needed to make the diagnosis, are dacryocystography and tomography. Obstruction with forward and lateral displacement of the lachrymal sac and canaliculi may be demonstrated on dacryocystography. Coronal tomography will show expansion of the anterior ethmoid cells in most cases, particularly those in which the

mucocele is covered by a well-defined bony margin, but tomography in the axial plane is by far the most accurate method of defining the expansion of an ethmoid mucocele both in the ethmoid labyrinth and in the soft tissues of the orbit (fig. 80).

Sphenoid mucoceles. Under this heading are included expansions of the posterior ethmoid cells in addition to sphenoid expansions; they are probably better designated as spheno-ethmoidal mucoceles (Takahashi, Jingu & Nakayama, 1973). Radiology plays the key role in the diagnosis of this condition and the correct surgical approach is determined by accurate interpretation of the films. Because of the proximity of the sphenoid sinus to the optic nerve, cavernous sinus and ocular motor nerves, mucocele expansion of the sinus results in symptoms due to involvement of these structures, and the patients commonly present with headache combined with eye symptoms, such as blurred vision and diplopia. On x-ray they are liable to be

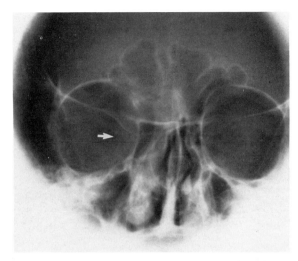

Fig. 79. Anterior ethmoidal mucocele. Occipito-frontal view showing the erosion of the orbital plate of the ethmoid associated with relatively slight changes in the translucency of this area.

misdiagnosed either as pituitary tumours or as a nasopharyngeal or sphenoid neoplasm (figs. 81, 82), often considered too extensive for surgery. In the former instance the patient may undergo craniotomy, which in this condition carries a high mortality (Nugent, Sprinkle & Bloor, 1970) or if sphenoid malignancy is mistakenly diagnosed the patient may be sent for radiotherapy (Neffson, 1957). When this is found to be ineffective exploratory surgery is usually undertaken and the true condition discovered. In most patients, adequate nasal drainage is all that is required for proper treatment.

In general, the radiological features become more emphatic as the lesion expands the sphenoid sinus. Early in the course of the disease the changes may be limited to the sinus itself (Minagi, Margolis & Newton, 1972) and may consist only of opacification of one or both sphenoid sinuses. At this stage certain radiological diagnosis is not

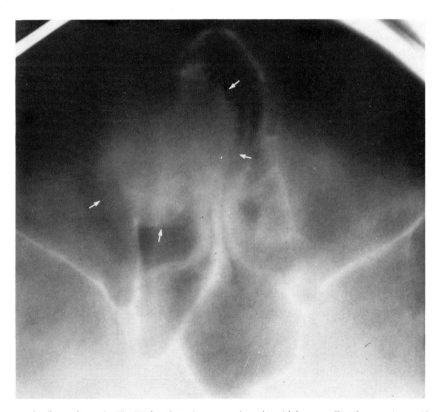

Fig. 80. Axial tomograph of case shown in Fig. 79 showing a large anterior ethmoidal mucocelle. The mass is considerably larger than would be anticipated from the occipito-frontal projection.

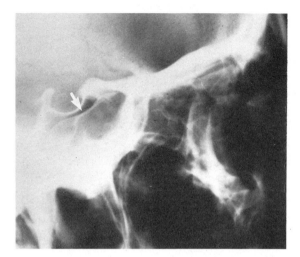

Fig. 81. Sphenoidal mucocele. Secondary spread of ethmoidal mucocele into the right half of the sphenoid sinus after previous external ethmoidal operation *(Courtesy of Dr. M. B. Denny)*.

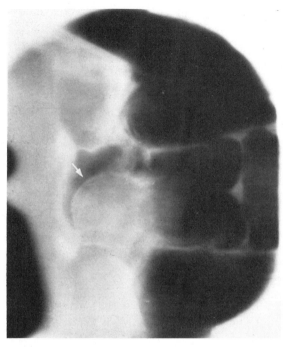

Fig. 82. Antero-posterior tomograph demonstrating the well-defined mass bulging into the sphenoid fossa (same case as Fig. 81).

always possible but as pressure within the sinus continues, an expansion of the cavity ensues, with bone destruction in the floor of the pituitary fossa, erosion of the medial wall of the optic canal and sometimes enlargement of the superior orbital fissure and elevation of the planum sphenoidale. The apex of the petrous pyramid and clivus may also be eroded (Phelps & Toland, 1969). In order to make the differential diagnosis from neoplastic invasion of the sphenoid it is essential to demonstrate expansion of the sinus, as opposed to destruction of bone *in situ,* characteristic of malignancy. A variety of skull projections should be used including optic canal and submento-vertical views. Tomography in three planes is an essential part of the investigation of these patients. These studies may demonstrate unmistakable evidence of sinus enlargement with discontinuous curvilinear expansions of the sinus walls. A diagnostic feature has been described by Takahashi *et al.* (1974). They reported the presence of multiple cyst-like expansions which appeared to be inter-communicating and were best seen on tomography. These result from expansion of compartments of the sinus or aberrant pneumatisations participating in the general expansion of the main sinus cavity. Carotid angiography should not be necessary to make the diagnosis but may show an upward and lateral displacement of the intra-cavernous segment of the internal carotid artery.

If infection persists or the mucocele becomes reinfected an empyema of the sphenoid sinus develops (figs. 83, 84).

Mucoceles of the maxillary antrum. The maxillary antrum is the least common site for mucocele formation. Clinically the symptoms are due to sinus expansion into the nose, mouth and orbit, displacing the turbinates, teeth and eye and causing proptosis. On plain x-ray the sinus is invariably opaque and expanded, encroaching upon the ethmoid cells. As in other sinuses enlargement with good preservation of the thin bulging walls is the clue to the diagnosis, but in some projections the changes may look very like early malignancy and tomography is usually needed to confirm the expansion.

Pneumosinus dilatans

This condition was originally described by Benjamins (1918) and more recently has been reviewed by Lombardi (1967). The term refers to an abnormal expansion of part of the paranasal

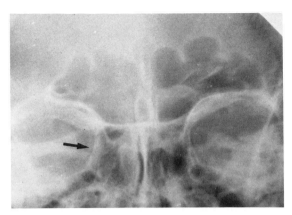

Fig. 83. Empyema of right sphenoid sinus plus right frontal sinus infection.

(Figs. 83 and 84 reproduced by permission from Seminars in Roentgenology, April, 1968).

sinuses. The dilatation is confined to one or to a few cells of a sinus cavity: it contains air only and is lined with normal sinus epithelium. Lombardi records 51 cases in the literature with a male predominance of 16 : 1 and an age incidence of 20 to 40 years. A similar phenomenon may occur in association with a meningioma and is then usually seen in the sphenoethmoid area, producing the so-called "blistering phenomenon". This hyperplastic growth of the sphenoid and ethmoid sinuses has been described in five patients by Wiggli & Oberson (1973) all of whom had surgically verified meningiomas.

A single example of this condition occurring in the orbit and affecting the ethmoid cells has been encountered. This was a 19-year-old female who presented with a six-year history of proptosis and lateral deviation of the eye. Radiologically, an exuberant pneumatisation of the right ethmoid cells was observed and was seen to be expanding into the right orbit. At surgical decompression the cells concerned were shown to be lined by normal mucosa, and after subsequent recurrence of the proptosis the underlying cause of the overgrowth of the ethmoid cells was shown to be due to an extradural meningioma in the medial part of the orbit.

Empyema

Infection of a mucocele results in an empyema of the affected sinus. Radiologically, an empyema of a sinus may be indistinguishable from a mucocele and the presence of infection usually results in a loss of sharpness of the bony outline of the sinus. Empyema of the antrum is not uncommon in adults but is rare in infancy (Kallay, 1940). In infancy such an empyema may be asymptomatic.

Whilst mucoceles of the sphenoid sinuses are rare, empyema is not infrequent and is associated with serious intracranial complications (Couroille & Rosenbald, 1938). The radiological features are bone erosion and destruction of the sella especially the dorsum sellae, associated with erosion and flattening of the pituitary fossa (Rongetti & Daniels, 1950; Grant, 1931).

Non-secreting cysts

As a sequel of infection or allergic manifestations in the paranasal sinuses, degenerative cysts may occur in the lining wall of the sinus. Lindsay (1942) has

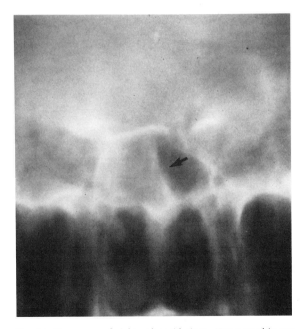

Fig. 84. Empyema of right sphenoid sinus. Tomographic cut showing complete opacity of right sphenoid sinus and normal translucency of left sphenoid sinus.

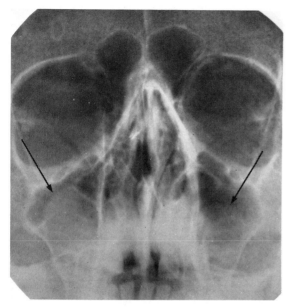

Fig. 85. Non-secreting cysts of antrum. Note normal mucosa in remaining portion of both antra.

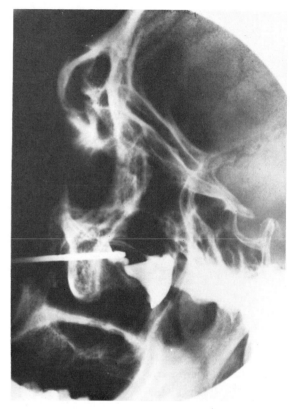

Fig. 87. Lateral view of case shown in Fig. 86 showing the convex upper border.

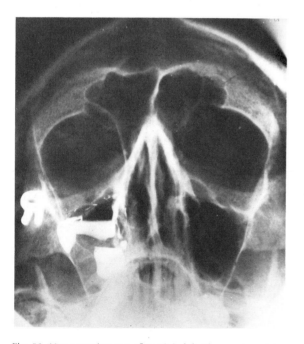

Fig. 86. Non-secreting cyst after Lipiodol. The opacity arising from the floor of the right antrum is outlined by Lipiodol injected into the sinus.

termed these non-secreting cysts as they do not have an epithelial lining and appear to be formed by dehiscence of the mucous membrane. They are generally unassociated with any change in the mucosa in any other part of the antrum so that they must be regarded rather as a sequel of infection or allergy (fig. 85).

With ordinary cultural methods the cyst fluid is usually sterile and chemical analysis reveals that the fluid is an exudate. Their cholesterol content is high and on transillumination, by virtue of the doubly refracting property of this substance, the affected antrum appears clear. Cholesterol fluid absorbs x-radiation so that on radiological examination the cyst appears opaque. The combination of these findings, namely an antrum which is clear on transillumination and opaque to radiographic examination, should suggest the possibility of a cholesterol filled non-secreting cyst.

Radiological appearances:

(i) Non-secreting cysts appear as *convex rounded shadows* appearing from the floor or medial wall of the antrum.
(ii) The *remainder of the antrum shows normal translucency.*
(iii) Slight *alterations in the degree of convexity* of the cyst may occur with alterations in posture, but the level never assumes a horizontal level.

Differential diagnosis. Radiologically, these cysts have to be differentiated from:
(a) Polypi
(b) Mucoceles
(c) Areas of localised mucosal oedema
(d) Cysts of dental origin.

Although superficially their characteristics are indistinguishable from polypi their presence with normal mucosa over the remainder of the sinus is strong evidence in favour of a cyst. If cystic degeneration has occurred in a polyp it may not be possible to distinguish the two conditions. Allergic localised thickening of the mucosa may also give an appearance identical with non-secreting cysts and its differentiation may only be possible by confirming the transient nature of this condition by serial radiography.

Osteomyelitis

Osteomyelitis may occur in the bony walls of any of the nasal sinuses but it is most commonly seen in the frontal bone. Osteomyelitis of the frontal bone may occur as a manifestation of a haematogenous spread or secondary to trauma but its occurrence in the absence of a predisposing sinus infection is rare. This feature probably accounts for its extreme rarity before puberty. It may occur (Lewy, 1941) as a result of spread of infection from a sinus or it may be an unfortunate sequel to surgical intervention in sinus disease (Auston & Littlett, 1941). On rare occasions it occurs in the maxilla or zygoma following antral infection. More commonly osteomyelitis of the maxilla arises from apical infection around the teeth. It may also follow an antro-oral fistula subsequent to a dental extraction.

Osteomyelitis of the superior maxilla in newborn infants may arise from an infection of the unerupted first deciduous molar situated on the adjoining anterior wall of the maxilla. The

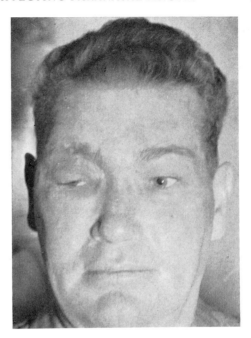

Fig. 88. Post-operative osteomyelitis showing oedema and swelling of soft tissue over the right eyebrow. The patient, a young male adult, had an external right frontal operation done several years previously. Obstruction of the right fronto-nasal duct follows colds and the present attack had resulted in fever and swelling of the soft tissues over the right frontal sinus. Operation revealed the frontal sinus contained pus and the bony wall showed osteomyelitic changes.

infection rapidly spreads superiorly to the orbit, anteriorly to the canine fossa and posteriorly to involve the antrum. The condition is rare and Asherson (1939) was only able to collect 70 case reports in the literature since Rees' original description in 1847. The condition arises in the first few weeks of life and the onset is sudden and heralded by a feverish attack and signs of meningism. The oedema of the eyelid and face on the affected side together with chemosis point to the diagnosis.

In the early stage of infantile osteomyelitis, radiology can offer little help in diagnosis as the small size of the antrum makes radiology of little value in excluding antral or ethmoidal infection. In the later stages, radiography may demonstrate the extent of bone involvement and size and number of sequestra that have formed (McKenzie, 1913; Stevens, 1941). Osteomyelitis following paranasal sinus infection may be acute or chronic. In the early

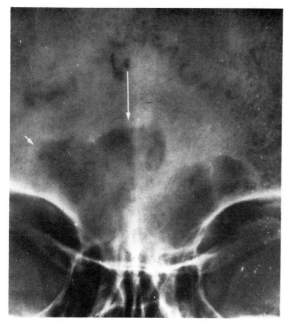

Fig. 89. Osteomyelitis of frontal bone. Note the loss of the well-defined bony outline and the patchy motheaten appearance of the surrounding bone.

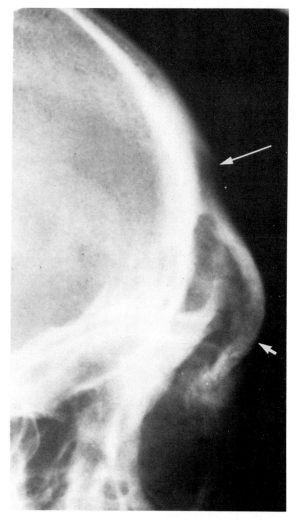

Fig. 90. Lateral view of same case shown in Fig. 89. Note erosion through outer table of frontal bone (long arrow), and patchy outline of anterior wall of frontal sinus (small arrow).

stages of the acute disease no radiological changes can be detected until some decalcification of bone has taken place. Even when such changes have occurred they are extremely difficult to recognise owing to the blurring of the bone detail by the overlying thickened mucosa.

In the frontal bone, which is by far the most commonly involved, the technical difficulties of recognising osteomyelitis are less, but even so it should be remembered that quite extensive bone involvement may exist without radiological changes. Radiological evidence is often lacking in the acute stage. Bone changes can seldom be detected until four or five days after the onset of osteomyelitis (Apffelstaedt, 1938; Schmidt, 1937). In 10 to 14 days after the onset of the disease radiological changes are generally well established. Osteomyelitis of the frontal bone may occur in the absence of frontal sinuses (Lewy, 1941).

The system of veins (Breschett's plexus) which extends through the diploe of the frontal bone and freely communicates both with the venous plexuses in the scalp and in the dura, makes the spread of infection in the frontal bone easy. Consequently osteomyelitis of the frontal bone is always associated with thrombo-phlebitis with the result that metastatic osteomyelitic foci may occur at sites away from the original infection.

Radiological appearances:

(a) *Dilatation of the diploetic veins.* Laskiewicz (1939) demonstrated a dilatation of the diploetic veins in the radiograph in a case of frontal osteomyelitis. Although dilatation of the veins of the frontal bone may be an early sign of frontal osteomyelitis the variation in the size and number of

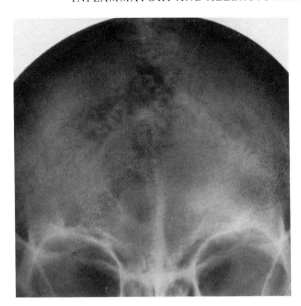

Fig. 91. Osteomyelitis of frontal bone secondary to bilateral frontal sinus infection. The patchy motheaten appearance of the frontal bone is readily seen in this occipito-frontal view.

diploic veins in the frontal sinus makes the value of this sign doubtful. This author found that conditions which obstructed the drainage of the sinus, *e.g.* septal deviation *etc.,* greatly enhanced the development of osteomyelitis.

(b) *Irregular moth-eaten appearance of the sinus walls.* In the postero-anterior view the irregular moth-eaten appearance of the bony walls may be detected. This moth-eaten appearance is brought about by a loss of sharpness of the spongy bony framework of the diploe due to decalcification of the bony trabeculae. Unfortunately, swelling of the soft tissues may also produce unsharpness of the bony trabeculae. Destruction of the bony trabeculae when it can be demonstrated is, however, diagnostic of osteomyelitis of the frontal bone. Stereoscopic lateral films may show spotty decalcification of the walls of the frontal sinuses together with coincident swelling of the soft tissues of the forehead. The lateral views are of increased value as confusing shadows due to overlying soft tissue oedema are avoided.

(c) *Loss of the normal pencil-line outline of the sinus walls.* In the early stages the most useful radiological sign is decalcification and a loss of the normal pencil-line outline of the sinus wall (Brown,

1944; MacMillan, 1940). As the white line disappears decalcification of the bone outside the sinus will appear and this feature indicates considerable involvement of the frontal bone. As the osteomyelitis becomes chronic, irregular areas of decalcification mixed with areas of sclerosis become apparent. In this stage, radiology is of considerable assistance in visualising the extent of bone involvement and in detecting sequestra. Lateral or tangential views accurately localised with a small cone to improve detail are the best method of detecting sequestra. As these generally originate from the inner or outer tables of the frontal bone, they are best seen in the lateral views, and postero-anterior views are disappointing in detecting sequestra. Tomography may be of considerable assistance in diagnosing the extent of an osteo-myelitic process in the frontal bone (Chamberlain, 1942). It should be remembered that on an average the disease process extends 1 to 2 cm further than the maximum limit of changes detected on the radiograph.

Osteomyelitis involving the sphenoid bone is very uncommon. Ballenger (1939) emphasises the difficulties of diagnosis before intracranial complications have supervened. The clinical features are those of a sphenoiditis. The radiological information is helpful but not diagnostic. Calcification in the ligaments around the sphenoid is regarded by Ballenger as indicating chronic infection of the sphenoid bone. The frequency of calcification in the petro-clinoid and inter-clinoid ligaments as a normal finding makes the value of this observation as a diagnostic sign highly speculative.

Extra-dural and cerebral abscesses

A spread of infection from a frontal sinus backwards through the posterior wall results in the most dreaded of all complications, namely the development of an intra-cranial abscess.

Sjöberg (1939) found eight cases of frontal abscess in an analysis of an extensive series (3,364) of acute and chronic frontal sinusitis, a frequency of 0·4% in acute and 0·2% in chronic cases.

Plain radiographs give no indication of the development of this complication unless gas is present in the cavity. Pyograms, *i.e.* radiographs taken after the injection of 2 ml of contrast medium into the abscess cavity, are of great assistance in

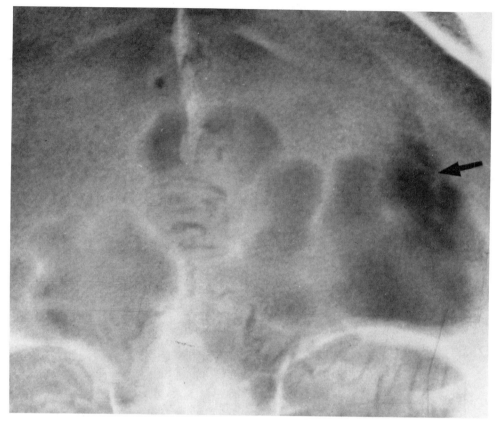

Fig. 92. Osteomyelitis of left frontal bone with sequestrum formation. A sequestrum was removed at surgical exploration. Tomography is usually necessary to confirm the presence of a sequestrum.
(By permission of W. B. Saunders Company, Philadelphia from Radiology of the Orbit by G. Lloyd.)

determining the extent of the cavity and as a guide to therapeutic control (Tutton & Shepherd, 1949). Pyograms also give an indication of the track along which infection has spread from the paranasal sinuses. They are equally helpful in determining the presence or absence of loculi in the abscess cavity.

Sphenoidal fissure syndrome

Kretzschmar & Jacot (1939) describe cases of sphenoidal fissure syndrome due to spread of an osteo-periostitis from the sphenoid sinus. The clinical features of retro-bulbar pain, limitation of extreme eye movements and temporal hemi-dyschromatopia are due to the pressure on the nerve structures passing through the fissures.

The radiological findings are those of blurring of the medial margin of the superior orbital fissure with indistinct margins of the fissure. Decalcification of the bone around the fissure may also be present.

REFERENCES

ADAMS, W. S. (1944) A Case of Senile Tuberculosis of the Maxillary Antrum. *J. Lar. Otol.*, **59**, 250.

AGAR, J. S. & CAZORT, A. (1939) Pathological Nasal Conditions Affecting Clinical Allergy. *Sth. med. J.*, **32**, 1063.

APFFELSTAEDT, O. (1938) Beitrag zum Krankheitsbilde der Osteomyelitis cranii rhinogenen ursprungs. *Arch. Ohr.-Nas.-u. KehlkHeilk.*, **144**, 335.

ASHERSON, N. (1939) Acute Osteomyelitis of the Superior Maxilla in Young Infants. *J. Lar. Otol.*, **54**, 691.

AUSTON, P. N. & LITTLETT, A. (1941) *Proc. Staff Meet. Mayo Clin.*, **16**, 761.

BALLENGER, H. C. (1939) Osteomyelitis of the Sphenoid Bone. *Ann. Otol. Rhinol. Lar.*, **48**, 95.

BENJAMINS, C. E. (1918) Pneumosinus Frontalis Dilatans. *Acta otolar.*, **1**, 412.

BROWN, L. A. (1944) Osteomyelitis of the Frontal Bone. *Archs Otolar.*, **39**, 485.

CHAMBERLAIN, D. (1942) Occupational Deafness. *Archs Otolar.*, **35**, 595.

CHIDEKEL, N., JENSEN, C., AXELSSON, A. & GREBELIUS, N. (1970) Diagnosis of Fluid in the Maxillary Sinus. *Acta radiol.*, **10**, 433.

COUROILLE, C. B. & ROSENBALD, L. K. (1938) Intracranial Complications of Infections of the Nasal Cavities and Accessory Sinuses. *Archs Otolar.*, **27**, 692.

CULLOM, M. M. (1941) Operative Technique for Traumatic Cataract (Ozena). *J. Am. med. Ass.*, **117**, 987.

FRIEDMAN, I. (1971) *J. Lar. Otol.*, **85**, 631.

GRANT, A. L. (1931) Acute Abscess in the Body of the Sphenoid, Ruptured into the Pituitary Fossa. Autopsy Report. *Laryngoscope*, **41**, 842.

HANSEL, F. K. (1936) Allergy of the Nose and Paranasal Sinuses. London: Kimpton.

HARRINGTON, F. T. (1938) Investigation and Conservative Treatment of Nasal Factor in Asthma. *Indian Med. Gaz.*, **73**, 725.

HERSH, J. H. (1945) Primary Infection of Maxillary Sinus by Actinomyces Necrophorus. *Archs Otolar.*, **41**, 204.

IBSEN, B. (1945) Basal Convex Shadows in Maxillary Sinus. *Nord. méd.*, **27**, 148.

KALLAY, F. (1940) Empyema of Antrum in Ten-day-old Infant. *Gyógyászat*, **80**, 58.

KERN, R. A. & SCHENCK, H. P. (1933) Chronic Paranasal Sinus Infection; Relation to Diseases of Lower Respiratory Tract. *Archs Otolar.*, **18**, 425.

KRETZSCHMAR, S. & JACOT, P. (1939) Des Symptomes Precoces et d'une de la Fente Sphenoidale. *Schweiz. med. Schnschr.*, **69**, 1103.

LAFF, H. I. (1939) Deforming and Recurring Polyps of Youth. *Archs Otolar.*, **30**, 795.

LASKIEWICZ, A. (1939) Les Osteomyelitis de Os Plats du Crane d'Origine Nasale et Otique. *Revue Lar. Otol. Rhinol.*, **60**, 185.

LEWY, R. B. (1941) Osteomyelitis of the Frontal Bone in the Absence of Frontal Sinuses. *Archs Otolar.*, **33**, 425.

LINDSAY, J. R. (1942) Non-secreting Cysts of Maxillary Sinus Mucosa. *Laryngoscope*, **52**, 84.

LOMBARDI, G. (1967) *Radiology in Neuro-Ophthalmology*. Baltimore: Williams & Wilkins.

LLOYD, G. (1975) *Radiology of the Orbit*. Philadelphia: Saunders.

LLOYD, G., BARTRAM, C. I. & STANLEY, P. (1974) Ethmoid Mucoceles. *Br. J. Radiol.*, **47**, 646.

LUCAS, H. A. (1952) Histopathology of Sinusitis. *J. Lar. Otol.*, **66**, 480.

McKENZIE, D. (1913) Diffuse Osteomyelitis from Nasal Sinus Suppuration. *J. Lar. Otol.*, **28**, 6.

MacMILLAN, E. A. (1940) Acute Disseminated Encephalomyelitis. *N. Carol. med. J.*, **1**, 382.

MINAGI, H., MARGOLIS, M. T. & NEWTON, T. H. (1972) Tomography in the Diagnosis of Sphenoid Sinus Mucocele. *Am. J. Roentg.*, **115**, 587.

NEFFSON, A. H. (1957) Mucocele of the Sphenoid Sinus. *Archs Otolar.*, **66**, 157.

NUGENT, G. R., SPRINKLE, P. & BLOOR, B. M. (1970) Sphenoid Sinus Mucoceles. *J. Neurosurg.*, **32**, 443.

OSBORNE, D. A. (1963) Mycotic Infection of the Frontal Sinus. *J. Lar. Otol.*, **77**, 29.

PALUBINSKAS, A. I. & DAVIES, C. H. (1959) Roentgen Features of Nasal Accessory Sinus Mucoceles. *Radiology*, **72**, 576.

PHELPS, P. D. & TOLAND, J. (1969) Mucocele of Sphenoidal Sinus Eroding Petrous Temporal Bone. *Br. J. Radiol.*, **42**, 845.

POTTER, D. G. (1972) Tomography of the Orbit. *Radiol. Clin. N. Am.*, **10**, 21.

REES, G. A. (1847) On Uncommon Forms of Abscess in Childhood. *Lond. med. Gaz.*, **4**, 859.

RONGETTI, J. R. & DANIELS, J. T. (1950) Treatment of Empyema of the Sella Turcica of Sphenoid Origin. *Archs Otolar.*, **52**, 166.

RUSSELL, H. G. B. (1939) Observations upon the Nasal Aspect of Asthma. *St Bart's Hosp. Rep.*, **72**, 23.

SCHMIDT, H. (1937) Osteomyelitis der Platten schadelknochen insbesondere des Stirnbeins. *Arch. Ohr.-Nas.-U. KehlkHeilk.*, **143**, 115.

SJÖBERG, A. A. (1939) Contribution to Prognosis and Treatment of Rhinogenous and Otogenous Brain Abscesses. *Acta oto-lar.*, **27**, 638.

STEVENS, J. B. (1941) Osteomyelitis of the Frontal Bone. *Archs. Otolar.*, **33**, 694.

TAKAHASHI, M., JINGU, K. & NAKAYAMA, T. (1973) Roentgenologic Appearances of Spheno-ethmoidal Mucocele. *Neuroradiology*, **6**, 45.

TUTTON, G. K. & SHEPHERD, W. H. T. (1949) Thorotrast Pyograms in Cerebral Abscess. *Br. J. Surg.*, **36**, 240.

VUORINEN, P., KAUPPILA, A. & PULKKINEN, K. (1962) Comparison of Results of Roentgen Examination and Puncture and Irrigation of the Maxillary Sinuses. *J. Lar. Otol.*, **76**, 359.

WIGGLI, U. & OBERSON, R. (1973) *Schweiz. med. Wschr.*, **103**, 1492.

WILSON, C. P. (1946) Personal communication.

ZIZMOR, J. & NOYEK, A. (1968) Cysts and Benign Tumours of the Paranasal Sinuses. *Seminars in Roentgenology*, **3**, 172.

CHAPTER 5

Cysts and new growths involving the paranasal sinuses

Cysts and neoplasms arising from the mucosa or the bony walls may affect any of the paranasal sinuses. The maxillary sinuses, however, owing to their close proximity to the teeth, additionally may be involved by cysts or tumours of dental origin. Cysts or tumours involving the paranasal sinuses may be classified as follows:

Benign tumours

(a) Fibroma, and ossifying fibroma
(b) Osteoma, cancellous or ivory
(c) Localised manifestations of a general bony disease, *e.g.* leontiasis ossea, Paget's disease, or polyostotic fibrous dysplasia
(d) Osteochondroma
(e) Haemangioma
(f) Osteoclastoma
(g) Osteoid osteoma.

Cysts and tumours of developmental origin

(a) Dermoids
(b) Meningoceles.

Malignant tumours

(a) Sarcoma
  (i) Fibrosarcoma
  (ii) Osteogenic sarcoma
(b) Carcinoma – squamous celled or adenocarcinoma
(c) Melanoma
(d) Secondary invasion from growths in adjoining structures
(e) Metastatic deposits from distant primary growths.

Granulomas

Cysts

Cysts involving the paranasal sinuses may be classified as follows:

(a) Cysts of non-dental origin
  (i) Retention cysts (*secreting cysts*)
  (ii) Non-secreting cysts of the sinus mucosa
  (iii) Mucoceles
  (iv) Traumatic bone cysts
  (v) Haemorrhagic cysts
(b) Cysts of dental origin
  (i) Dental (radicular, root) cysts
  (ii) Dentigerous (follicular) cysts
  (iii) Cystic odontomes
  (iv) Tuberosity cysts
  (v) Primordial cysts
(c) Fissural cysts (developing from embryonal defects)
  (i) Globulo-maxillary cysts
  (ii) Incisive canal cysts
(d) Dermoids and cholesteatomas.

Benign tumours

Fibroma and ossifying fibroma. These tumours arise from the fibrous stroma of the mucosa. They have the same histological features as fibromas occurring in other sites, being composed of masses of tightly packed spindle or oval cells.

Radiologically, they appear as rounded solitary soft tissue shadows often indistinguishable from a polypus or cyst, projecting from the wall of the sinus. Fibromas are rare and usually occur in the frontal sinuses.

Fibromas may also arise from the ethmoidal capsule and project into the nasal cavity causing

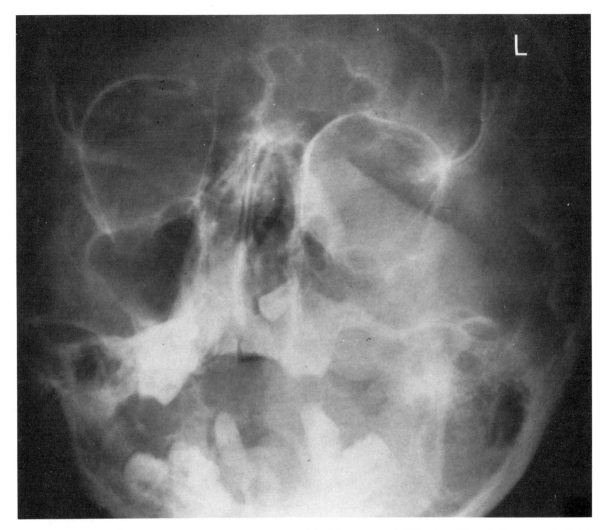

Fig. 93. Neurofibromatosis of facial bones. Note the distortion of the left antrum and thickening of the soft tissues over the facial skeleton. Differentiation from fibrous dysplasia can be made by the fact that the antral walls although distorted are not involved and thickened as in fibrous dysplasia.

considerable displacement of the nasal wall or of the nasal septum. Such fibromas frequently grow to considerable size and may be mistaken for sarcomas from their size and the thinning of the nasal walls they produce. From the fact that they frequently ulcerate and cause post-nasal bleeding and discharge, clinical differentiation from malignant growths may be difficult. Fibromas of the paranasal sinuses may arise as a part of a generalised neurofibromatosis (Uffenorde, 1939) (fig. 93).

Fibromas may also undergo ossification (Crowe & Baylor, 1923; Woodruff, 1945; Ball, 1951; Welin, 1948). Ossifying fibromas may completely obliterate the affected sinus. In some cases differentiation from sarcomas may not be possible even on histological examination. Ossifying fibromas may also be confused with odontomes. Hara (1944) reporting a case of ossifying fibroma of the superior maxilla, claimed that the pathological nature of the tumour was a secondary osteoma since it appeared as a result of secondary ossifica-

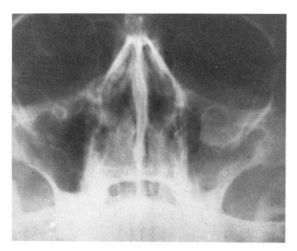

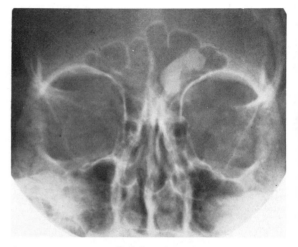

Fig. 94. Neurofibroma of left antrum (inferior orbital division, 5th nerve). The expanded inferior orbital canal is seen.

Fig. 96. Ivory osteoma of left frontal sinus shows uniform dense bone with a well-demarcated outline occurring in a frontal sinus showing normal translucency.

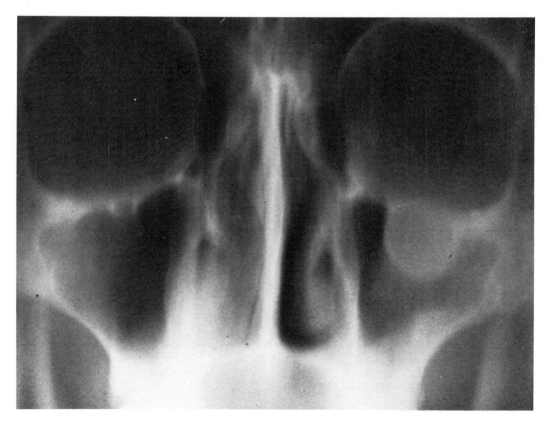

Fig. 95. Postero-anterior Tomograph of case shown in Fig. 94 showing enlarged left inferior orbital canal.

tion of massive fibromas of the maxillary antrum.

Fibromas occur equally in either sex and are most frequently found in young adults; they may show a familial tendency (Rosedale, 1945) (fig. 93). The commonest site of origin is the horizontal ramus of the mandible and the next is the antral walls. Radiologically antral fibromas present as small round swellings projecting into the antral cavity. Massive fibromas appear as expanding tumours involving the maxillary antrum. Pressure atrophy of part or the whole of the antral walls may occur (figs. 94, 95). Recognition of the atrophy of the antral wall as distinct from malignant invasion is of utmost importance in differentiating a fibroma from a carcinoma of the antrum. Features which aid this differentiation are the patchy change which occurs with malignant invasion as opposed to smooth uniform loss of bone seen in pressure atrophy.

Papilloma (inverting papilloma). Papillomas may occur in the maxillary antra and grow to form soft tumours filling the antrum. They may cause expansion of the antrum with thinning of the walls and may be mistaken for antral carcinoma with bone destruction (figs. 97 and 98).

Osteoma. Osteomas are either composed of hard, dense bone similar to cortical bone, when they are known as ivory (cortical) osteomas (fig. 96), or they may be composed of cancellous bone (fibrous osteomas) (fig. 103) (Eden, 1939).

Frequency. Childrey (1939) found 15 cases in a series of 3,570 radiographs of the sinuses and consequently felt that these tumours were far commoner than generally recognised. Twelve of the 15 cases involved the frontal sinuses. Osteomas of the other nasal sinuses are less common. Only 55 examples of osteomas of the ethmoidal bones had been recorded in the literature up to 1939 (Scholz, 1939). Duydal (1939) felt that the infrequent appearance today of the large massive osteomas reported in past literature was a direct consequence of the more widespread use of radiology (fig. 103). Ivory osteomas occur most frequently in the frontal sinus, where they grow to a considerable size, deforming the sinus itself (fig. 104). In a review of 200 cases of osteomas affecting the paranasal sinuses Fetissof (1929) found that the incidence of osteomas was as follows: frontal sinus 50%, ethmoidal labyrinth 40%, maxillary sinus 6·2%, sphenoidal sinus 3·6%. Malan (1938) found that 38·95% of osteomas involved the frontal sinuses.

All authors are agreed that osteomas pre-dominantly occur in males (Dowling, 1944) and their major occurrence is between the second and third decades. The aetiology of osteomas is obscure but Gatewood & Settel (1935) believe that these tumours have their origin in an embryonal rest.

If the osteoma obstructs the ostium of a sinus super-added infection with a loss of translucency of the sinus occurs; otherwise the sinus is normally translucent. In the frontal sinus the majority of ivory osteomas appear to arise from the anterior wall or floor of the frontal sinus. The osteoma may extend down into the ethmoidal cells (fronto-ethmoidal osteoma) (fig. 102) when the growth may increase to a considerable size and be associated with infection. Cancellous osteomas on the other hand may occur in any sinus and they are covered with a thin bony cortex – the density of the calcification may be extremely low and may be such that the osteoma has the appearance and density of a fibroma. Various writers have described osteomas in association with unerupted teeth or with dentigerous cysts; it is highly probable, however, that such cases are really atypical examples of odontomes.

Radiological appearances. Radiologically, ivory osteomas appear as dense rounded masses with clear-cut outlines and are composed of an amorphous structureless mass, hence the analogy to ivory (figs. 96 and 100). Cancellous osteomas on the other hand are generally of three types (Worth, 1939).

(a) The type occurring in young adults which has an appearance not unlike orange skin.
(b) A second type occurring in the adult patient which appears as a dense mass (structureless) of new bone.
(c) A third type produces an ill-defined swelling with a ground-glass appearance and small cyst-like cavitites.

Apart from the changes of infection complicating osteomas, ethmoidal osteomas are particularly prone to the development of spontaneous pneumocephalus (Kessel, 1939). Erosion of the ethmoidal cells and the frontal bone allows the development of a fistulous communication (Malan, 1938).

Leontiasis ossium. Leontiasis ossium is an overgrowth of the facial bones with considerable encroachment on the paranasal sinuses. The entity was originally described by Knaggs (1923) as a

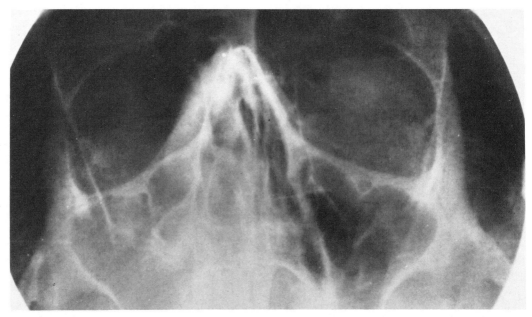

Fig. 97. Inverting papilloma. Occipito-mental view showing opaque right antrum with thinning of lateral wall suggesting infiltration.

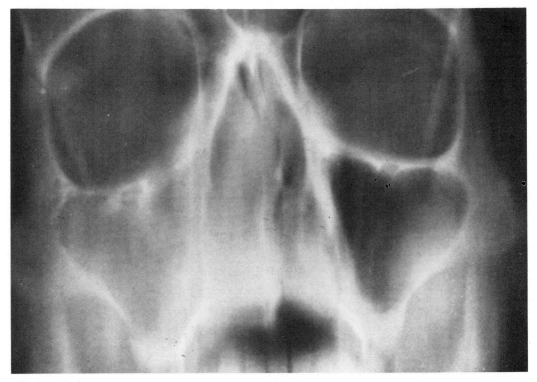

Fig. 98. PA tomograph showing thinning of lateral wall of antrum and "erosion" of the zygoma mimicking a malignant tumour. (Same patient as Fig. 97.)

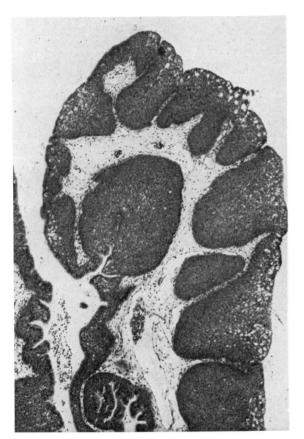

Fig. 99. Inverting papilloma (Schneiderian).
The polyp-like frond with thickened epithelium with darkly staining cells (low power magnification).
(Courtesy of Pathology Department, University of Edinburgh.)

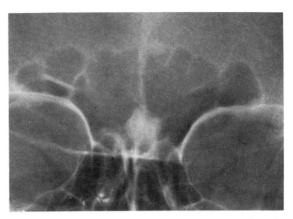

Fig. 100. Ivory osteoma of left frontal sinus. A male aged 32 who had complained of frontal headaches for several months. The occipito-frontal view shows a homogenous bony shadow occupying the medial half of the left frontal sinus. Obstruction of the fronto-nasal duct can be deduced from the diminished translucency of the outer half sinus. At operation the osteoma arose from the ethmoidal cells around the fronto-nasal duct and projected into the left frontal sinus.

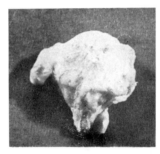

Fig. 101. Photograph of the osteoma shown in Fig. 100 after operative removal. The small nodule which projected into the fronto-nasal duct can be seen inferiorly.

creeping periostitis of the facial bones but there is now considerable doubt as to the validity of this assumption. Other authorities (Eden, 1939) consider that the condition is one of localised fibrous dysplasia occurring in the facial bones. Likewise, it has been thought to represent a localised form of Paget's disease occurring in the facial bones. Both inner and outer aspects of the facial bones are involved in the thickening and the condition histologically resembles Paget's disease or fibrous dysplasia.

Collins (1939) regarded leontiasis ossium as a symptom complex and classified the aetiological causes into non-inflammatory and inflammatory.

Non-inflammatory. Paget's disease. Although Paget's disease most frequently affects the vertex of

the skull, in the more advanced stages the disease process may actually extend into the facial bones. Rarely the disease may actually start in the facial bones producing a leonine appearance (Kernan, 1942). In the early stages the typical diphasic changes seen in Paget's disease may be seen in the facial bones but in the later sclerotic stage it may not be possible to distinguish the Paget form of leontiasis ossium from the other types. Some authorities maintain that in Paget's disease there is no encroachment in the actual lumen of the paranasal sinuses but, in our experience, except in the earliest stages, encroachment on the lumen of the maxillary or frontal sinus is almost always present.

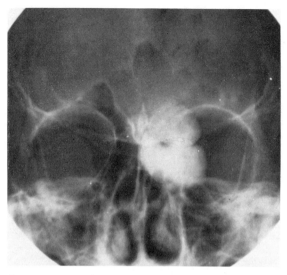

Fig. 102. Fronto-ethmoidal osteoma (ivory). Dense lobulated homogenous bony mass projecting downwards into the ethmoid region. The left frontal sinus is opaque due to obstruction of the left fronto-nasal duct. The patient, a middle-aged Indian lady, had complained of proptosis and obstruction of the lachrymal duct for two years.

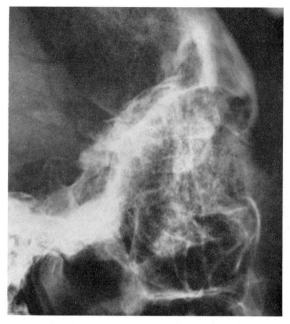

Fig. 104. Lateral view of case shown in Fig. 103 showing the extensive nature of the osteoma.

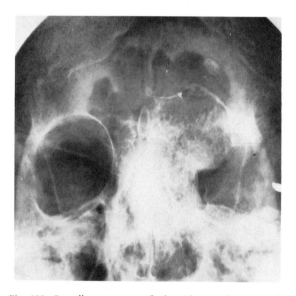

Fig. 103. Cancellous osteoma of ethmoids extending upwards into frontal sinus. Cancellous osteoma may contain such a loose bony structure that it may be mistaken for a fibroma. At operation however, it is frequently far more solid in character than appears from the radiograph.

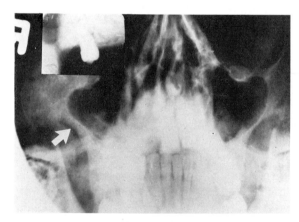

Fig. 105. Dental film of right molar region showing the dysplastic character of the bony change in Paget's disease (insert). Occipito-mental view shows early thickening of lateral wall of right maxillary antrum with decrease in the size of the antral cavity.

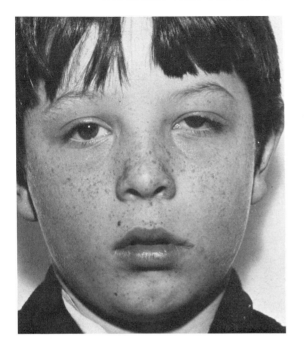

Fig. 106. Fibrous dysplasia. Swelling of soft tissue around left orbit and prominence of left maxilla in an early case of fibrous dysplasia. A young boy who complained of painless swelling of left maxilla.

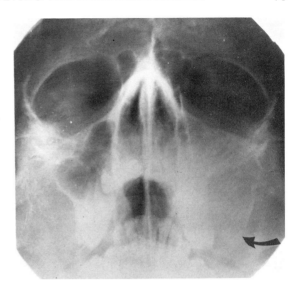

Fig. 107. Occipito-mental view of same case showing homogenous opacity of left antrum with expansion of the lateral wall of the antrum. The medial wall of the antrum is not involved.

Radiologically leontiasis ossium presents as a thickening of the facial bones. In the early stages the new bone produced does not radiologically differ in any way from the normal bone. Encroachment on the lumen of the sinus occurs at an early stage and displacement of the infra-orbital canal may occur. This latter feature is not seen in Paget's disease even in the later stages when almost complete obliteration of the infra-orbital canal may be present. In more advanced Paget's disease the actual texture of the bone changes and sclerosis may occur with localised areas of overgrowth of bone (fig. 105). When this stage has been reached dense bosses of bone occur over the affected areas. The spread of the disease process is always temporarily arrested at the suture lines. In the later stages of leontiasis grotesque deformities of the face occur and encroachment on the orbital cavities may produce advanced degrees of exophthalmos. Other generalised bone diseases which give rise to leontiasis are:

Acromegaly. There is a generalised enlargement of the frontal sinuses but there is none of the over-growth of bone seen in true leontiasis ossium. The leonine appearance when it occurs in this condition is due to overgrowth of soft tissues and not to increase in thickness of the facial bones although the mandible itself may be prognathic.

Fibrous dysplasia. Polyostotic fibrous dysplasia may give rise to a leontiasis ossium syndrome (figs. 106, 107, 108). The bone change may be associated with changes in other parts of the skeleton. In other cases there may be no evidence of generalised disease and, as already stated, some authorities (Eden, 1939) regard localised fibrous dysplasia of the facial bones as one of the commonest causes of leontiasis ossium. Kernan (1942) has described an example of fibrous dysplasia occurring in the frontal sinuses. The radiographs showed that a cystic bony swelling involved the frontal sinus and extended backwards to encroach on the anterior cranial fossa. The condition has to be differentiated from chronic osteomyelitis secondary to sinus infection which may be associated with considerable bone overgrowth.

Inflammatory. The inflammatory varieties of leontiasis ossium may be grouped as follows:

CREEPING PERIOSTITIS. Knaggs (1923) in his original description of leontiasis ossium regarded creeping periostitis as one of the causes of the

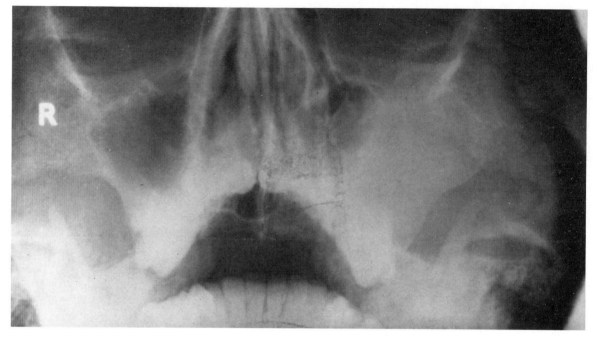

Fig. 108. Advanced fibrous dysplasia involving left maxilla. The cavity of the left antrum is partly obliterated and the lateral wall of the antrum is grossly thickened. Some of these cases were originally mistaken for osteosarcoma. They have to be differentiated from an ossifying fibroma of the maxilla.

condition. Radiologically, this process is characterised by subperiosteal deposits of new bone spreading to other parts of the facial bones. The relentless spread of the process is temporarily held up at the suture lines.

CIRCUMSCRIBED OSTEITIS. Westmacott (1933) has described a localised osteitis causing a leonine appearance of the face. In both cases described by this author there was dental suppuration. Collins (1939) preferred to regard these cases as a nodular form of creeping periostitis. Another condition which is intimately connected with the circumscribed osteitis is obliterative sinusitis (Skillern, 1936). This condition is regarded as a proliferative osteitis of the sinus wall secondary to infection. Skillern (1936) believed that this represented a protective mechanism to infection. The condition was extremely prone to occur after surgical drainage of a sinus had been undertaken.

Osteo-chondroma. This forms an extremely rare form of benign tumour occurring in the paranasal sinuses. Radiologically, it most frequently resembles a cancellous osteoma and the differentiation from this tumour can generally only be made on histological examination.

Haemangioma. Haemangiomas arising in the walls of the antra may give rise to an appearance not unlike a cancellous osteoma. Otty (1940) has described a haemangioma of the superior maxilla which had radiological appearances very similar to a cancellous osteoma. The presence of dilated vessel markings in the surrounding bone wall should suggest the possibility of a haemangioma. Haemangiomas may also occur in the frontal bones. Keleman & Holmes (1948) and Kaplan & Kanzer (1939) remark that prior to 1939 no report on a correct pre-operative diagnosis of a haemangioma of the antrum had been made. Recently the radiological picture has been more clearly appreciated and angiography with selective catheterisation of the external carotid artery has made the diagnosis more accurate and the outlining of the supplying vessels more readily identifiable.

Radiological features:

(1) The *radiological features* are a sun-ray or sun-burst pattern which radiates from a common centre and is mostly angled from the plane of the bone (Bucy & Capp, 1930).

(2) Characteristic of these tumours are *perpendicular striations caused by delicate radiating spicules,* the long axis of striation pointing towards the periosteum.

(3) At other times, haemangiomas tend to show a *honeycomb or soap-bubble effect.*

(4) *Dilated vascular grooves* caused by the dilated and hypertrophied supplying vessels may be seen in the adjoining normal bone.

Osteoclastoma. Osteoclastomas occurring in relation to the nasal cavities are rare (Handousa, 1951); only 13 cases are recorded. The radiological features are:

(a) A shadow similar to a bone cyst, *i.e.* uniform opaque or translucent. ,

(b) Trabeculation is rare and was not seen in seven out of eight cases (Handousa, 1951).

(c) Osteoclastoma arising in the ethmoid or sphenoid sinuses gives rise to opaque cyst-like swellings. Superimposition of the shadows of the ethmoid cell walls mimic trabeculation within the tumour. These tumours may occur as part of hyperparathyroidism.

Cysts and tumours of developmental origin

DERMOID CYSTS. The origin and appearances of the dermoid cyst have already been discussed in Chapter 3.

MENINGOCELE. The importance of frontal meningoceles as a diagnostic problem lies in similarity, both clinically and radiologically, between a meningocele and a mucocele of the frontal sinuses. The vast majority of meningoceles are of congenital origin but on rare occasions may be traumatic (Stuart, 1944). Symptoms do not necessarily arise soon after birth and the difficulties of diagnosis are greater when they present in adolescence. Hypertelorism (Greig, 1924) may be the presenting clinical symptom and may be associated with a swelling in the frontal region.

Radiological appearances:

(1) A *circumscribed mid-line bony* defect in the frontal bone.

(2) The *outline of the bony defect* is smooth and clear-cut and may even show sclerosed margins.

(3) The condition *is generally associated with an absence of one or both of the frontal sinuses.*

Frontal meningoceles have to be differentiated from mucoceles of the frontal sinuses and from cholesteatoma (epidermoid tumour) involving the frontal sinuses.

Malignant tumours

Malignant tumours of the paranasal sinuses originate in the mucosal lining. The maxillary antra are most frequently involved, less commonly the ethmoidal cells and most infrequently the sphenoids or frontal sinuses. As the mucosal lining of the sinuses is composed of columnar epithelium containing mucous glands, the growth is an adeno-carcinoma. This is not invariably so as under the influence of chronic irritation metaplasia to a squamous epithelium may occur, consequently when malignant change supervenes the growth may be squamous-celled carcinoma.

In a series of 127 cases of growths of the paranasal sinuses Watson (1942) found that in 102 instances the maxillary antrum was involved. In a series of 112 cases studied, x-ray examination revealed bone destruction in 83 cases. In 108 of the cases the histological nature of the growth was a squamous-celled or epidermoid carcinoma.

Sarcoma

FIBRO-SARCOMA. These arise from the fibrous stroma of the lining mucosa and are generally of the small round or spindle cell type and on the whole are extremely rapid growing. Rhabdo-myosarcoma of the antra have also been described (Pastore, Sahyoun & Mandeville, 1950). They occur at a younger age than carcinoma and tend to metastasise early. Both round and spindle celled types of sarcomas have extremely bizarre symptoms. Many patients arrive with edentulous jaws which tell of futile dental extraction for an ill-defined pain in the upper jaw. Sarcomas occurring in children usually present with swelling of the affected cheek.

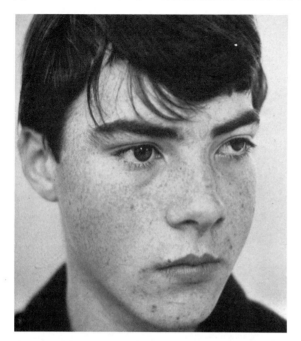

Radiological appearances. Radiologically, fibro-sarcomas present as:

(i) *A soft tissue tumour.* As the most frequent site of a sarcoma of any type is the maxillary sinus, it appears opaque but the degree of antral opacity may be less dense than that seen in infective conditions.

(ii) *Invasion of the surrounding structures.* Sarcomas tend to occur in the region of the alveolus and displacement of the teeth with an alteration in their alignment may be an early sign of the growth (fig. 109). Expansion and thinning of the sinus walls may occur. The thinning is usually mainly due to pressure atrophy and invasion of the antral bony walls is not as marked a feature as in carcinoma.

OSTEOGENIC SARCOMA. The radiological features of an osteogenic sarcoma arising from the bony walls of the paranasal sinuses do not differ materially from osteogenic sarcoma arising in flat bones in other parts of the skeleton. Brünner (1953) recorded an osteogenic sarcoma of the frontal sinus in which some sclerosis was the presenting feature.

Carcinoma. Carcinoma of the antrum is a slowly growing tumour which may remain asymptomatic

Fig. 109. Myxo-sarcoma of left maxillary antrum. Showing swelling of left cheek, more apparent in tangential view. The 13-year-old schoolboy was relatively symptom-free.

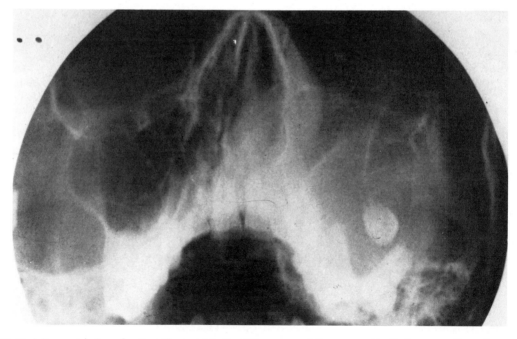

Fig. 110. Occipito-mental view of patient illustrated in fig. 109 – opaque left antrum with displacement of a molar toothbud. Differentiation from fibrocystic disease and a dentigerous cyst cannot be made on radiological grounds.

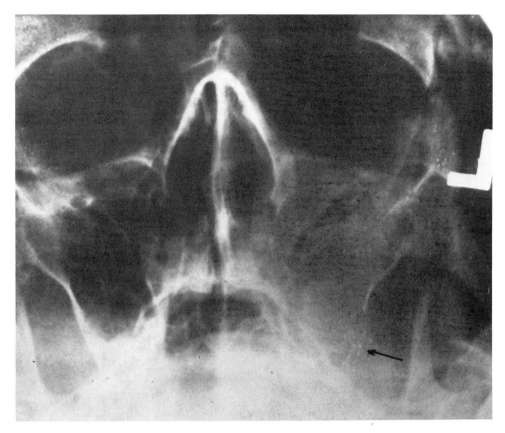

Fig. 111. Sarcoma of the maxillary antrum. Occipito-mental view of a female aged 52 years who had noticed pain and swelling in the left cheek for a few months. Bloodstained discharge had also occurred from the nose and post-nasally. The radiograph shows complete obliteration of the air space of the left antrum with expansion and destruction of the lower parts of the medial and lateral walls of the left antrum. Radiologically the growth was regarded as a carcinoma of the left antrum but histological examination showed a fibrosarcoma.

for an unusually long period. Pain is generally a prominent feature and this again is frequently referred to the teeth. The inferior aspect of the medial wall and floor of the antrum are the commonest sites for the origin of these growths (Windeyer, 1944). Tumours arising in these sites tend to involve the nasal cavity early with the rapid development of nasal obstruction or bleeding.

Radiological appearances. Radiologically the features of an antral carcinoma are:

(i) *General cloudiness of the maxillary antra* with a loss of the normal translucency. The density of the maxillary antrum tends to be less than the opacity produced by infection or retained secretion, but

this difference is inconstant and has no diagnostic significance.

(ii) *Erosion of the antral walls.* The invasive nature of the lesion forms the cardinal differentiating feature from a chronic sinusitis. The medial wall of the antrum is most frequently affected but unfortunately erosion of this wall is less easily detected than of the other antral walls (figs. 113(A), 113(B)). Early bony erosion of the floor or lateral wall of the antrum is more readily seen in the occipito-frontal view than in the occipito-mental view usually used to demonstrate the antra. Extensive loss of the lateral wall is necessary in the occipito-mental view before it can be appreciated. Tomography is the most useful method of determining early bone

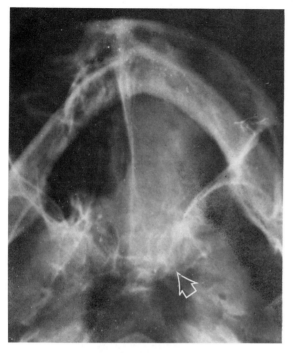

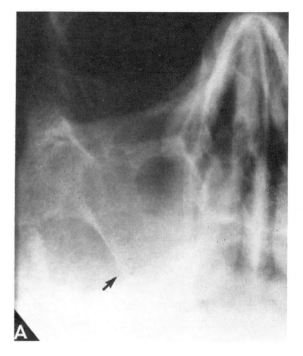

Fig. 112. Submentovertical view of case shown in Fig. 111 showing a large soft tissue mass projecting to the right side of the nasal cavity and destroying bone. There is a backward extension of the soft tissue mass into the nasopharynx.

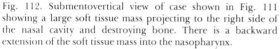

erosion. Too great care cannot be expended in searching for the early speckled appearance of the bony wall which is the first sign of malignant invasion (figs. 113(A), 113(B)). Estimation of recurrence of tumour after radiotherapy in the light of bone loss is an extremely difficult problem (figs. 114, 115, 116) and may not be possible without recourse to biopsy.

(iii) *Bulging of the antral walls.* Associated with the infiltration of the antral wall there is often a bulging of the antral wall caused by infiltration of the growth (fig. 117).

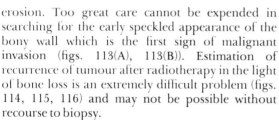

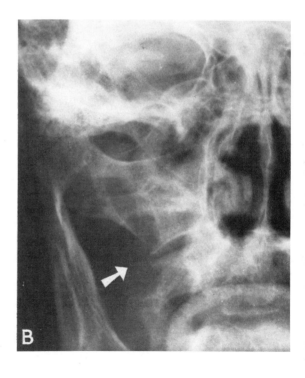

Fig. 113. (A) Carcinoma of right maxillary antrum. The extensive destruction of the right lateral antral wall is barely appreciated in the occipito-mental view.

(B) The occipito-mental projection shows the extent of bone destruction quite clearly although the lateral wall is partly covered by the cervical spine.

(By permission of Churchill-Livingstone Ltd., Edinburgh from Textbook of Radiology edited by D. Sutton.)

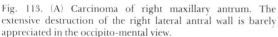

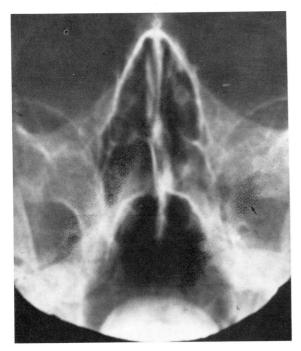

Fig. 114. Occipito-mental view showing loss of bony wall over outer part of left antrum. Differentiation of bone necrosis after radiotherapy from recurrent growth poses great diagnostic difficulties. Radiograph of case shown in figs. 115 and 116.

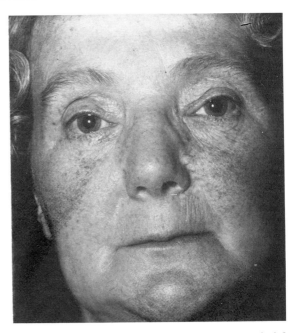

Fig. 115. Clinical photograph showing telangectasis over the left cheek with loss of soft tissues over the left cheek.

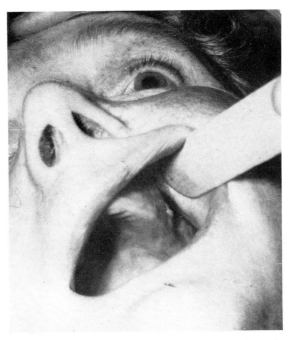

Fig. 116. Intra-oral view demonstrating an ulcerative lesion in alveolar sulcus after radiotherapy (see fig. 114).

Unfortunately bony invasion is a relatively late sign (Berger, 1945) and indicates that the growth is advanced. Berger maintains that the vast majority of early carcinomas of the antrum are discovered accidentally at operation for sinusitis. O'Keefe & Clerf (1946) in a study of 47 cases of carcinoma of the maxillary antra contradicted this view, finding that x-rays were more accurate in the diagnosis of cancer than biopsy, 61% as compared with 44%.

The medial wall of the antrum further forms a source of confusion as this structure is sometimes apparently absent in the radiograph in normal people. This apparent absence of the medial wall is probably due to the combination of an obliquity of the wall and its thin structure. In such cases, care must be taken not to confuse this normal variation with bony destruction. Bone destruction consequent on spread of the tumour to the ethmoid-orbital region may be extremely difficult to recognise. Link (1938) records such a case of antral carcinoma where pre-operative radiology and exploratory biopsy both revealed negative

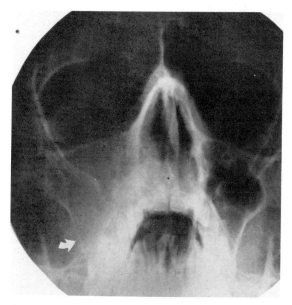

findings. In other instances radiography may demonstrate destruction of the orbital floor, indicating an upward spread. Backward spread of the growth outside the limits of the antrum may result in destruction of the greater and lesser wings of the sphenoid, and in more advanced cases involvement of the sella turcica and clinoid processes (figs. 117, 118). Axial tomography is particularly valuable in determining the posterior limits of extension of the growth. Computerised axial tomography which is a recent development in the investigation of growths of the antrum, may prove an invaluable method of detecting and assessing posterior spread of growth into the pterygo-maxillary fossa (figs. 119, 120).

Invasion of the nasal cavity and orbit. When the growth breaks beyond the confines of the antrum the surrounding structures become involved. Thus, the floor of the orbit may be eroded and the eyeball displaced upwards and forwards whilst the spread of the growth outwards through the lateral wall of the antrum may give rise to a large soft tissue swelling in the cheek. Posteriorly, the growth may extend backwards into the pterygoid fossa with

Fig. 117. Carcinoma of right maxillary antrum showing opacity of the antrum and extensive destruction of bony lateral wall of maxillary antrum. The upward extension of the growth has thinned the roof of the antrum.

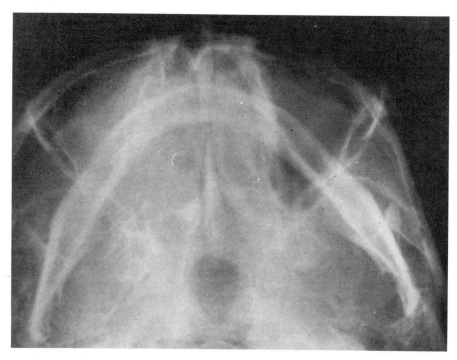

Fig. 118. Carcinoma of right maxillary antrum – same case as fig. 117. Submento-vertical view showing backward extension of tumour into the pterygo-maxillary fossa.

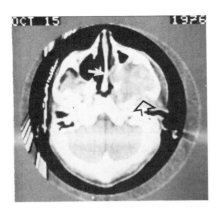

Fig. 119. Computerized axial scan (EMI) showing invasion of pterygoid space posteriorly (black arrow) and the nose medially (white arrow) by a large malignant tumour involving the right maxillary antrum.

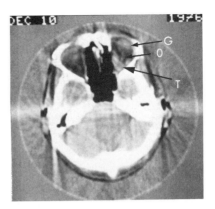

Fig. 120. EMI scan showing value of this method in demonstrating soft tissue invasion. There is an extension into the right orbit from a malignant tumour of the palate which has spread up through the right ethmoid bone. The globe (G) and the optic nerve (O) are quite clearly visible and surrounded by the tumour (T).

involvement of the cranial nerves as they leave the skull. Inferiorly, the growth may cause considerable bulging of the palate and may even ulcerate through the palate (figs. 121, 122). The evaluation of the extent of spread of the tumour is of utmost importance in determining the type of therapy to be instituted. Posterior extension into the pterygoid fossa may be difficult to assess. Conventional axial tomography and computerised axial tomography are the optimum methods of showing this change.

Selective arteriography of the internal maxillary artery has also been used to detect spread of the tumour. The branches of the internal maxillary artery form the "surgical circle around the maxillary sinus" (Lamarque et al., 1971) and displacement of these vessels may be an early sign of extension outside. The arteriographic signs are; posterior displacement of the internal maxillary artery, rigidity and stretching of its branches and encasement leading to narrowing, obstruction and rigidity of the branches. More direct arteriographic signs are pathological hypervascularisation and persistence of contrast within the tumour.

Carcinoma involving both maxillary antra has been described by Berger (1945). It is exceedingly rare and Berger's case is the only recorded case in the literature. In this case the lesions from their histological characters appeared to be separate but radiologically the features of each tumour were no different.

Carcinoma of the ethmoid cells. Carcinoma arising in the ethmoid and frontal sinuses also have the same

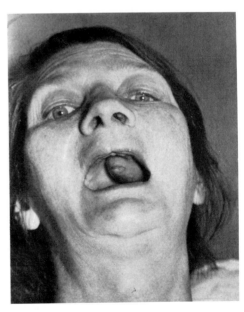

Fig. 121. Carcinoma of the antrum. A female aged 58 years who had noticed a swelling in left half of the palate for six months. The swelling had rapidly increased in size during the last two months. Two months prior to this examination the swelling had increased to such a size as to render it impossible for her to wear her dentures. 14 days prior to admission the swelling had been incised under the mistaken diagnosis of an abscess. The photograph shows a large soft tissue swelling with a superficial ulcer projecting into the roof of the mouth. The diagnosis of a carcinoma of the left antrum with a downward extension through the palate was made.

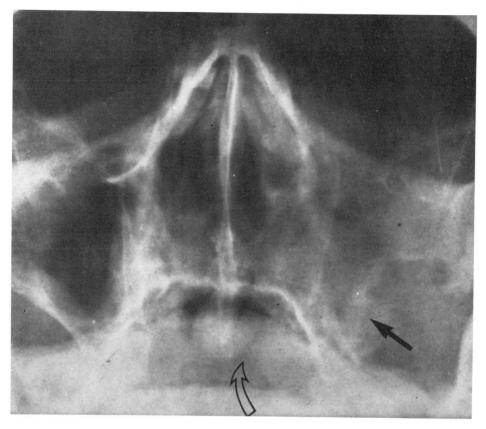

Fig. 122. Occipito-mental view of case shown in Fig. 121 showing the extension of the tumour laterally and also into the mouth.

histology as those arising in the maxillary antrum. The radiological diagnosis of carcinoma of the ethmoid is extremely difficult in its early stages as destruction of the bony walls may be easily overlooked (fig. 123). The diagnosis can only be made when opacity of the affected sinus is associated with invasion and destruction of the cell walls (fig. 124), and postero-anterior tomography is essential for early diagnosis.

Carcinoma of the frontal sinus. Carcinoma of the frontal sinuses is excessively rare. In most cases of carcinoma involving the frontal sinuses it is a secondary spread from the ethmoidal region. Destruction of the surrounding bone is an early and prominent feature in carcinoma of the frontal sinus.

Carcinoma of the frontal sinuses produces early obstruction of the fronto-nasal duct; the differentiation of the growth from superadded infection secondary to an obstructed fronto-nasal duct is extremely difficult. Haas (1951) has reported alterations which may occur in the frontal sinus secondary to carcinoma in other sites in the para-nasal sinuses as follows:

(i) Irregular opacity consistent with a secondarily invading tumour (difficult to differentiate from the homogenoeous haziness produced by secondary infection).

(ii) Uncommonly secondary invasion of the sinus with infiltrative destruction of bony walls. Differential diagnosis is from primary carcinoma of frontal sinus.

(iii) Bony change is restricted to margin of sinus (benign secondary osteitis).

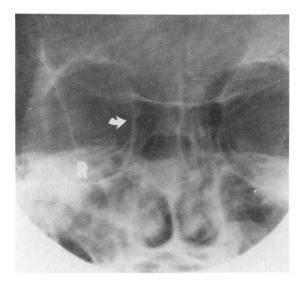

Fig. 123. Carcinoma of ethmoid cells. Relatively little changes are seen in the occipito-frontal view with the exception of a small degree of bone destruction.

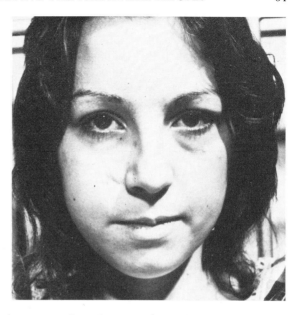

Fig. 125. Swelling of right maxillary region in a young patient suffering from myeloid leukaemia. Infiltration of the right maxillary antrum by leukaemic tissue.

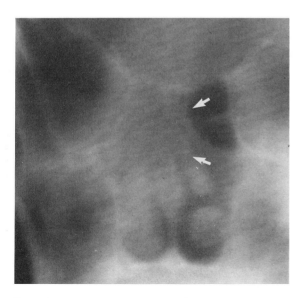

Fig. 124. Anteroposterior tomogram of case shown in Fig. 123 shows the extensive soft tissue tumour present and the considerable degree of bone destruction.

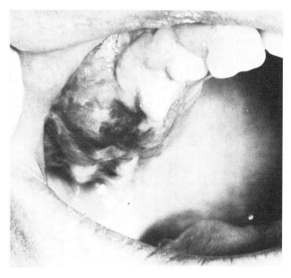

Fig. 126. Intra-oral view showing soft tissue bleeding mass projecting into mouth. An epulis-like mass lies in the molar region.

The x-ray features of this group are:

(i) Demineralisation or disappearance of the white line representing the normal compact bony wall of the frontal sinus.

(ii) Later smaller or larger sections of the outline of the sinus attain a blurred appearance.

(iii) The findings resemble a low-grade secondary osteitis which can be found occasionally in cases of long-standing infective sinusitis with intermittent or constant occlusion of the sinus either by polypus or other alterations of the sinus membrane.

Carcinoma of the sphenoid sinus. Carcinoma of the sphenoid is rare and the tumour spread is principally in two directions, anteriorly into the spheno-ethmoidal recess and upwards into the sella turcica. In advanced cases it may be difficult to determine whether the primary growth was in the sphenoid sinus itself or whether the sinus was secondarily invaded from a nasopharyngeal or pituitary tumour.

Adnexal tumours. These tumours are characterised by extensive bone invasion without comparable soft tissue swelling. They are frequently mistaken for carcinoma of the sphenoid sinus. Invasion of bone is extensive and considerable destruction of the wings of the sphenoid bone may occur.

The aetiology of these tumours is thought to be from the basal cells of the developmental track of Rathkes pouch.

Tumours of Rathke's pouch or the pituitary gland may produce an invasion of the roof and anterior walls of the sphenoid sinus and the translucency of the sinus may be obliterated by an extension of the tumour into the sphenoid sinus. Supra-sellar tumours and cysts frequently calcify, a feature which is of assistance in diagnosis from a primary carcinoma of the sphenoid sinus.

Chordoma. Muller (1858) first identified the tumour as a growth of the notochordal remnants. The tumour arises in the basi-occiput and basi-sphenoid and in 92 out of 253 cases reported in the literature the tumour appears in the nasopharynx (Halper, 1949).

The tumour may arise in the body of the sphenoid bone when its principal feature is destruction of the basi-sphenoid. Calcification in the tumour occurs but the degree of calcification is generally slight and the predominant radiological feature is bone destruction. Mixter & Mixter (1940)

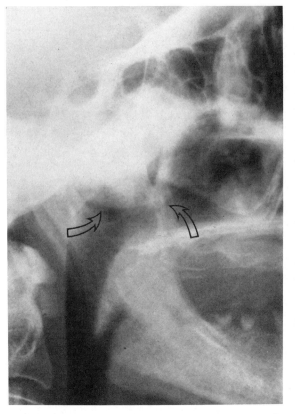

Fig. 127. Chordoma showing soft tissue mass projecting into the nasopharynx.

found that small well defined areas of bone destruction and coarse mottling were the characteristic features. Chordoma may grow into the nasopharynx with the development of a large soft tissue swelling (figs. 127, 128). The tumour is seldom midline in position contrary to published accounts and may grow to a large size before producing symptoms. In the nasopharynx the tumour may produce dysphagia. Arteriography is seldom of use in diagnosis as the lesions are avascular and their arterial features are mainly displacement of the vessels. Tumour staining does not occur.

Melanoma. Melanomas arising in any part of the paranasal sinuses are exceedingly rare tumours. Smith (1939) reporting two cases of his own was only able to find 12 similar cases in the literature. Radiologically such tumours are indistinguishable from carcinoma and the correct diagnosis can only

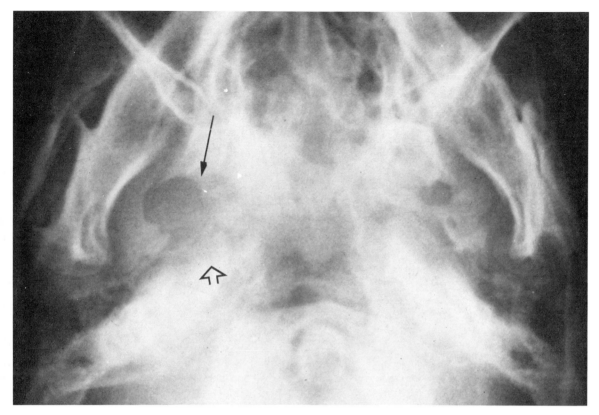

Fig. 128. Chordoma showing bone erosion of middle cranial fossa.

be made on histological examination. Mayoux & Perron (1939) were able to find 38 cases of melanoma of the sinuses in the literature. They emphasise the essential epithelial origin of these tumours.

Cysts of non-dental origin

Retention cysts. Following infection of the sinus mucosa cicatricial contraction of the necks of the glands may occur with the development of retention cysts. The vast majority of these cysts are small but occasionally they attain the size of an acorn. They are formed by obstruction to the outflow of secretion from the mucous glands lining the sinuses, and consequently they are lined by columnar epithelium. They seldom give rise to symptoms and most frequently, though not invariably, they are associated with a previous sinus infection. In a routine autopsy study of the antra in

100 cases, 13% were found to contain cysts (Tunis, 1910). Less frequently the cyst may enlarge and produce pressure deformities of the antral wall (Hardy, 1939).

Radiologically, these cysts appear as rounded opacities with a smooth outline projecting into the antral cavity (fig. 129). These cysts are opaque both to transillumination and x-rays in contrast to non-secreting cysts which transilluminate normally and are opaque only to x-rays.

Non-secreting cysts. These cysts are formed by oedematous dehiscence of a connective tissue plane. Their walls are formed by the crowding and packing of the connective tissue as the cyst enlarges (McGregor, 1928) and they show no epithelial lining and are post-inflammatory in origin (Lindsay, 1942). They are thin walled and contain a clear amber fluid which generally shows a high percentage of cholesterol. In virtue of the doubly refracting property of cholesterol, they often show

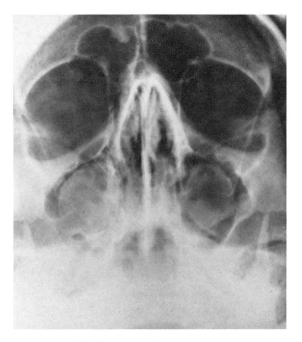

Fig. 129. Calcified cysts in both maxillary antra. These appearances had followed injections into the maxillary antra for therapeutic purposes. No expansion of the antral cavities has occurred.

(Courtesy of Dr. G. Green and Seminars in Roentgenology.)

normal translucency on light transillumination of the antrum.

Radiologically the cyst appears as a smooth-walled, dome-shaped opacity often associated with an apparently normal mucosa over the remainder of the antrum. These cysts never attain sufficient size or degree of tension to distort the bony antral walls. Non-secreting cysts have to be differentiated from localised mucosal thickenings and polypi of the antral walls (fig. 85).

Mucoceles. Mucoceles are not true cysts, as their lumen is that of the sinus itself. They are formed by blockage of the ostium of the sinus and by the accumulation of mucoid material in the sinus. They are commonest in the frontal sinus.

The thinning of the bony walls due to pressure atrophy is such that the translucency of the mucocele may be greater than that of the normal sinus and many appear hypertranslucent. In addition there is loss of scalloping of the bony outline and bulging of the intersinus septum in the frontal sinus.

Traumatic cysts. These are uncommon and the result of a haematoma in the soft tissues which undergoes liquefaction and then becomes sur-rounded by a wall of fibrous tissue.

Haemorrhagic cysts. Lillie & Pastore (1941) described two examples of such cysts occurring in the frontal sinuses and were unable to find any other references to such cysts. The radiographs revealed a more circumscribed mass than seen in a mucocele although the symptoms resembled a mucocele. These authors believe that trauma may have played a part in the development of such cysts. Operation revealed a definite cyst-like mass containing amorphous material, cholesterol crystals and calcium deposits.

Cysts of dental origin

Dental (radicular, root) cysts. The dental cyst is primarily an infected granuloma of a devitalised tooth or root which has acquired an epithelial lining. The tooth itself may have been removed before the development of the cyst.

The origin of the epithelial lining is doubtful. According to some authors it is derived from the epithelium of the gum, whilst according to others it is developed from epithelial cell rests (Malassez, 1885). Whatever the source of the epithelium the net result is a cystic cavity with a well defined outline. These cysts may bulge into the antrum filling it completely, or bulge the palate producing pressure atrophy of the adjoining bone.

Radiological appearances. The features of dental cysts largely depend on their size. Small cysts cause a pressure erosion of the surrounding bone with the result that a clear area with a well-defined outline is produced in the alveolar process. If the tooth has not been extracted the root projects into the cyst and partial or complete absorption of the root may occur. When the cyst projects into the antral cavity it produces a rounded opacity in the antrum itself (fig. 130). With an increase in size of the cyst, it may bulge into the antrum completely filling it and causing an expansion of the walls of the antrum. Small dental or follicular cysts in the canine region have to be differentiated from an enlarged alveolar recess of the antrum. This can be done by tracing the inverted Y formed by the floor of the nose and the anterior wall of the antrum, the main stem of the Y being formed by the medial wall of the antrum. Dental cysts arising anteriorly characteristically separate both limbs of the Y (fig. 131).

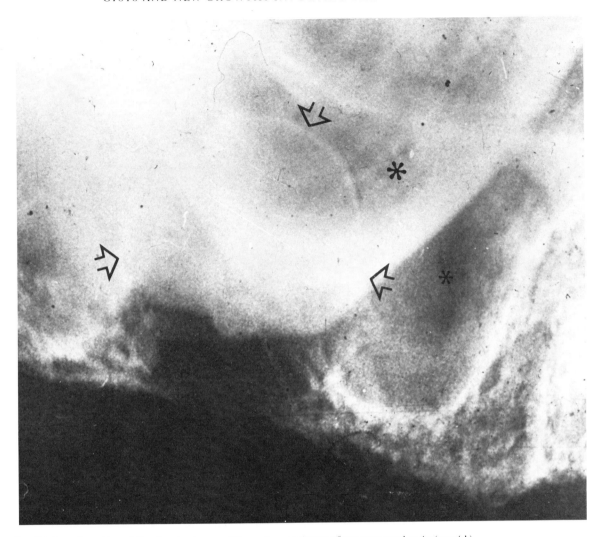

Fig. 130. Dental cyst. Dental film showing bony wall (arrow) separating cyst from true antral cavity (asterisk).

Dentigerous cysts (follicular odontomes). These are derived from the developing tooth bud of the second dentition and as such may contain a rudimentary or completely developed tooth. When the tooth is absent the correct diagnosis can be made by noting the gap in the dentition. As with dental cysts, the follicular cysts have a well-defined bony wall without any bone sclerosis around the clear-cut wall. They are more frequently found in the mandible than the maxilla. They generally grow to a much larger size than dental cysts and consequently often cause considerable expansion of the maxilla. The misplaced tooth generally lies in one portion of the cyst. In the maxilla the floor of the antrum may be elevated by the cyst which may encroach on the antrum to such an extent that the whole antrum is obliterated. In approximately 20% of cases where the cyst has grown into the antrum varying sized defects of the lateral bony wall of the antrum occurred (fig. 131) (Sonesson, 1950). Such a cyst has to be distinguished from a mucocele of the antrum. In such cases, the presence of an

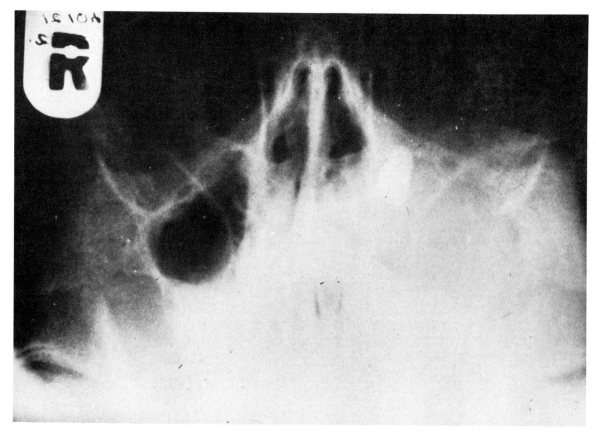

Fig. 131. Dentigerous cyst. The opaque antrum and the displaced tooth is clearly seen. The lateral bony wall of the antrum has apparently disappeared but actually is merely thinned by pressure atrophy.

uncrupted tooth is of diagnostic importance (Weaver, 1939). The follicular cyst arises from an uncrupted or undeveloped tooth of the second dentition. This tooth may be fully or partially developed or completely absent. If the tooth is present, its crown is directed towards the centre of the cyst and its root is embedded in bone. This is an important point in the radiological differentiation from a dental cyst as in the latter, the root not the crown is directed towards the cyst.

Primordial cysts are more frequently met with in the mandible than in the maxilla. All types, however, may occur in the maxilla. Such cysts tend to displace the floor of the antrum upwards and may closely simulate a tumour arising from the antrum. Determination of the precise nature of such a cyst is of importance in planning treatment (Shear, 1976).

Epithelial odontomes (Adamantinoma). These have to be distinguished from dentigerous cysts which they closely resemble. Such differentiation may not be possible until histological examination of the tumour has been undertaken. Eighty per cent of epithelial odontomes occur in the mandible and 15% in the maxilla. The average age at which it is first recognised is a little past 30 years. When the tumour develops in the maxilla the adamantinoma is usually of a solid glandular character and cystic types are less common. Mosher (1944) recorded an epithelial odontome of the maxillary sinus occurring in a male aged 61 years. Radiograms showed a large mass involving the maxillary antrum and eroding the bony walls. Phelps (1939) reported a case of epithelial odontome of the upper jaw in which there was extensive invasion of bone.

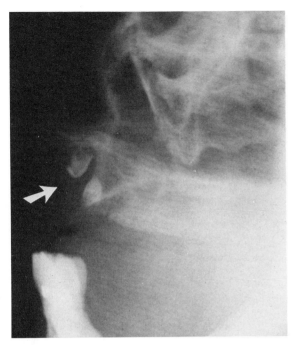

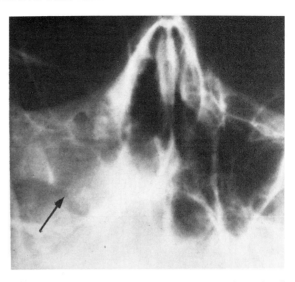

Fig. 134. Dentigerous cyst showing apparent loss of lateral wall of antrum and a bony rim medially.

Fig. 132. Simple dental cyst. Lateral view showing two tooth roots present in the cyst. The cyst lies anteriorly in the maxilla.

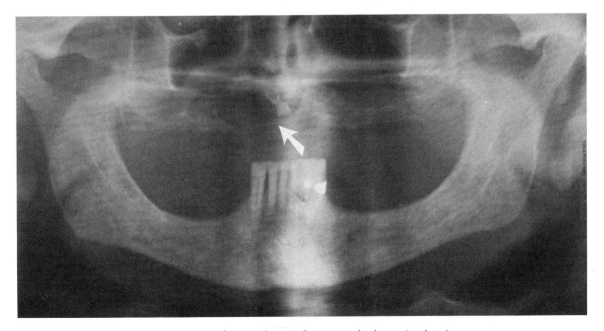

Fig. 133. Pantomograph reveals the full extent of the cyst shown in fig. 132 not clearly seen in other views.

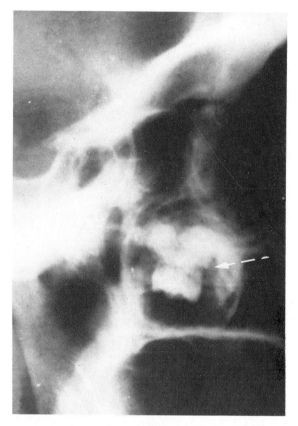

Fig. 135. Compound odontome showing the conglomerate portions of the dental mass lying over the antrum in the lateral view.

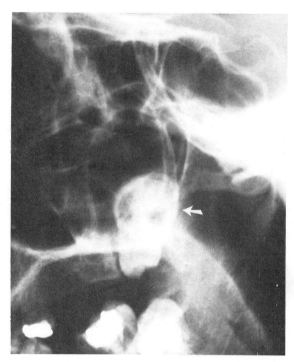

Fig. 136. Compound odontome. The calcified mass of the odontome is seen to lie outside the antral wall.

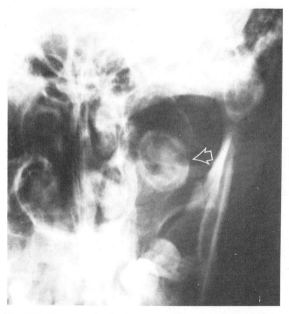

Fig. 137. Compound odontome. P.A. view demonstrating the calcification in the wall of the mass and the amorphous central calcification.

Radiological features. The radiological features vary with the type of the odontome.

EPITHELIAL ODONTOMES. These are by far the commonest. They appear as multilocular cystic areas or as solid tumour and may encroach on the antral cavity itself. The actual tumour may appear as a cystic cavity with coarse trabeculae crossing the cavity. Some degree of expansion of bone is present but seldom to the degree seen in osteoclastoma. In other cases the cysts may be so small and the trabeculation so dense that the whole mass appears solid.

COMPOUND ODONTOMES. These are formed by aggregation of masses of the various elements, dentine and enamel, which form teeth. Radiographically, they appear as dense masses in which various components of teeth may be identified. When they occur in the maxilla they tend

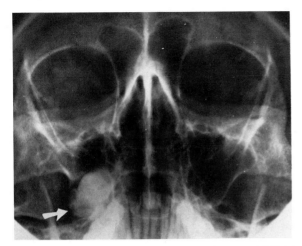

Fig. 138. Tomographic view of case shown in fig. 139. Relatively dense homogenous mass of the dental structures with no form.

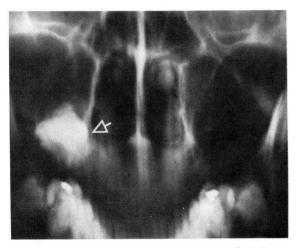

Fig. 139. Composite odontome – mass in floor (alveolus) of right maxilla projecting into right antrum. No change in mucosa of right antrum.

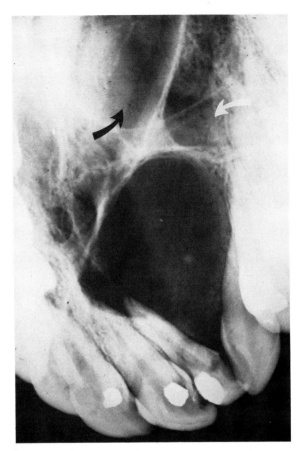

Fig. 140. Globulo-maxillary cyst. Occlusal film showing separation of lateral incisor and canine tooth by the smooth outline of the cyst. The nasal cavity is shown by black arrow and the antrum by white arrow.

to push the floor of the antrum upwards and bulge into the cavity of the antrum (figs. 136–139).

COMPOSITE ODONTOMES. These are composed of several teeth formed into a conglomerate mass. The individual teeth may be recognised and the mass causes the floor of the antrum to be pushed upwards (fig. 135).

Tuberosity cysts. Cysts of the maxillary tuberosity are of dental origin and may give rise to considerable confusion as they have to be dis-

tinguished from a large tuberosity recess of the maxillary antrum. The maxillary tuberosity is frequently composed of cancellous bone and this wide lattice work of bone must not be mistaken for a cyst. Careful examination with dental films and the absence of any true expansion of the tuberosity will enable a cancellous tuberosity to be distinguished from a true cyst.

Fissural cysts

(i) Globulo-maxillary cysts. These cysts are of developmental origin and represent cystic involutions from a failure of complete fusion between the lateral aspect of the premaxilla and

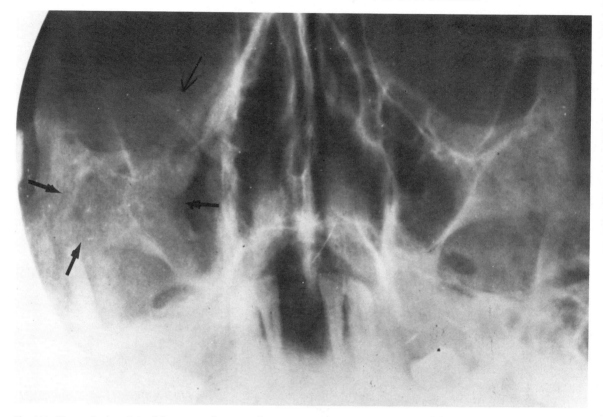

Fig. 141. Metastatic deposit in right zygoma showing infiltration into right antrum and extension into antral cavity. The site of the primary tumour was in the breast. The distinguishing radiological features are the disproportionate destruction of bone with relatively little soft tissue mass extending into the antrum.

maxilla. According to Thoma (1934) this is the most common type of the fissural developmental cyst. Consequently such cysts are always found in the region of the canine teeth and they tend to displace the canine and lateral incisor teeth (fig. 140). Radiographically, they may be confused with an enlarged alveolar recess of the antrum.

With occipito-mental and lateral views it is generally possible to distinguish this cyst from an extension of the true antral cavity. Oblique occlusal views may also greatly aid in the separations of the cyst from the true cavity of the antrum. In doubtful cases tomographic films will generally enable the cyst outline to be fully shown.

(ii) **Incisive canal cysts.** Cysts involving the premaxilla are generally the result of failure of both halves of the premaxilla to fuse (Huizinga, 1925). Incisive canal cysts reveal themselves as midline cysts lying in the region of the incisive canal. They seldom grow to a large size, and indeed, the smaller ones have to be distinguished from excessively large incisive canals. A characteristic feature (Rosenberger, 1944) is that the cyst lies in a depression on the bone surface instead of developing within the bone itself. It is also situated in the midline although projection may suggest it is one sided and the incisive canal is invariably expanded to some degree. The actual size of the normal incisive canal varies considerably and the differentiation of a small cyst from a large normal canal may occasion some difficulty.

The anatomical outlines of the cyst are best shown by means of occlusal films but in some cases tomographs in the postero-anterior position may better outline the topographical relations of the cyst to the nasal cavity and palate.

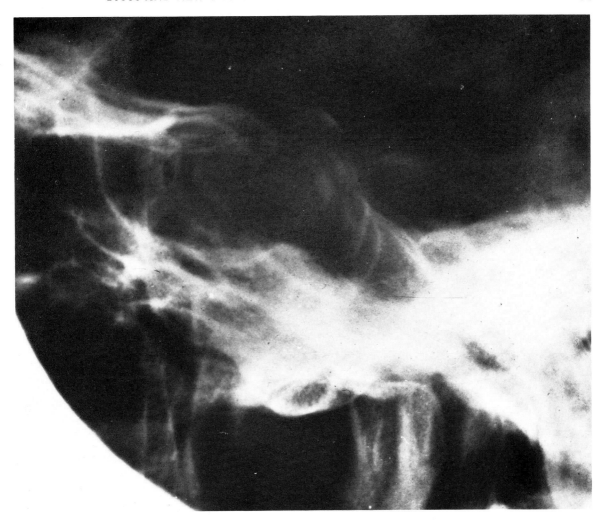

Fig. 142. Direct invasion of the sphenoid sinus by a pituitary tumour.

Secondary involvement of the paranasal sinuses

ORAL TUMOURS. Secondary involvement of the paranasal sinuses by tumours arising elsewhere is usually the result of contiguous spread of a growth. Blood-borne metastatic deposits from tumours arising elsewhere in the body only occur on extremely rare occasions (Concetti, 1949). In such cases the extent of bone destruction is usually greater than the extent of changes in the antral cavity itself. Secondary invasion of the antrum usually results from a direct spread of a carcinoma of the alveolus or palate (Brunner, 1949). An antro-oral fistula develops rapidly and the differentiation of such a carcinoma from an antral carcinoma invading the mouth may be difficult.

Radiological appearances:
(i) Destruction of bone may be more marked on the oral side of the alveolus.
(ii) Loss of translucency of the maxillary antrum is almost invariably present due to the associated infection of the antrum and the spread of growth.

Benign tumours arising in the nasal fossae may cause pressure atrophy of the walls of the sinuses and the tumour mass may bulge into and cause an opacity of the affected sinus.

Primary malignant tumours of the nasal cavity are generally carcinomas and they almost invariably involve the antrum by direct spread.

REFERENCES

BALL, S. (1951) Ossifying Fibroma of the Frontal Sinus. *Archs Otolar.,* **53,** 460.

BERGER, M. D. (1945) Neoplasms of Both Maxillary Sinuses. *Archs Otolar.,* **42,** 397.

BRUNNER, H. (1949) Involvement in the Paranasal Sinuses in Tumours Originating from the Mucous Membrane of the Cheek. *Oral Surg.,* **2,** 1235.

BRUNNER, H. (1953) Primary Tumours of the Frontal Bone. *Archs Otolar.,* **57,** 2.

BUCY, P. C. & CAPP, C.S. (1930) Primary Haemangioma of Bone. *Am. J. Roentg.,* **23,** 1.

CHILDREY, J. H. (1939) Osteoma of the Sinuses, the Frontal and the Sphenoid Bone. *Archs Otolar.,* **36,** 63.

COLLINS, E. G. (1939) Osseous Affections of the Maxillary Sinus. *J. Lar. Otol.,* **54,** 121.

CONCETTI, F. (1949) Su due casi di metastasi dell'anteipofisi da carcinoma del collo dell'utero e da carcinoma mammario. *Clinica ostet.,* **51,** 101.

CROWE, S. J. & BAYLOR, J. W. (1923) Benign and Malignant Growths of the Nasopharynx and their Treatment with Radium. *Archs Surg., Chicago,* **6,** 429.

DOWLING, J. R. (1944) Osteoma of the Frontal Sinus. *Archs Otolar.,* **41,** 99.

DUYDAL, S. I. (1939) Osteoma of Right Frontal Sinus. *Annls Otolaryng.,* p. 461.

EDEN, K. C. (1939) The Benign Fibro-osseous Tumours of the Skull and Facial Bones. *Br. J. Surg.,* **27,** 323.

FETISSOF, A. G. (1929) Pathogenesis of Osteoma of Nasal Accessory Sinuses. *Ann. Otol. Rhinol. Lar.,* **38,** 404.

GATEWOOD, W. L. & SETTEL, N. (1935) Osteoma of the Frontal Sinus. *Archs Otolar.,* **22,** 154.

GREIG, D. M. (1924) Hypertelorism. *Edinb. med. J.,* **31,** 560.

HAAS, L. L. (1951) Secondary Alterations of the Frontal Sinus in Cancer of the Paranasal Sinuses. *Am. J. Roentg.,* **66,** 797.

HALPER, H. (1949) Chordomata. *Br. J. Radiol.,* **22,** 88.

HANDOUSA, A. B. (1951) Osteoclastoma in Relation to the Nose. *J. Lar. Otol.,* **65,** 549.

HARA, H. J. (1944) Ossifying Fibroma of the Superior Maxilla. *Archs Otolar.,* **40,** 180.

HARDY, G. (1939) Benign Cysts of the Antrum. *Ann. Otol. Rhinol. Lar.,* **48,** 649.

HUIZINGA, E. (1925) On Cysts Near the Nose Entrance. *Acta otolar.,* **8,** 505.

KAPLAN, A. & KANZER, M. (1939) Sunray Haemangioma of Skull. *Archs Surg., Chicago,* **39,** 269.

KELEMAN, G. & HOLMES, E. M. (1948) Cavernous Haemangioma of the Frontal Bone. *J. Lar. Otol.,* **62,** 577.

KERNAN, J. D. (1942) Osteitis Fibrosa Cystica of the Left Frontal Sinus. *Archs Otolar.,* **36,** 385.

KESSEL, F. K. (1939) Orbito-ethmoidal Osteomata with Intracranial Complications. Report of a Case. *Guy's Hosp. Rep.,* **89,** 337.

KNAGGS, L. (1923/24) Leontiasis Ossea. *Br. J. Surg.,* **11,** 347.

LAMARQUE, J. L. et al. (1971) *J. Radiol. Electrol.,* **52,** 357.

LILLIE, H. I. & PASTORE, P. N. (1941) Haemorrhagic Cysts of the Frontal Sinus which Simulated Mucocele. *Ann. Otol. Rhinol. Lar.,* **50,** 544.

LINDSAY, J. R. (1942) Non-secreting Cysts of Maxillary Sinus Mucosa. *Laryngoscope,* **52,** 84.

LINK, R. (1938) Maligner tumor der ethmo-orbitalen region. *Arch. Ohr., Nas.-u. Kehlk Heilk,* **145,** 259.

McGREGOR, G. W. (1928) How and When the Mucous Membrane of the Maxillary Sinus Regenerates. *Archs Otolar.,* **8,** 647.

MALAN, E. (1938) Chirurgia degli osteom delle comta pneumaticle perifacciali; contributo-anatomo clinice. *Arch. ital. Chir.,* **48,** 1.

MALASSEZ, L. (1885) Sur l'existence d'a mas epitheliaux autour de la racine des dents chez l'homme adulte et a l'etat normal (debris epitheliaux paradentaires). *Archs Physiol. norm. Path.,* **3/5,** 129.

MALASSEZ, L. (1885) Sur le role des debris-epitheliaux paradentaires. *Archs Physiol. norm. Path.,* **3/5,** 309; **3/6,** 379.

MAYOUX, R. & PERRON, R. (1939) Les tumeurs melaniques du nez. *Revue Lar. Otol. Rhimol.,* **60,** 245.

MIXTER, C. G. & MIXTER, W. (1940) Surgical Management of Sacrococcygeal and Vertebral Chordoma. *Archs Surg., Chicago,* **41,** 408.

MOSHER, W. F. (1944) Adamantinoma of the Maxillary Sinus. *Archs Otolar.,* **40,** 61.

MULLER, H. (1858) *Z. rat. Med.,* **2,** 202.

O'KEEFE, J. J. & CLERF, L. H. (1946) *Ann. Otol. Rhinal. Lar.,* **55,** 312.

OTTY, J. H. (1940) Tuberculoma of Nose. *J. Lar. Otol.,* **55,** 115.

PASTORE, P. N., SAYHOUN, P. F. & MANDEVILLE, F. B. (1950) Rhabdosarcoma of the Maxillary Antrum. *Archs Otolar.,* **52,** 942.

PHELPS, K. A. (1939) Case of Malignant Adamantinoma of Right Maxillary Sinus. *Trans. Amer. Lar. rhinol. otol. Soc.,* **45,** 393.

ROSEDALE, R. S. (1945) Massive Fibroma of the Maxillary Antrum as a Part of Multiple Neurofibromatosis in Siblings. *Archs Otolar.,* **42,** 208.

ROSENBERGER, H. C. (1944) Fissural Cysts. *Archs Otolar.,* **40,** 288.

SCHOLZ, W. (1939) Isoliertes siebbeinosteom in der orbits. *Z. Hals-Nasen-u. Ohrenheilk.,* **45,** 86.

SHEAR, M. (1976) *Cysts of the Oral Region.* Bristol: John Wright & Sons.

SKILLERN, S. R. (1936) Obliterative Frontal Sinusitis. *Archs Otolar.,* **23,** 267.

SMITH, A. T. (1939) Primary Melanoma of Nasal Cavity. *Archs Otolar.,* **29,** 437.

SONESSON, A. (1950) Odontogenic Cysts and Cystic Tumours of the Jaws. *Acta radiol.,* (Suppl.), **81,** 48.

STUART, E. A. (1944) An Otolaryngologic Aspect of Frontal Meningocele. *Archs Otolar.,* **40,** 171.

THOMAS, K. H. (1934) *Clinical Pathology of the Jaws.* Springfield: Thomas., p. 262.

TUNIS, J. P. (1910) Inflammation of the Sinus Maxillaris with Special Reference to Empyema. *Laryngoscopy,* **20,** 931.

UFFENORDE, H. (1939) Seltene Geschwulstbildungen im Stirnhöhlengebiet. *Hals-Nas.-u. Ohrenarzt,* **30,** 246.

WATSON, W. L. (1942) Cancer of Paranasal Sinuses. *Laryngoscope,* **52,** 22.

WEAVER, D. F. (1939) Infected Dentigerous Cyst of Antrum of Highmore. *Proc. Staff Meet Mayo Clin.,* **14,** 135.

WELIN, S. (1948) Fibro-osteomas of the Paranasal Sinuses, Roentgenologically Simulating Malignant Neoplasms. *Acta radiol.,* **30,** 457.

WESTMACOTT, F. H. (1933) Localised Osteitis. *Int. Congr. Med.,* Sect. 15, **17,** 243.

WINDEYER, B. W. (1943/44) Tumours of the Maxilla. *Br. J. Radiol.,* **16,** 362; **17,** 18.

WOODRUFF, G. H. (1945) Ossifying Fibroma of the Ethmoid Cells and Frontal Sinus. Report of a Case. *Ann. Otol. Rhinol Lar.,* **54,** 582.

WORTH, H. M. (1939) Radiological Findings in Some Less Common Jaw Affections. *Proc. R. Soc. Med.,* **32,** 331.

CHAPTER 6

Traumatic lesions involving the paranasal sinuses

FOREIGN BODIES

Foreign bodies in the antra may gain entrance through the nose or through the antral walls by direct trauma (Schroder, 1937). Glass from a shattered windscreen in motor car accidents is one of the commonest foreign bodies entering the sinuses by direct trauma (figs. 143, 144). Foreign bodies in the antra give rise to suppuration and this usually persists as long as the foreign body remains in the sinus. The foreign body may serve as a nucleus and become encrusted with salts giving rise to the development of an antral rhinolith (see Chapter 3). Richardson (1946) records such a case where a metal pin was driven into the left antrum.

A completely different type of foreign body that may occur in the antrum is a misplaced tooth. Such teeth are generally surrounded by fibrous capsules and as they do not actually lie free in the antrum they seldom form rhinoliths. Exceptions do occur and such a case is described by Noonan (1946).

The commonest foreign body found in the antrum is a tooth root, usually the result of displacement during extraction. The root usually is a molar one but a premolar root or several roots may be displaced into the antrum.

An antro-oral fistula develops as a sequel of this accident and if it is of any size prolapse of the antral mucosa into the mouth may occur. At other times, granulation tissue growing from the fistula may present a polypoid appearance on the gum simulating prolapsed antral mucosa. The antrum invariably becomes infected through an antro-oral fistula but owing to dependent drainage through the fistula a fluid level seldom forms in the antrum.

Radiological features

The radiological diagnosis of an antro-oral fistula depends upon:

(a) The demonstration of an infected antrum,

(b) A defect in the floor of the antrum, and

(c) The presence of a tooth root or roots in the antrum.

(a) *Infected antrum.* The infected antrum usually shows as localised thickened mucosa over the floor or complete opacity of the antrum. No fluid level can be seen and the opacity is produced by the inflamed mucosa and mucopus. Films taken with a higher penetration should be used if a tooth root is to be demonstrated in the thickened mucosa (figs. 145, 146). In other antro-oral fistulae the antral mucosa may show remarkably little change. Tomography in the postero-anterior plane may be of greatest value in demonstrating the tooth root.

(b) *Defect in the floor of the antrum.* The defect in the floor of the antrum can be best visualised by intra-oral or occlusal films of the suspected portion of the alveolus. An unhealed tooth socket, with a defect at its apex indicates an antro-oral fistula (figs. 145 and 146). The extent of mucosal thickening is probably dependent on the size of the fistula. Many of these antro-oral fistulae heal spontaneously and recurrence only follows a cold or nasal infection when the ostium of the antrum becomes blocked. Other fistulae remain permanently open from the inception of the fistula. If the fistula is large, antral mucosa may prolapse into the mouth. More frequently granulation

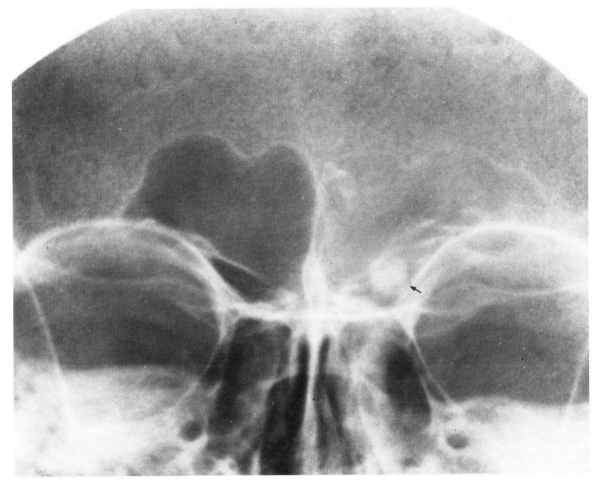

Fig. 143. Foreign body in frontal sinus. Occipito-frontal view of a middle-aged male who had suffered a slight head injury in a road traffic accident five weeks previously. He presented with frontal headaches. The occipito-frontal view shows an opacity over the left frontal sinus associated with a denser opacity in the lower part of the left frontal sinus.

tissue forms a mass projecting through the fistula into the mouth.

(c) *Tooth roots.* Special techniques are necessary if the tooth root in the antrum is to be demonstrated. Films utilising a higher kilovoltage than normal should be employed to penetrate the thickened mucosal lining of the antrum (fig. 146). Tomographic films in the postero-anterior plane using thin sections are the most accurate means of demonstrating tooth roots lying in the antrum. Intra-oral dental films often fail to demonstrate the tooth root presumably because once in the cavity of

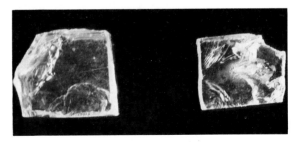

Fig. 144. The dense opacity in Fig. 143 consisted of a small fragment of windscreen glass (about 5 mm wide) that had directly penetrated into the left frontal sinus.

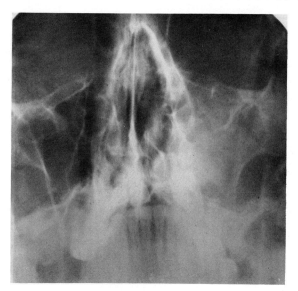

Fig. 145. Antro-oral fistula showing complete opacity of left antrum. No tooth root can be seen in the occipito-mental view.

the antrum, the roots may be outside the range of dental films.

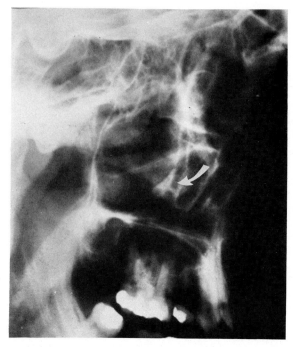

Fig. 146. Lateral view of case shown in Fig. 145 – showing the dental root lying within the antral cavity. Tomographic studies in the postero-anterior position may be necessary to demonstrate the tooth root when the antrum shows complete opacity.

TRAUMA

Traumatic lesions affecting the paranasal sinuses result from two types of injury:

(a) Associated with fractures of the bony walls of the sinuses – generally the result of direct violence applied to the facial bones.
(b) Changes in the paranasal sinuses which are associated with variations in atmospheric pressure (barotrauma).

Fractures involving the paranasal sinuses

The maxilla from its prominent position is most liable to trauma and consequently fractures of the walls of the maxillary antrum are relatively common.

The frontal sinus may be injured by direct violence or by a spread of a fracture from the anterior cranial fossa or the vertex of the skull. Fractures of the facial bones are often associated with other injuries of the skull and cervical spine and for this reason and because co-operation of the patient is essential for accurate radiography of these parts, radiographic examination of fractured facial

bones is best delayed until the patient is able to co-operate.

Fractures of the maxillary antra

The common fracture of the maxilla is the "tripod fracture" (triple fracture) and is the result of direct violence to the cheek bone. Three easily detectable fracture lines make up this fracture (fig. 147). One running through the roof of the antrum, which may be medial or lateral to the infra-orbital groove. In other cases, it may run across the infra-orbital canal and involve the infra-orbital nerve. The resulting displacement of the fractured maxilla is dependent on the force applied. Generally the displacement is not marked, but any displacement is important as this results in a disturbance of the floor of the orbit with a downward displacement of the eyeball and diplopia (King & Samuel, 1944; Radcliffe, 1949). Herniation of orbital tissues into the antrum may give a tear drop appearance in the roof of the antrum (fig. 151).

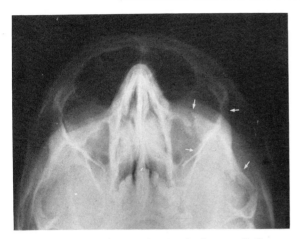

Fig. 147. Lateral face fracture showing the features of a fracture of the zygomatic tripod (infra-orbital margin, zygomatic arch, lateral wall of antrum and widening of the fronto-malar synchondrosis).

In searching for the infra-orbital portion of the triple fracture, care must be taken not to confuse the maxillo-nasal suture with the fracture. This suture line usually lies medial to the infra-orbital fracture and its longitudinal direction is downwards and outwards. Comparison with the opposite side will enable the diagnosis to be made. It is seldom affected in fractures involving the facial bones. The second fracture line extends through the outer wall of the antrum. Care must be taken not to confuse the normal vascular marking "pseudo fracture lines" (Dolan & Haydon, 1973) caused by the posterior superior alveolar artery with a fracture line (fig. 60). The third fracture line involves the zygomatic arch and this may be single when the break generally occurs at the convexity of the zygoma or may be multiple when the fracture occurs through either root of the zygoma.

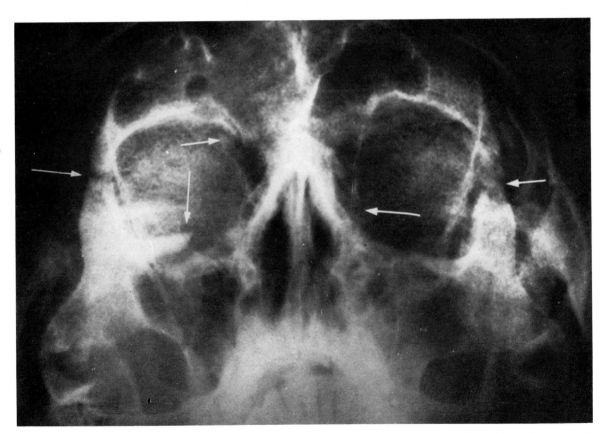

Fig. 148. Middle third face fracture showing fractures through the ethmoids, maxilla and nasal bones with backward displacement of the middle third of the facial bones.

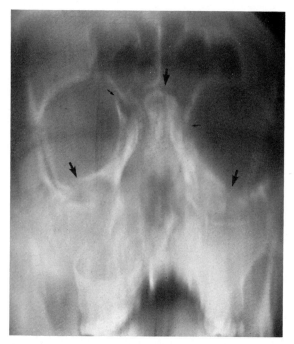

Fig. 149. Tomographic views of middle third face fractures showing the fracture lines far more clearly than in the routine occipito-frontal views.

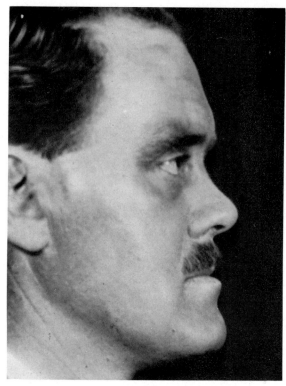

Fig. 150. Clinical photograph showing profile view of unreduced middle third face fracture showing the dish face appearance caused by the backward displacement of the fracture.

The separated fragment of the zygoma may be displaced downwards and backwards with a widening of the fronto-zygomatic synchondrosis (fig. 147).

As the tripod fracture of the maxilla often results in a backward displacement of the whole body of the maxilla with some impaction, the fracture lines already mentioned may be difficult to visualise. In such cases, tomography may be of considerable assistance in demonstrating the fracture lines and this method of examination is extremely useful in assessing post-operative reduction. On the plain films the widening of the fronto-zygomatic synchondrosis may be of the utmost value in drawing attention to the possibility of a fractured maxilla. The value of the exaggerated occipito-mental view (the incident beam is tilted at an angle of 30° caudally and centred through the antrum) in the diagnosis of antral fractures cannot be over-emphasised. The displacement of fractured fragments can be better visualised in this view.

Fractures involving the middle third of the face also involve the antra or ethmoids. The detection of these fractures in the early stages after injury when they are most easily reduced presents a radiographic problem as such patients frequently have other fractures and are not ambulatory, and only bedside radiography is possible.

Accurate lateral views of the skull are, however, possible with a bedside unit and careful study of the posterior walls of the maxillary antra and of the pterygoid laminae will show buckling of these structures indicating posterior displacement of the middle third of the facial bones (fig. 150).

The changes produced in the maxillary antra by these fractures are:

(a) *Generalised oedema of the mucosa.* This results in a generalised haziness of the whole sinus with an appearance indistinguishable from sinusitis. It is important not to mistake oedema of the soft tissues overlying the injured area for mucosal changes within the antra. Opacities due to overlying soft

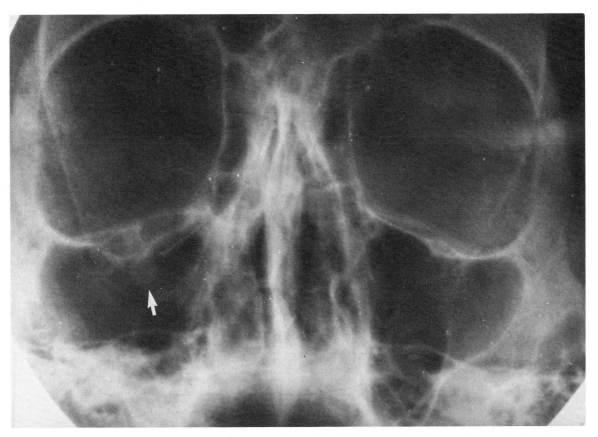

Fig. 151. Blow-out fracture of right orbit showing "tear-drop" in roof of right antrum caused by prolapse of the orbital contents through the fracture line into the roof of the antrum.

tissue bruising can generally be seen to extend beyond the confines of the antra and submento-vertical views will differentiate between soft tissue changes and those within the antrum.

(b) *Localised swelling of the mucosa.* This is a more common finding and represents a mucosal or submucosal haemorrhage. It is localised to the site at which the fracture line involves the antral mucosa. Radiologically, it appears as a rounded opacity projecting into the air sinus; the appearances may closely simulate a polyp or a localised cyst of the antral wall. Normal markings such as caused by the ala nasi or upper lip, especially if swollen due to associated trauma, may cause considerable confusion and their features have already been described (Chapter 2).

(c) *Fluid levels.* A fluid level associated with mucosal thickening may appear in the maxillary antrum. The fluid is generally pure blood or a bloodstained exudate. Fluid levels in the antra following trauma are uncommon and a generalised or localised oedema of the mucosa is a far commoner radiological finding. Fluid levels can be most frequently seen in radiographs taken a few days after the fracture.

Blow-out fractures of the maxillary antrum and orbital floor

Antral blow-out fractures are classically caused by violent contact with a round hard object such as a cricket ball or baseball, but in fact the vast majority are the result of a blow in the eye from a closed fist. The essential mechanism of this type of injury was described by Pfeiffer (1943) when considering the cause of traumatic enophthalmos. In the same year

Linhart (1943) postulated a similar mechanism for fractures of the medial wall of the orbit through the lamina papyracea of the ethmoids. Smith and Reagan (1957) produced experimental evidence on the cadaver to support Pfeiffer's original observations. According to these authors the mechanism of injury is as follows: part of the impact of the blow is absorbed by the orbital rim, which remains intact, but the force of the blow causes a backward displacement of the eye and an increase in intra-orbital pressure, with a resultant fracture of the orbital floor, de-compressing the orbit and causing a herniation of orbital soft tissues into the maxillary antrum. The inferior rectus muscle or the inferior oblique muscle or both may be caught in this herniation resulting in impairment of ocular mobility and diplopia. It is the impairment of muscle function which constitutes the particular gravity of the blow-out fracture. Early surgical intervention is required to release the trapped muscle and restore free movement of the globe. Unless this is done the diplopia will persist, and the patient may have a permanent enophthalmos. The latter sign is not always immediately apparent until the oedema and bruising have subsided and, indeed, there may be an initial proptosis if there is orbital emphysema or an intra-orbital haematoma. Clinically, vertical diplopia is the most important feature and may be accompanied by parasthesia or anaesthesia of the cheek and upper lip in the distribution of the infra-orbital nerve, which may be involved in the fracture. When these signs are present and accompanied by x-ray evidence of a blow-out fracture there is often need for early surgery. A traction test of the inferior rectus may show restriction of passive ocular elevation, and confirm the need to free the trapped muscle.

The characteristic radiological appearance is that of a small, soft tissue shadow in the roof of the maxillary antrum, due to the herniated soft tissues from the orbit; this is associated with a depressed bony fragment, which is nearly always visible on plain x-ray at the fracture site. Sometimes oblique views are necessary to show the depressed fragment convincingly, or it may be seen on the lateral film. The projection which consistently shows these fractures even when only minimal changes are present, is the occipito or 30° occipito-mental view of the orbits. Tomography in the postero-anterior plane may confirm the fracture, but is not always needed to make the diagnosis. However, lateral tomography is important if surgery is indicated, to show the backward extent of the fracture. Difficulty may arise if the antrum concerned is completely opaque due to haemorrhage, and in these cases it may be justified to carry out contrast orbitography, as described by Milauskas, Fueger & Schulze (1966) if a blow-out fracture is suspected clinically. These authors use an injection of water-soluble contrast medium outside the muscle cone. Films taken after the injection may demonstrate contrast medium within the herniated soft tissues, or in the cavity of the maxillary antrum itself, thus confirming the presence of a break in the floor of the orbit. Blow-out fractures are easily missed on routine skull films unless a nose/chin view is taken, and it should be a standard practice always to take this view on a patient who has received an upper facial bone injury, especially when associated with a clinical "black eye".

Frontal sinus fractures

Fractures involving the frontal sinuses may be the result of direct trauma or result from an extension of a fracture of the cranium. Fracture lines may involve one or both walls of the frontal sinus. Fractures of the posterior wall of the frontal sinus are rare and are generally extensions of fractures of the floor of the anterior cranial fossa. Fractures involving only the anterior wall of the sinus are far commoner and are usually the sequel of direct violence.

Fractures involving the outer wall of the frontal sinus are especially prone to be depressed and may be easily overlooked. The postero-anterior views are of little use in demonstrating fractures of the anterior wall of the frontal sinus and lateral and tangential views are of greatest value. Tomographs in the postero-anterior and lateral planes may also be of considerable assistance in demonstrating such fractures and evaluating the extent of depression of the fractured fragments. The changes occurring in the frontal sinuses following a fracture are similar to those seen in the antra. A fluid level following any injury is extremely rare and a general haziness of the sinus is by far the most frequent finding. Indeed, if a fracture line involves the frontal bone, and the sinus on the same side as the fracture is hazy, the appearances are probably due to blood or thickened mucosa in the sinus. Stab wounds and

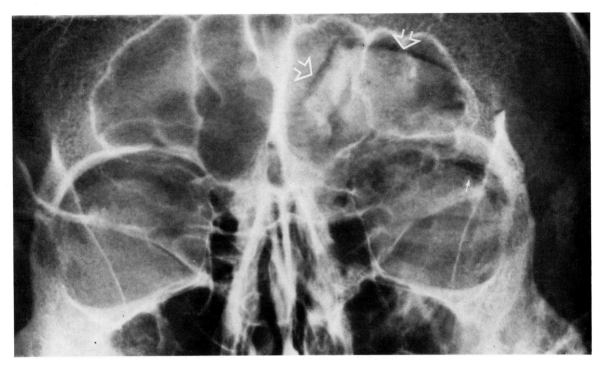

Fig. 152. Fracture of frontal bone. Comminuted fracture of posterior wall of left frontal sinus (hollow arrow) with air in left orbit indicating opening of frontal sinus with air in the supra-orbital tissues (white arrow).

gunshot wounds affecting the frontal and ethmoidal sinuses present diagnostic problems for the radiologist.

The development of a traumatic pneumocephalus after facial injury is important as, although in some cases the air may be extradural, in the early stages it may not be possible to differentiate it from subdural air. The importance of the early recognition of pneumocephalus with its implied tear of the meninges cannot be overestimated. Raider (1951) has classified pneumocephalus anatomically as follows:

(i) Extracranial (associated with brain hernia).
(ii) Intracranial.
    (1) Extradural.
    (2) Subdural.
    (3) Extraventricular.
        (a) Cortical, (b) Cisternal.
    (4) Ventricular.

The prognostic significance of pneumocephalus worsens as the air passes deeper into the cerebral substance.

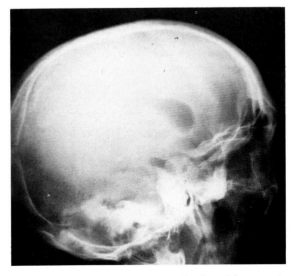

Fig. 153. Spontaneous ventriculogram after frontal fracture. Air lies in lateral ventricle and in subarachnoid spaces.

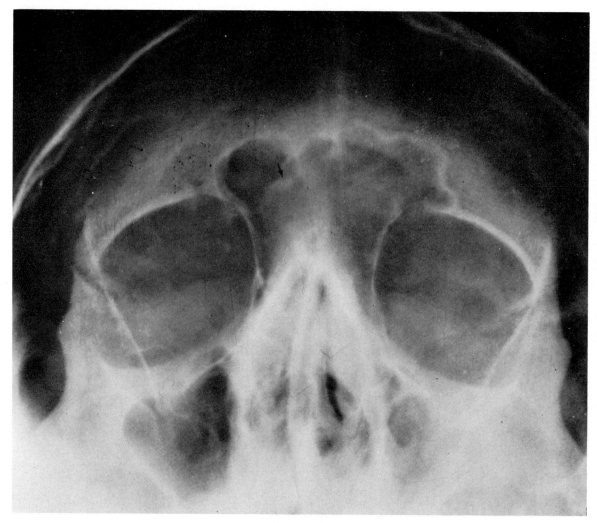

Fig. 154. Occipito-mental view showing a round opacity in the left frontal sinus in a patient who complained of frontal headaches after a road traffic accident. Surgical exploration revealed a herniation of brain tissue through a fracture into the left frontal sinus.

Pneumocephalus may also develop as a sequel to surgical removal of orbito-ethmoidal osteomas (Cushing, 1927) and may even occur after removal of nasopharyngeal fibromas (Hill, 1942). Both these conditions may produce such a degree of pressure atrophy of the surrounding bone that damage to the thinned atrophic walls readily occurs during surgical removal of these tumours.

The extent of bone erosion associated with fronto-ethmoidal osteoma is such that spontaneous pneumocephalus may develop (Kessel, 1939).

Brain herniation may follow a frontal fracture (fig. 154).

Fractures of the ethmoids and sphenoids

Fractures of the ethmoids occur as part of a Le Fort III injury and when severe may involve the cribriform plate. They have a sinister significance related to the frequency with which dural tears are associated with cribriform plate fractures and fractures of the roofs of the middle ethmoidal cells.

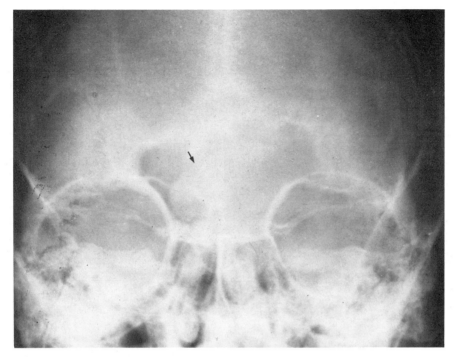

Fig. 155. Occipito-frontal view of case shown in Fig. 154 shows the outline of the "polyp" more sharply.

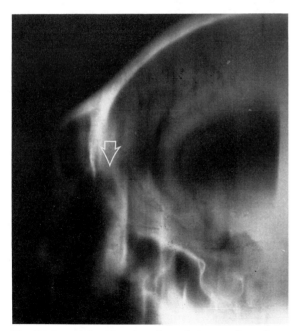

Fig. 156. Lateral decubitus view of encephalogram of case shown in fig. 155 showing the tracking of air down into the mass present in the frontal sinus.

Fractures involving the ethmoidal (cribriform plate) bone may be classified as follows:

(a) Discrete fractures.
(b) Fissured fractures.

Discrete fractures. In the anterior and middle cranial fossa the moulding of the skull by the convolutions of the brain results in the production of small hillocks of thick bone and a more thin peripheral bone. When fissured fractures reach the thickened prominence of bone, the fracture either runs around the boss or the thickened fragment of bone is splintered off and may perforate the dura (fig. 155).

Fissured fractures. The direction taken by the fracture is determined partly by the direction and force which produces the fracture. The fractures tend to run around and isolate the thickened ridges of bone and it is at this site that dural laceration may occur. The sites at which the fractures tend to involve the ethmoidal plate are:

(i) The roof of the anterior ethmoidal cell at the point where it forms the lateral wall to the olfactory groove.

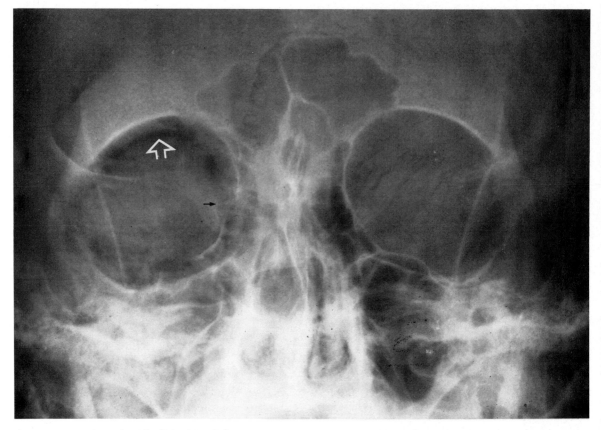

Fig. 157. Fracture into ethmoid cells (right) with free gas present in orbital tissues and opacification of right group of ethmoid cells.

(ii) The prominent blister of the ethmoidal roof.
(iii) The part of the posterior ethmoidal roof in the region of the posterior ethmoidal foramen.

Fractures of the ethmoidal plate are relatively harmless when confined to the plate itself but when they spread laterally in the region of the middle ethmoids or posteriorly where they meet a ridge of bone overlapping the posterior ethmoidal foramen, they are very liable to cause splintering and dural laceration.

Ethmoidal blow-out fractures

These are caused by a similar mechanism to that described for antral blow-out fractures and follow the same type of eye injury. Combined antro-ethmoidal fractures are common in severe blow-out injuries, but the ethmoidal fracture may often occur in isolation. They present radiologically in many patients as orbital emphysema, associated with clouding of the ethmoid cells on the injured side. The actual site of the fracture is seldom directly visible on plain x-ray. The injury is usually not of any clinical significance, and only rarely is there any interference with muscle function so that more detailed radiological investigation is seldom required. If it does become necessary to show the exact site of fracture and its extent, then axial tomography is the procedure of choice, and is the optimum method of showing the full extent of the fracture.

Demonstration of dural tears associated with fractures of the cribriform plate and anterior cranial fossa can be investigated (Jefferson &

Lewtas, 1963) by the introduction of air into the subdural space and tomography in the sagittal and antero-posterior planes.

Detection of such tears is of utmost importance as they are not necessarily associated with immediate cerebrospinal rhinorrhoea and later may form a source for the development of an infective meningitis. Isotope studies may be useful to confirm the presence of a tear.

Sphenoid sinus fractures

A fluid level in the sphenoid sinus may be the only sign of a fracture of that bone or of the base of the skull. Films should be taken in the erect position or supine with a horizontal beam to detect such levels.

Aero-Sinusitis (Barotrauma)

Rapid alterations in barometric pressure may produce changes in the sinuses particularly if there is any obstruction to the ostium of the sinus.

Polypoid or hypertrophied mucosa is the most common cause of obstruction. Haematoma appearing as localised rounded opacities may occur in the mucosa but more frequently a generalised opacity of the sinus appears due to thickened mucosa. Fluid levels seldom occur in the sinus unless infection is superimposed.

In addition, alteration in barometric pressure may force infected material from the nasal cavities into the sinus, producing an infective sinusitis with typical clinical symptomatology and radiological findings.

REFERENCES

CUSHING, H. (1927) Experiences with Orbito-ethmoidal Osteomata having Intracranial Complications, with Report of 4 Cases. *Surgery Gynec. Obstet.*, **44**, 721.

DOLAN, K. D. & HAYDON, J. (1973) Maxillary Pseudofracture Lines. *Radiology,* **107**, 321.

HILL, F. T. (1942) Nasopharyngeal Fibroma with Report of Case with Secondary Pneumocephalus. *Trans. Amer. Lar. rhinol. otol. Soc.*, **48**, 154; *Ann. Otol. Rhinol. Lar.*, **51**, 105.

JEFFERSON, A. & LEWTAS, N. (1963) Value of Tomography and Subdural Pneumography in Subfrontal Fractures. *Acta radiol.*, **1**, 119.

KESSEL, F. K. (1939) Orbito-ethmoidal Osteomata with Intracranial Complications. *Guy's Hosp. Rep.*, **89**, 337.

KING, E. F. & SAMUEL, E. (1954) Fractures of the Orbit. *Trans. Ophthal. Soc. U.K.*, **64**, 134.

LINHART, W. O. (1943) Emphysema of the Orbit: A Study of 7 Cases. *J. Am. med. Ass.*, **123**, 89.

MILAUSKAS, A. T., FUEGER, G. F. & SCHULZE, R. R. (1966) Clinical Experiences with Orbitography in Diagnosis of Orbital Floor Fractures. *Trans. Am. Acad. Ophthal. Oto-Lar.*, **70**, 25.

NOONAN, P. E. (1946) Anomalous Antral Tooth. *Archs Otolar.*, **43**, 134.

PFEIFFER, R. L. (1943) Traumatic Enophthalmos. *Archs Ophthal.*, **50**, 25.

RADCLIFFE, A. (1949) Fractures Involving Air Sinuses. *J. Lar. Otol.*, **63**, 453.

RAIDER, L. (1951) Spontaneous Pneumocephalus. *Am. J. Roentg.*, **66**, 231.

RICHARDSON, G. A. (1946) Foreign Body Involving Maxillary Antrum. *Archs Otolar.*, **43**, 508.

SCHRODER, G. W. (1937) *Fumdkopper in der Kuferhohle.* Wurzburg:

SMITH, B. & REAGAN, W. F. (1957) Blow-out Fractures of the Orbit: Mechanism and Correction of Inferior Orbital Fracture. *Am. J. Ophthal.*, **44**, 733.

CHAPTER 7

Radiological methods of investigation of the ear, mastoid process and temporal bone

Historical

The application of x-ray examination to the investigation of disease of the mastoid process followed soon after the discovery of x-rays and as early as 1904 the use of oblique views to demonstrate the mastoid process was reported.

A year later, 1905, Schüller described his lateral projection, which avoided overlap of the opposite mastoid process and which is still widely used today. Later Sonnenkalb (1913) described a variation of Schüller's positions. In 1913 Law described a lateral oblique projection combining 25° sagittal plane rotation and 25° caudal angulation of beam, and in 1923 Meyer described another lateral oblique projection where both angles are increased to 45°.

In 1925 Grashey described a technique for obtaining a tangential picture of the petrous bone and in 1917 Stenvers' oblique postero-anterior projection was described and it has been widely accepted and extensively used since that time.

In 1920, the technique for examination with the patient in the sitting position rather than in the supine position was described. In 1950, Chaussé reported three separate projections, II, III, and IV, for investigation of the mastoid bone and these projections are still widely used.

In Scandinavia Runstrom (1929) described projections for demonstrating the anatomy of the temporal bone in cases of chronic discharge from the middle ear. Runstrom advocated two lateral oblique positions (I and II), an oblique position (III) and an axial projection (IV). The widespread acceptance of hypocycloidal tomography in the investigation of mastoid disease followed the introduction of the polytome (Massiot).

General considerations

The same technical considerations governing radiography of the paranasal sinuses apply equally to the mastoid process. The need for maximum detail and contrast is more necessary than in most other parts of the body as the structures examined are minute and pathological changes that cause gross clinical disturbances may only produce minimal radiological changes.

Rotating anode tubes with ultra fine focus (0·3 mm) capable of dealing with heavy exposures are an advantage for good radiography of the mastoid process. The use of enlargement technique (macroradiography) has not proved as useful as was anticipated and is not used as a routine method.

Potter Bucky grids are only needed in mastoid radiography when the area covered is more than a 9 cm diameter circle. The Bucky diaphragm is used for the lateral oblique, the submento-vertical and Towne's views, when both temporal bones are included in one film. For the Chaussé III, Stenvers' and transorbital views coning and accurate localisation of the beam produces the necessary detail and contrast.

However, in children and unco-operative patients motional blur rather than lack of contrast is responsible for films lacking diagnostic quality and the Bucky grid is discarded to allow the exposure time to be shortened.

Too great emphasis cannot be placed on the use of coning and the secret of good contrast is accurately coned films. Certain of the newer apparatus, specially designed for skull and mastoid radiography, have greatly facilitated accurate centering by keeping the film and incident-beam central and thus enabling very small cones to be used.

It is hardly necessary to emphasise that both mastoid processes must be radiographed as it is by this means that developmental variations are recognised. Prior to radiography the auricle should be strapped in a forward-bent position by adhesive tape although there are objections as the folded auricular cartilage throws an increased soft tissue shadow over the mastoid process. It is our opinion that variations in translucency caused by the fossae in the helix when the auricle is left in position make interpretation more difficult.

Tomography is now accepted as a major method of investigation of the temporal bone and, for the demonstration of fractures and bone erosion, is certainly the method of choice. Whether circular, polycycloidal or the older established linear tomographic section applied obliquely to the mastoid process is the most universally acceptable has yet to be determined but there is agreement that whatever tomographic method is used fine focal tubes and accurate coning are necessities.

Special apparatus for mastoid radiography

In keeping with the rapid development of x-ray equipment much of the older equipment has fallen into disuse and is only of historic interest.

The craniotome type of apparatus, which has been evolved from the basic concept of the Lysholm skull table (Lysholm, 1925) has greatly facilitated radiography of the mastoid process. This original craniotome concept has undergone considerable modifications in different countries, but the modern units – Mimer (Elema), Princeps (CGR), etc. represent specialised units which are invaluable in the study of the temporal bone. Whilst these costly specialised units are not essential for good radiography of the mastoid process, they certainly lighten the burden of the technician and are invaluable when a large volume of mastoid radiography is undertaken.

As every skull varies in shape, it follows that set angles will not reproduce exactly identical views in different individuals, and the principle of serial views of the temporal bone propounded by Dulac (1962), and readily achieved by his Princeps unit, has much to commend it.

The advances in tomographic equipment have seen the development of several units capable of circular, ellipsoid, hypocycloidal or even more complex movements. The Polytome (Massiot) is the most complex of these units and can produce tomographic cuts of the temporal bone of 1 mm thickness. The hypocycloidal movement obliterates the disturbing summation linear shadows of the conventional linear tomograph. Other units such as the Stratomatix and the Multiplanigraph (Siemens) can also produce circular or elliptical tomographic sections.

Whether the inherent unsharpness of a tomographic cut is more than offset by the obliteration of overlying structures is sometimes questionable but, in the detection of fractures, bone erosion and sequestrum formation, tomography is undoubtedly superior to conventional radiography.

Standard positions

The last decade has seen major advances in conservative surgery of mastoid infection and in the treatment of deafness. Equally the development of efficient antibiotics has lessened the need for surgery in acute mastoid infections. With these major developments emphasis has been on the assessment of pathological changes in the middle ear, and the radiological focus has naturally shifted from the mastoid process to the middle ear.

Standard positions are equally essential for the investigation of the mastoid as for the paranasal sinuses. As the demonstration of fluid levels in the mastoid cells is seldom possible (unlike the paranasal sinuses) whether radiography is conducted in the erect or horizontal position is a matter of individual preference.

The standard projections which may be used for the mastoid and temporal bone can be grouped according to the pathological states under investigation, and the projection used must depend on the condition under investigation.

(a) *General survey – general anatomy, and cellular development*
  (i) Lateral (Schüller)
  (ii) Lateral oblique (Law)
  (iii) Submento-vertical views (Hirtz)
  (iv) Oblique postero-anterior (Stenvers)

(b) *Middle ear and ossicles*
  (i) Localised Towne's views
  (ii) Chaussé III projection
  (iii) Transorbital oblique views (Guillen)
  (iv) Submento-vertical view

(c) *Petrous apex and internal meatus*
  (i) P.A. views (transorbital)
  (ii) Stenvers' views
  (iii) Chaussé III projection

(d) *Oval window*
  (i) Rossi's position

Lateral view. As the temporal bones are symmetrically placed on both sides of the skull it follows that a true lateral view can only be obtained by superimposing the mastoid processes. The so-called "lateral" view is obtained with the sagittal plane of the skull rotated by 15° to the horizontal so that the mastoid processes are not superimposed. The same result may be achieved by angling 15° and directing the incident beam through the mastoid process nearest the film (figs. 158). Schüller's lateral projection angles the tube to 25°

or rotates the sagittal plane of the skull to the same degree to obtain the separation of the mastoid processes.

Boards which can be angled to 20° assist in positioning the head but have the disadvantage that the Potter Bucky grid cannot be used.

The incident beam is centred 2 in (5 cm) above the uppermost external auditory meatus. The cone should be just large enough to cover the mastoid area.

This view gives a general survey of the mastoid process, but as the incident ray passes along the length of the petrous bone this is superimposed on the mastoid process. The internal meatus is superimposed on the external meatus in this view. The mastoid antrum can be seen and the position and depth of the lateral sinus and mastoid emissary vein can be clearly seen. This view is valuable as a general survey view in determining generalised haziness or loss of translucency in the cells throughout the mastoid process (fig. 159).

Lateral oblique (Law's position). This position attempts to project the petrous bone anterior to the mastoid process so that a view of the mastoid antrum and the cells around the mastoid antrum can be obtained (fig. 160).

A double inclination is placed on the tube, the incident beam is angled 15° caudally and at the same time 15° towards the face. Exact duplication of the position is difficult owing to the double

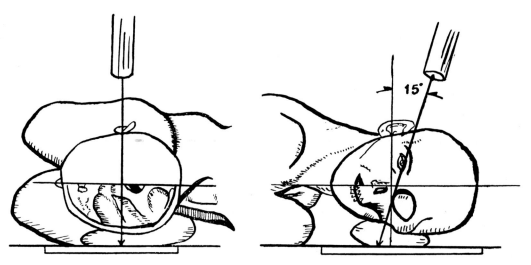

Fig. 158. Line drawing showing the position and the incident ray for lateral views of the mastoid process. The sagittal and coronal planes in relation to the film are shown and the caudal inclination of the beam prevents superimposition of the mastoid processes.

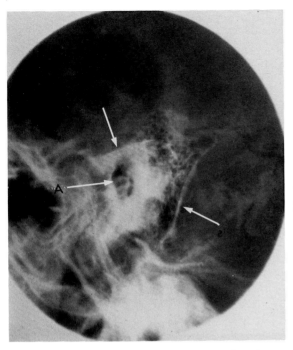

Fig. 159. Lateral radiograph of mastoid showing lateral sinus plate (S), superimposed internal and external meatus (A), tegmen tympani (T).

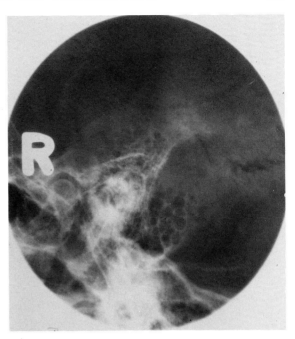

Fig. 160. Lateral oblique view. The mastoid cells can be "opened" either by rotating the sagittal plane 15° towards the cassette or by angling the incident beam forwards by the same angle.

inclination of the tube but some assistance can be obtained by discarding the use of the Potter Bucky grid and using an angle board to obviate the second angulation.

The lateral oblique position allows the mastoid antrum and the cells around the sinodural angle to be fully investigated. Early breakdown of cell walls around the mastoid antrum can be visualised (fig. 160). The lateral oblique projection is superior to the lateral view in demonstrating the mastoid antrum and the attic.

Meyer's projection. The patient lies in the horizontal position and the sagittal plane is turned at an angle of 45°. The incident ray is angled 45° caudally and centred through the mastoid process nearest the film.

The resulting radiograph shows the mastoid antrum and cells around the lateral sinus clearly. Unfortunately, replication of the position is difficult and for this reason the projection has not been as widely used as those already mentioned. The attic and the ossicles can be seen clearly in this view.

The oblique postero-anterior position (Stenvers' view). This view demonstrates the whole length of the petrous bone, the incident ray passing at right angles to it.

The patient lies in the prone, or sits in the erect position facing the film. The radiographic base line is horizontal and the sagittal plane of the skull is rotated through 35° and tilted 15° away from the side to be examined. This latter tilt prevents the shadow of the occipital bone overlying the mastoid bone.

The incident ray is inclined at an angle of 12° cranially and is centred on a point 1 in medial to the tip of the mastoid process (fig. 161).

The radiograph in Stenvers' position shows the length of the petrous bone and the mastoid tip. Usually when the mastoid tip is clearly seen, the apex of the petrous bone is under-exposed, but usually when the exposure is used to demonstrate the apex the details of the mastoid tip can be seen by viewing under strong illumination. Some investigators prefer to make two exposures – one for the mastoid process itself using a lower kilo-voltage

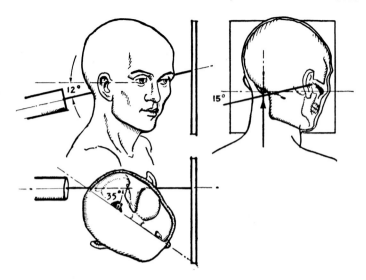

Fig. 161. Line drawing to illustrate position for Stenvers' view. The sagittal plane is rotated through 35°. The sagittal plane is tilted 15° away from the mastoid to be radiographed. The incident beam inclined at an angle of 12° cranially is centred through the mastoid process.

and a second using a higher kilo-voltage to show the apex of the petrous bone.

A radiograph in this position should demonstrate the internal auditory meatus and the semicircular canals. With an accurately centred radiograph the superior semi-circular canal is vertical and viewed end on, the horizontal semi-circular canal is also projected so that both limbs are superimposed (fig. 162).

The internal auditory meatus and the tip of the petrous bone can be seen in this position and this view can be usefully employed to demonstrate early widening of the internal meatus by tumours.

The mento-vertical or submento-vertical position. Essentially this position is the same as used for demonstrating the sphenoid sinus (see Chapter 1).

Examination of each temporal bone individually with localised views, although more time consuming greatly improves the quality of the radiograph. The incident beam is centred so that it passes through the external auditory meatus.

Views of both mastoid processes are taken on a single film to facilitate comparison and to allow both exposures to be developed under identical conditions and thus obviate possible differences due to different processing techniques.

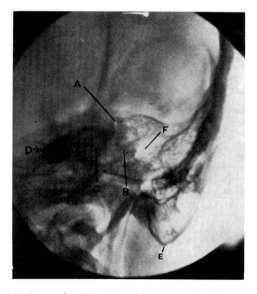

Fig. 162. Stenvers' position. Normal anatomical markings.
A. Superior semicircular canal.
B. External semicircular canal.
C. Cochlea.
D. Internal auditory meatus.
E. Tip of petrous bone.
F. Mastoid antrum.

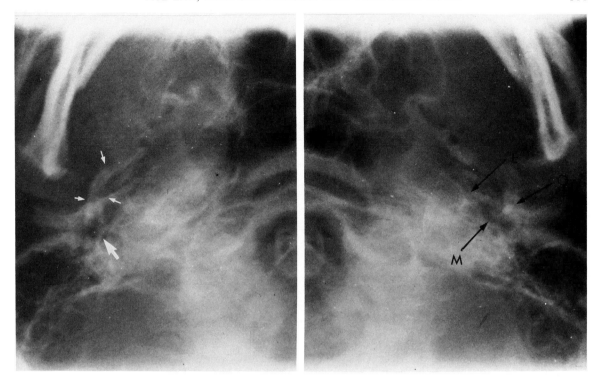

Fig. 163. Anatomical variation in the right stylo-mastoid process (small arrows) overlying the middle ear (broad arrow) in the submentovertical projection and obscuring the detail of that structure. The left side shows the normal appearances:
O—ossicles (combined shadow of malleus and incus)
E —bony Eustachian tube
M—middle ear cavity.

Whether the films are taken in a submento-vertical or mento-vertical position depends on the patients' comfort, and the flexibility of the cervical spine may determine the projection used. Angulation of the incident beam can compensate for lack of tilt of the skull consequent on cervical stiffness.

The radiograph demonstrates the middle ear, tympanic tube and mastoid antrum (fig. 163). This view is also of considerable value in assessing an anteriorly placed lateral sinus, and the malleus and incus can be seen. It is also valuable in assessing forward extension of cholesteatoma.

If the centering point is too far anterior the angle of the jaw is projected over the middle ear and obscures that structure. To avoid this difficulty Etter and Cross (1963) have suggested that the incident beam should be at an angle of 105° rather than 90° to the base line.

Towne's position (30° fronto-occipital). With this view the patient sits or lies with the occiput against the film and the radiographic base line horizontal or vertical.

The incident ray is angled 30° towards the feet and directed through the occiput so that the incident beam passes through the external auditory meatus (fig. 164).

The radiograph in Towne's position shows the middle ear and the internal auditory meatus. This view is also one of the most useful views for estimating enlargement of the internal auditory meatus (fig. 165). Erosion and widening of the aditus ad antrum can also be seen by this method.

Chaussé III projection. To assess the integrity of the ossicular chain and pathological processes developing in the middle ear, the Chaussé III projection is invaluable.

The incident beam is angled along a line from

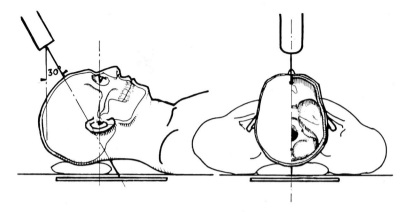

Fig. 164. The "reverse Towne's" view should be used in young patients as the radiation dose to the eyes is only one-sixth of that produced when an A.P. view is taken. The "reverse Towne's" view is more difficult to achieve and in the older patient where radiation dosage is less important the conventional position as illustrated is generally used.

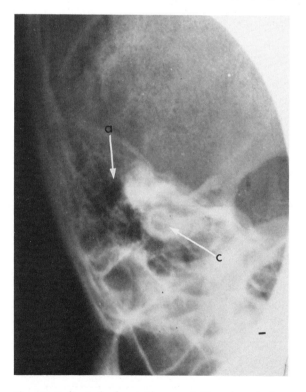

Fig. 165. Radiograph of mastoid process in Towne's projection. c. Cochlea. a. Mastoid antrum.

the supraorbital margin to the external meatus, the radiographic base line being at right angles to the film. The sagittal plane is rotated to 5°–10° towards the opposite side and the film is placed behind the mastoid. The incident beam is centred through the mid point between the external orbital margin and external meatus (fig. 166). In this position the radiograph shows the ossicular chain and also the medial wall of the middle ear.

This view is also useful in assessing changes around the oval and the round windows. The facial canal in the region of the genu is also well seen. Erosions and fistulae of the lateral semicircular canal can be clearly seen in this view.

Transorbital view (Guillen). The transorbital view of the temporal bone is performed in the prone position by projecting the incident beam through the ipsilateral orbit, the line of the incident ray passing through the level of the mid point of the external auditory meatus and emerging through the mid point of the orbit. The ossicles and the internal wall of the middle ear can be seen in this projection and it is an improvement on the Chaussé III as the ossicles are thrown clear of the external semi-circular canal (fig. 167). The production gives a good comparative view of both internal auditory canals (figs. 167 and 168). Although the antero-posterior projection is technically superior to the postero-anterior, the orbital cavity being enlarged in the former position, it must not be used as the radiation dose to the lens of the eye is six times that

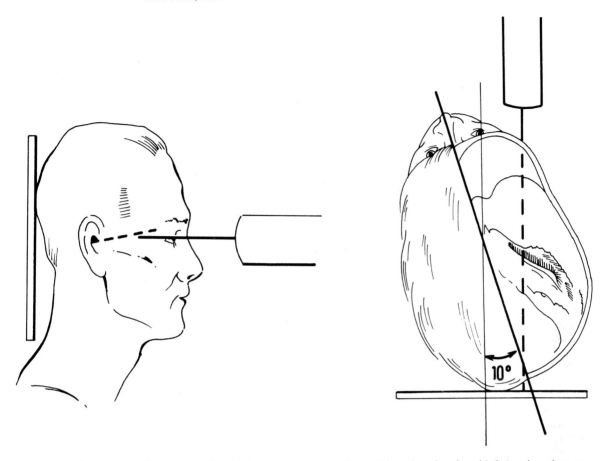

Fig. 166. The Chaussé III position projects the middle ear structures on to the vault bone lateral to the orbital rim where there are relatively few extraneous bony markings.

The angles of the sagittal plane are shown and the incident ray is to the mid-point of a line drawn between the outer end of the eyebrow and the external meatus.

in the postero-anterior projection (Dahlin, Nylen & Wilbrand, 1973).

Special views

Certain other views are used to demonstrate special aspects of the temporal bone and it is readily appreciated that no single view will show all the intricate anatomical details of the petrous bone.

(1) *Chaussé II*. This projection is of greatest value in the investigation of the jugular foramen and the posterior aspect of the temporal bone. The incident ray is directed through the open mouth with the incident beam passing through the upper part of the external auditory meatus, and the mouth between the superior and inferior molars. The chin is rotated towards the affected side to 25° and the incident beam shows a 10° upward tilt.

(2) *Tomography*. Tomographic examination of the middle ear and mastoid process has become an essential method of radiological examination (Agazzi, Cova & Senaldi, 1958; Brünner, Petersen & Stoksted, 1961). In all tomographic projections carried out in the antero-posterior plane eye shields must be used to minimise the lens dosage (Chin, Anderson & Gilbertson, 1970).

The essential requirements are a fine focus tube to obtain the maximum detail and a tomograph capable of sections of 1 mm thickness. Linear tomographs need an angle of cut of 60° to produce

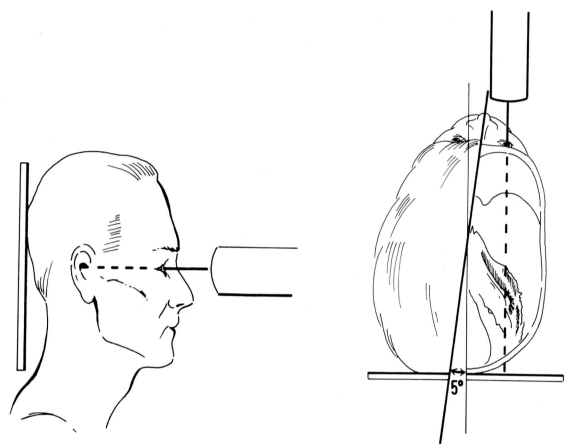

Fig. 167. Transorbital view.
    The sagittal plane is angled towards the side to be radiographed.
    The transorbital view projects the ossicular shadows clear of the bony wall of the middle ear.
    Again in younger age group the reverse P.A. position should be used to minimize dosage to the eye.

a cut of 1 mm thickness (Littleton, Runbaugh & Winter, 1963), a range outside the normal linear tomographs. In practice a 40° linear tomographic cut has produced a cut nearer 2 mm (Agazzi et al., 1958). In addition parallel shadows, linear and other summation shadows (parasitic shadows) cause considerable difficulties in interpretation of films (Reichman, 1972). In the postero-anterior plane cuts through the "cochlear plane" which lies anterior to the external auditory meatus demonstrate the external auditory canal, the post-meatal spur, the lateral attic wall, the malleus and the tympanic cavity, the cochlea and carotid canal. The "vestibular plane" about 4 mm posterior to the cochlea plane shows the external auditory

canal, meatal spur, the incus, mastoid antrum, vestibule, oval window, lateral and superior semi-circular canals, the jugular fossa, internal auditory canal, jugular foramen, hypoglossal canal and occipital condyle (figs. 174, 175).

Hypocycloidal movement can produce cuts of 1 mm thickness with an angle of cut of 48° with minimum unsharpness (Mündich & Frey, 1959; Valvassori, 1963; Brünner et al., 1961; Jensen & Rovsing, 1968) and are considered superior to the linear tomograms.

The planes of cut are either lateral (fig. 176), postero-anterior, axial and half axial (Brünner et al., 1961) or submentovertical (Hanafee & Gussen, 1974). As in routine mastoid radiography the

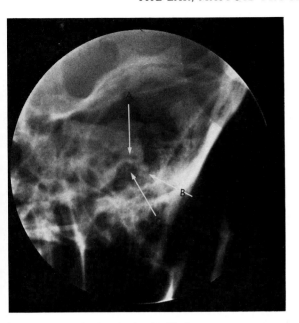

Fig. 168. Transorbital projection (Guillen).
A. Horizontal semicircular canal
B. Ossicles
C. Facial canal just below the horizontal (lateral) semicircular canal.
(By permission of Churchill Livingstone, Edinburgh from Textbook of Radiology edited by D. Sutton.)

planes of cut depend on the type of pathology and the structure being investigated.

By the use of an inclined board if a tilting polytome is not available satisfactory tomograms of the temporal bone in the submento-vertical position can be obtained. This position may be invaluable in detecting early erosions of the internal auditory meatus by acoustic neuroma before any true expansion has occurred.

The anatomical course and variations in the course of the facial nerve can be identified in lateral tomographs (Wright & McKay, 1967). Such information may be vital in the pre-operative assessment of a case. The course of the facial nerve in the middle ear may show dehiscence of the bony canal. Wilbrand & Bergstrom (1976) have undertaken an experimental study which shows that only the large dehiscences (Dietzel, 1961) equal to one third of the canal's circumference can be seen on tomography. These findings should be borne in mind when reporting on the integrity of the bony walls of the facial canal.

The axial, pyramidal, and semi-axial tomographic cuts are particularly useful in investigating the bony labyrinth for evidence of otosclerosis (Rovsing, 1974).

Contrast examination

Lumbar puncture and the instillation of 6 to 10 ml of pantopaque in the spinal theca will enable the internal auditory meatus to be filled and studied. This is preferably done under fluoroscopic control to prevent the contrast media reaching the middle cranial fossa and to obtain the best view of the internal auditory meatus (usually in Stenvers' position). Careful control of extension of the head will prevent the pantopaque reaching the middle cranial fossa. Tomography can be used to enhance detail and has been used without fluoroscopic control (Britton & Fluitsman, 1974). The contrast medium should be removed from the spinal theca after completion of the examination. The normal variations in the filling of the internal auditory meatus are described in Chapter 12.

REFERENCES

AGAZZI, C., COVA, P. L. & SENALDI, M. (1958) Seneiotica stratigrafica dell'osso temporale. In *Relazione al XVI Raduno del gruppo Otorinolaringologico dell'alta Italia Dic.*

BRITTON, B. H. & FLUITSMAN, B. (1974) Iophendylate Examination of the Posterior Fossa. *Radiol. Clin. N. Am.,* **12/3,** 431.

BRÜNNER, S., PETERSEN, Ø. & STOKSTED, P. (1961) Tomography of Auditory Ossicles. *Acta radiol.,* **56,** 20.

CHAUSSE, C. (1950) Trois Incidences pour l'examen du rocher. *Acta radiol.,* **34,** 274.

CHIN, P. K., ANDERSON, W. B. & GILBERTSON, J. W. (1970) Radiation Dose to Cortical Organs during Petrous Temporal Radiography. *Radiology,* **94,** 623.

DAHLIN, H., NYLEN, O. & WILBRAND, H. (1973) Radiation Dose Distribution in Temporal Bone Tomography. *Acta radiol. (Diagn.),* **353,** 14.

DIETZEL, K. (1961) Uber die dehnzangen des fazialiskanals. *J. Lar. Rhinol.,* **40,** 316.

DULAC, G. L. (1962) Exploration Tomographique du Temporal. In *Encyclopedie Medico-Chirurgicale (Oto-Rhino-Laryng), No. 20047C10.*

ETTER, L. & CROSS, L. C. (1963) Projection Angle Variations Required to Demonstrate the Middle Ear, Antrum and Mastoid Process. *Radiology,* **80,** 255.

GRASHEY, R. (1925) *Atlas typischer röntgenbilder von normalen menschen.*

HANAFEE, W. N. & GUSSEN, R. (1974) Correlation of Basal Projection Tomography in Clinical Problems. *Radiol. Clins N. Am.,* **12,** 419

JENSEN, J. & ROVSING, H. (1968) Tomographic Visualisation of Labyrinthine Fistula. *Radiology,* **90,** 261.

LAW, F. M. (1913) Radiography as an Aid in the Diagnosis of Mastoid Disease. *Ann. Otol. Rhin. & Lar.,* **22,** 635.

LITTLETON, J. T., RUNBAUGH, C. L. & WINTER, F. S. (1963) Polydirectional Body Section Roentgenography – a New Diagnostic Method. *Am. J. Roentg.,* **89,** 1179.

LYSHOLM, E. (1925) Apparatus for Precise Radiography. *Acta radiol.,* **4,** 507.

MEYER, E. G. (1923) *Fortschr. Röntgenstr.,* **31,** 12/1.

MÜNDNICH, K. & FREY, K. (1959) *Das rontgenschichtbild des ohres.* Stuttgart: Georg Thieme Verlag.

RUNSTROM, G. (1929) Projections for Demonstrating Anatomy of Temporal Bone in Chronic Discharge. *Acta radiol.,* Suppl.

REICHMAN, S. (1972) Development of Spurious Contours of Spherical and Cylindrical Objects in Tomography. *Acta radiol. (Diag.),* **12,** 317.

ROVSING, H. (1974) Otosclerosis: Fenestral and Cochlear. *Radiol. Clin. N. Am.,* **7/3,** 505.

SCHÜLLER, A. (1905) *Die shadenbasis in rontgenbild.* Hamburg: Lucas Grafe u Sillern.

SONNENKALB, G. (1913) Die darstellung des pneumatisation systeme beim lebenden. *Verh. dt. otol. Ges.,* **22,** 367.

STENVERS, H. W. (1917) Roentgenology of Os Petrosum. *Archs Radiol. Electrother.,* **22,** 97.

VALVASSORI, G. E. (1963) Laminography of the Ear. *Am. J. Roentg.,* **89,** 1155.

WILBRAND, H. F. & BERGSTROM, B. (1976) Multidirectional Tomography of Defects in the Facial Canal. *Acta radiol. (Diagn.),* **16,** 223.

WRIGHT, J. T. (1968) Cycloidal Tomography of Temporal Bone. *Australas. Radiol.,* **12,** 302.

CHAPTER 8

Development and anatomy of the ear and auditory apparatus

Development of the temporal bone

The temporal bone consists of four portions: the squamous, tympanic, petro-mastoid and the styloid process.

The squamous portion of the temporal bone is developed from a single ossific centre in membranous bone in the eighth week of foetal life, further growth is by the spread of ossification into the ascending portion of the temporal bone.

The tympanic bone forms the second part of the temporal bone developed in membrane bone. It grows in conjunction with the external auditory meatus which is developed from the petro-mastoid portion. The single centre for the tympanic portion appears in the third month of foetal life and at birth development has grown to form almost a complete bony ring.

The petro-mastoid bone is developed in cartilage and the mastoid process, although separate, is developmentally part of the petrous bone. It develops from four separate ossific centres:

(a) One originating near the eminentia arcuata. Ossification spreads in front and around the internal auditory meatus to the apex of the bone.
(b) A second surrounds the fenestra rotunda and forms the floor of the tympanum and vestibule.
(c) The third centre forms the roof of the antrum and tympanic cavity.
(d) The fourth centre arises near the posterior semi-circular canal and forms the mastoid process.

The petrous bone at birth is cancellous but as growth proceeds it gradually changes to the dense ivory hardness of adult bone enveloping the cochlea, vestibule, and semi-circular canals forming the membranous labyrinth.

The bony labyrinth formed from the petro-mastoid has three zones, the inner (endosteal) a middle (enchondral) and an outer (periosteal) layer. The endochondral layer has a unique structure consisting of primary skin-like fibre bundles mixed with cartilage remnants. It remains in an embryonic phase of development throughout life and the vital processes of constant resorption and bone deposition are absent. Vascularisation is relatively nil and this layer has no new bone-forming capacity, a factor of importance in the healing of fractures involving the bony labyrinth. Its avascularity makes it, however, extremely resistant to infection.

Because of the unalterability of the endochondral layer the bony labyrinth is of adult size at birth and it is because of the relatively large size and the cancellous character of the bone surrounding it that the labyrinth can be seen with great clarity in skull radiographs of young children.

Although the labyrinth itself is of adult size at birth, the petrous bone itself undergoes the normal growth and increases in size from infancy to adult life. At birth the bony labyrinth lies superficially but as the petrous bone develops it becomes more deeply embedded. Certain portions produce bony projections on the surface of the bone, *e.g.* the superior semicircular canal (the eminentia arcuata), the lateral semicircular canal (the medial wall of the aditus), and the basal turn of the cochlea (the promontory) on the medial wall of the middle ear.

The mastoid process is underdeveloped at birth and the styloid process entirely cartilaginous (Tremble, 1934). The stylo-mastoid foramen lies on the lateral side of the mastoid process. As the mastoid process grows this foramen comes to lie in its adult position on the inferior surface of the petrous bone.

The styloid process is developed from the cartilaginous skeleton of the second branchial arch and consists of two parts, the tympanohyal, developed from an ossific centre which appears from before birth and a distal portion stylohyal, which appears after birth.

The mastoid antrum is invariably present at birth and its development is independent of the growth of the external meatus and auricle. The mastoid cells are developed as outgrowths budding from the mastoid antrum. These cells invade the mastoid process and pneumatisation of the petrous bone occurs to varying degrees.

The various component parts of the tympanic bone fuse together as follows: the tympanic ring unites with the squama just before birth, the petro-mastoid and squama join during the first year of life. The tympanohyal portion of the styloid process also unites with squamous temporal during the first year but the styloid process remains ununited until puberty, and in some instances may remain ununited throughout life. An ununited suture line may be mistaken for a fracture of the styloid.

In 8% of infants under the age of one month radiological evidence of commencing pneumatisation of the mastoid process can be seen. At six months there is clear-cut evidence of mastoid pneumatisation. The extent of pneumatisation is more proportionate to the infant's general development rather than the chronological age (Koiransky, Ettman & White, 1949).

At birth the Eustachian tube, middle ear and mastoid antrum are filled with a mucoid material similar to Wharton's jelly but with the onset of breathing and crying this mucoid material is gradually discharged and these cavities become air-filled. The mastoid cells also contain similar material and whilst these cells adjacent to the mastoid antrum soon become air-filled, the more distal cells may remain persistently filled with a jelly-like substance.

The mastoid cells have been broadly grouped into pre- and post-labyrinthine groups or a more detailed classification relates to their anatomical site – petrosal, sub-labyrinthine, retro-facial, mastoid tip, lateral sinus, marginal cells (lying behind the lateral sinus), Eustachian (arising around and often opening into the Eustachian tube), zygomatic and squamous cells.

Extensive pneumatisation of the cells may on very rare occasions extend into the occipital or parietal bones and examples have been recorded of extensively pneumatised cells meeting cells from the opposite mastoid process at the occipital protuberance. The mastoid cells increase both in size and number with development of the petrous bone and whilst the bulk of pneumatisation is completed by puberty, some increase in the size of the cells may occur into old age.

There is great variation in the degree of pneumatisation of the individual mastoid process, probably determined by a genetic pattern. Wittmaack's view (1912) that deviations in such development are due to pathological processes is generally accepted. According to that author the mucous membrane of the attic gradually pushes into the mastoid antrum and surrounding bone, gradually displacing the marrow and giving rise to a honeycomb of connecting air cells. Early infection of the middle ear or a failure of discharge of the mucoid material present in the middle ear inhibits this pneumatisation process. Other authors contend that pneumatisation is dependent on genetic influences and on anatomical developments such as the position of the sigmoid sinuses, but all are agreed that early infection inhibits pneumatisation and the stage at which this occurs largely determines the ultimate degree of pneumatisation of the adult mastoid process.

The sclerotic mastoid either results from the inhibition of pneumatisation by infection followed by osteitis of the cellular septa leading to a sclerotic mastoid, or it is purely developmental in origin unrelated to infection resulting from a complete failure of the pneumatisation process. The consensus view is that the majority of sclerotic processes are usually the end result of an infective process.

That heredity plays a dominant part in the type of mastoid cellularity produced is undoubtedly confirmed by the work of Dahlberg & Diamant (1945) who showed that in twins (mono and dizygotic) the influence of hereditary factors was 1·56 times greater than environmental in determining the ultimate type of cellular development.

Auricle

Development. The auricle is developed from the tubo-tympanic recess formed between the first and third visceral arches and the first and second pharyngeal pouches (Frazer, 1914). The forward growth of the third branchial arch excludes the second arch and divides the tubo-tympanic recess into an inner portion later developing into the Eustachian tube and an outer portion which later forms the tympanic cavity. The tympanic antrum is developed as an upwards and backwards prolongation of the tympanic cavity. The external auditory meatus is developed from the dorsal end of the first branchial cleft. The intricate cartilaginous structure of the pinna is formed by the differentiation of six tubercles which appear around the margin of the hyomandibular cleft (Gray, 1973).

Anatomy. The external ear forming the structure for collecting sound waves consists of the auricle and the external auditory meatus. The auricle (pinna) has a characteristic shape and is composed of a cartilaginous frame-work covered by skin and subcutaneous tissue. The posterior edge (helix) which has a curved rolled appearance forms the most prominent part of the pinna and frequently casts confusing shadows in the lateral projections of the mastoid process.

The auricular cartilage funnels down to the concha which is attached to the cartilaginous external meatus. Arising anteriorly and to some extent covering the external meatus is the *Tragus* separated below by the sigmoid notch from the *Anti-Tragus* lying posteriorly. The lobule of the ear hangs from the inferior aspect and although it does not contain cartilage its projected shadow in the lateral view may suggest a soft tissue tumour in the naso-pharynx.

Especially deep fossae in the auricular cartilage may mimic areas of rarefaction in the mastoid bone and the ridges in the auricular cartilage may likewise cause increased densities suggesting bone infection.

Radiography of the auricle although seldom requested is best produced by turning the ear forward and inserting an occlusal film posteriorly (Fuchs, 1943) and using an antero-posterior projection. This projection allows the detail of the auricular cartilage to be seen and small deposits of calcified material such as found in gout can often be recognised in these films when they are not visible in conventional projections.

The external auditory meatus arises from the bottom of the concha and extends in a slightly curved course to the tympanic membrane. Approximately 2·5 cm in length, it runs a slightly curved course inwards, medially, forwards and finally upwards. Its outer third is cartilaginous and its inner two-thirds bony. It is oval in shape and at its outer end its greatest diameter is vertical but at its inner end its maximum depth is horizontal. The inner bony portion is considerably smaller than the outer cartilaginous portion.

The bony walls are formed by the temporal bone and the anterior wall separates the canal from the temporo-mandibular joint. The floor and the anterior wall are longer than the roof and posterior wall consequent on the oblique slope of the tympanic membrane. The tympanic membrane is attached to a groove in the bony wall known as the tympanic sulcus.

Radiographic anatomy. In the lateral oblique projections the external meatus appears as an oval shadow with its long axis vertical and a denser round shadow representing the internal meatus lying within it. Lying in the upper portion of the meatus the faint shadow of the tympanic process of the malleus and the long process of the incus can be seen. These, together with the shadows caused by the bodies of those bones give rise to the "molar tooth" appearance of these ossicles. They are most clearly seen in the lateral tomographic views (fig. 176).

In the lateral view the shadow of the mandibular condyle lies immediately anterior to the external meatus, the petro-tympanic fissure can be clearly seen crossing the anterior wall, and this suture may be mistaken for a fracture.

In the submento-vertical projection the anterior and posterior walls can be recognised and the site of attachment of the tympanic membrane (tympanic ring) appears as a linear area of increased density. In the transorbital view the superior and inferior walls of the external auditory meatus can be seen and the important inner end of the posterior and superior walls (post-meatal spine) can be seen as a harpoon-like shadow. This shadow respresents an important radiological landmark as it identifies the lateral wall of the aditus ad antrum.

The majority of changes occurring in the external meatus can be readily seen on direct inspection but, with stenotic lesions and atretic conditions, full radiological investigations, particularly tomography, are needed to assess the nature and extent of atresia.

Tomographic sections in the antero-posterior projection are the best methods of demonstrating the degree and extent of atresia of the meatus whilst lateral tomographs are better to demonstrate occlusions due to the development of exostosis of the auditory canal. Radiopaque foreign bodies can be seen in conventional views but it is well to remember that plastic beads and other such objects may be radiolucent.

The middle ear

The middle ear is a narrow air-containing cleft lying within the temporal bone and lined by mucous membrane. It consists of two parts: an upper epitympanic recess (attic) and a lower part representing the cavity of the middle ear proper.

The vertical and antero-posterior diameters measure approximately 1·5 cm whilst the narrowest portion, the transverse diameter measures only 6 mm in its widest portion and only 4 mm near its floor (Gray, 1973).

Laterally the tympanic cavity is bounded by the tympanic membrane and the lateral bony wall of the epitympanic recess. Anteriorly, the middle ear communicates with the pharynx by the Eustachian tube, posteriorly it communicates via the aditus with the mastoid antrum and indirectly via this with the mastoid air cells (fig. 169). The roof of the tympanic cavity is formed by the tegmen tympani which separates the middle ear from the middle cranial fossa. The floor is narrow and separates the tympanic cavity from the superior bulb of the internal jugular vein (fig. 170).

Dehiscence of the floor of the middle ear may allow a forward protrusion of the jugular bulb, mimicking a middle ear tumour. Incision of this unrecognised deformity may result in torrential bleeding but jugular venography should avoid this mistake (Overton & Ritter, 1973; Gejrot & Lauren, 1964).

The lateral wall of the tympanic cavity is formed

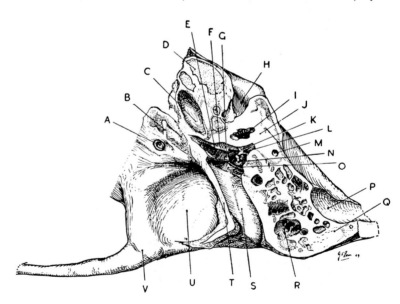

Fig. 169. Horizontal section through the middle ear demonstrating the topographical relationship of middle ear and the Eustachian tube.

A. Foramen spinosum
B. Styloid process
C. Carotid canal
D. Tip of petrous bone
E. Middle ear
F. Medial wall of middle ear
G. Tympanic process of malleus
H. Internal auditory meatus
I. Vestibule
J. Bony labyrinth
K. Stapes
L./N.   Incus and body of malleus
M. Posterior semicircular canal
O. Tympanic membrane
P. Sigmoid sinus
Q. Bony cortex of mastoid process
R. Mastoid air cells
S. External auditory meatus
T. Anterior wall of external meatus
U. Glenoid fossa
V. Root of zygoma.

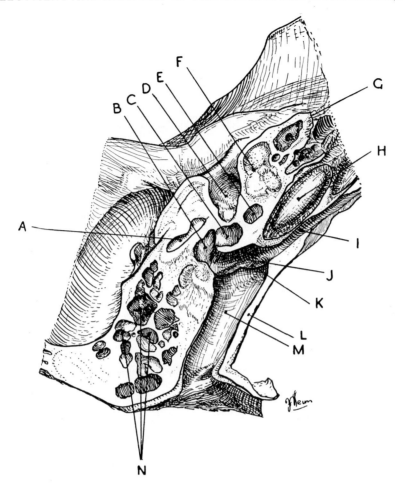

Fig. 170. Lower half of horizontal section.

A. Semicircular canal
B. Attic
C. Mastoid antrum
D. Internal auditory meatus
E. Internal ear

F. Tip cells
G. Tip of petrous bone
H. Carotid canal
I. Eustachian tube
J. Middle ear cavity

K. Tympanic ring and membrane
L. Anterior wall of external auditory meatus
M. External auditory meatus
N. Mastoid air cells.

by the tympanic membrane and the tympanic bony ring to which it is attached (fig. 171). The petro-tympanic fissure opens just anterior to the bony lip to which the tympanic membrane is attached. The medial wall of the tympanic cavity is formed by the bony wall of the cochlea (fig. 172).

The lowermost prominence (the promontory) is formed by the projection of the first turn of the cochlea. The oval window is situated above and behind the promontory and the round window more anteriorly. Both these windows can be recognised in postero-anterior tomographs.

The facial canal traverses the medial wall of the middle ear above the oval window and curves downwards at the genu towards the stylo-mastoid foramen. It lies in a thin bony canal but the walls are frequently incomplete. The horizontal portion of the facial canal can be best seen in the postero-anterior tomograms. It lies below the horizontal semicircular canal and lateral to the oval window.

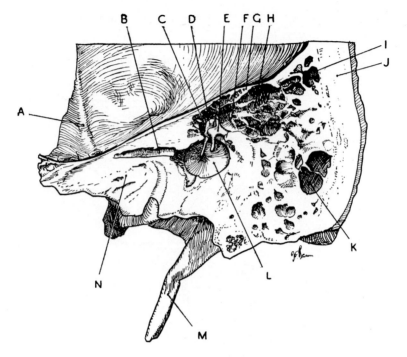

Fig. 171. Line drawing illustrating the lateral wall of the middle ear through the long axis of the middle ear.

A. Groove for middle meningeal artery
B. Bony Eustachian tube
C. Attic
D. Malleus
E. Incus
F. Aditus
G. Tegmen tympani
H. Mastoid antrum
I. Squamous group of mastoid cells
J. Bony cortex
K. Mastoid tip cells
L. Tympanic membrane
M. Styloid process
N. Petrous tip.

The descending limb is most readily identified in lateral tomograms (Brunner & Pedersen, 1970; Harrison & Burrows, 1969). The vertical segment can be demonstrated in 87% of subjects in good tomograms. There is considerable individual variation in the length of the facial canal. The vertical limb is shorter in females than males and may account for the increased prediliction of Bell's Palsy to occur in females (Pope, 1969).

The anterior wall of the middle ear is narrow consequent on the convergence of the lateral and medial bony walls. The larger lower portion is composed of the thin bony posterior wall of the carotid canal whilst the upper portion consists of two separate channels, the higher one carrying the tensor tympani and the lower one the Eustachian tube. The Eustachian tube in this part has bony walls, lies between the squamous and temporal portions of the temporal bone and is separated by a

thin plate of bone from the tensor tympani lying immediately above it. Detailed radiographic coverage of the middle ear is only possible by careful projections in the transorbital, submento-vertical and Towne's views.

The mastoid antrum is a small irregular air-containing cavity in the petrous bone. Its surface marking corresponds to McEwan's triangle. The size of the mastoid antrum varies considerably depending on the degree of pneumatisation of the mastoid process. The lateral wall of the antrum which is of varying thickness is formed by the squamous temporal bone; in infants, it lies relatively superficially but in the adult it may lie at a depth of 1 cm or more. Posteriorly the mastoid antrum lies in relationship to the sigmoid sinus separated by the group of mastoid air cells of varying degrees of development. The roof of the mastoid antrum is formed by a continuation of the

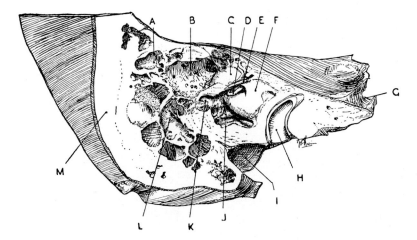

Fig. 172. Line drawing of medial wall of middle ear.

A. Mastoid cells
B. Mastoid antrum
C. Prominence of external semicircular canal
D. Stapes
E. Prominence of facial canal

F. Dome on vestibule
G. Groove for superior petrosal sinus
H. Groove of internal carotid artery
I. Jugular foramen
J. Middle ear

K. Aditus ad antrum
L. Mastoid cells
M. Bony cortex.

tegmen tympani. The anatomical features of the mastoid antrum are best seen in the lateral oblique, submento-vertical, and fronto-occipital projections.

The inclination and direction of the middle ear cleft inclined inwards at an angle of 45° to the sagittal plane is important in its radiographic visualisation. Only projections in which the incident ray passes along the long axis of the middle ear effectively demonstrate its walls. Its visualisation is to some extent dependent on the surrounding structures and a well-developed cellular mastoid seldom gives a clear view of the middle ear; cloudiness of the same cells due to infection may enhance the demonstration of the middle ear. Likewise in a sclerotic mastoid process the outlines of the middle ear may be more readily appreciated due to the density of the surrounding bone.

The aditus ad antrum which forms an important diagnostic landmark in assessing bone erosion due to a cholesteatoma (Welin, 1948) can be seen in the transorbital and lateral oblique positions. The tympanic membrane cannot be seen radiologically but the site of its attachment, the tympanic ring, can be seen in the submento-vertical position and this can be readily recognised in the tomographs.

Auditory ossicles

The three exquisitely shaped bones, the malleus, incus and stapes, provide the transmitting link for sound waves between the tympanic membrane and the inner ear. They are of immense importance as loss of continuity of this chain leads to conductive deafness. They stretch across the middle ear and are delicately held in place by ligamentous attachments. They are particularly vulnerable to trauma and disease processes involving the middle ear.

Malleus. The malleus lies with its head in the epitympanic recess and has two processes, the tympanic process directed downwards and backwards which is attached to the tympanic membrane and a small cone-shaped anterior process directed forwards.

The malleus can be seen in the lateral oblique projection when the head, manubrium and tympanic processes can be recognised comprising the anterior half of the "molar tooth" shadow. The head and body are, in virtue of their density, equally recognisable in the transorbital, submento-vertical (Larkin, 1944) and Towne's projection (Theron & Samuel, 1952). It is less well seen in the Stenvers' position. Tomographic sections in the posterior and lateral projections with the sagittal

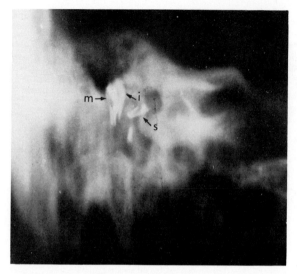

Fig. 173. P.A. tomograph of anatomical specimen after ossicles have been coated with lead. The inco-stapedial joint has been dislocated and a fragment of lead lies in the floor of the middle ear.
M—malleus
I —incus
S —stapes.

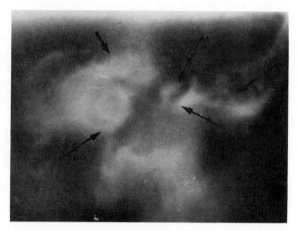

Fig. 174. P.A. tomograph through malleus.
A. Post meatal spur
B. Malleus
C. Cochlea
D. Mastoid cells.

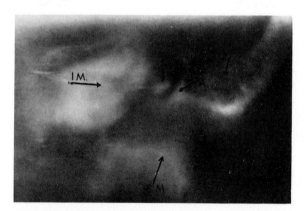

Fig. 175. P.A. tomograms through mastoid process (labyrinthine cut).
M.   Mastoid cells
I.   Incus
IM.   Internal auditory meatus
EM.   Inferior wall of external meatus
A.   Meatal spur

plane rotated are necessary to investigate the detailed anatomy of the malleus and the incudo-mallear joint (figs. 173, 174, 175, 176).

The radiological assessment of the development of the malleus and incus in atresia and of sequestration and necrosis of the bone with infection is of great importance but demands meticulous technique.

Incus. The incus is a cuboidal shaped bone with a long process projecting medially and a short conical process projecting backwards. The facet for articulation with the malleus lies on the anterior surface of the incus and separation of the malleal and incal shadow can only be clearly established in axial or lateral tomographs. In routine radiography the submento-vertical and lateral oblique views offer the best projections for separation of the shadows of the incus and malleus.

The long process runs parallel to the tympanic process of the malleus and in the lateral projection forms the posterior part of the composite "molar shadow" produced by both bones.

The incus because of its poor blood supply is particularly prone to necrosis associated with infections of the middle ear whilst its delicate ligamentous attachments make it particularly vulnerable to dislocations associated with skull injuries (fig. 203).

Stapes. This stirrup-like bone with its footplate fitting into the fenestra vestibuli and its head articulating with the os-articularis of the incus can only be visualised in antero-posterior tomographs of high quality. Even so congenital or pathological

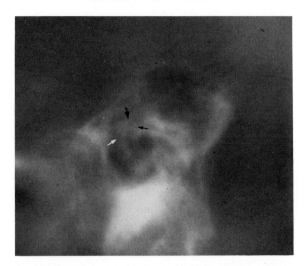

Fig. 176. Lateral tomograph showing ossicular shadows of both malleus (white arrows) and incus (black arrows). The sagittal plane of head must be rotated slightly so that the ossicles come to lie in the plane of the section. The inco-malleal joint can be seen (top arrow).

changes in the footplate and in the bony labyrinth surrounding the fossa ovale such as in otosclerosis can only be recognised when they are moderately advanced.

Eustachian tube

The Eustachian tube walled in its outer third by bone and in its inner two-thirds by cartilage connects the middle ear to the pharynx. Measuring approximately $1\frac{1}{2}$ in (3·8 cm) in length it is directed downwards and medially and is somewhat "S"-shaped and has an obtuse angle of 160° (Cunningham) at the junction of the cartilaginous and bony portions.

Medially it opens on the lateral pharyngeal wall below the Torus turbania in a slit-like opening 9 mm along its long axis. The pharyngeal opening is at a lower level than the tympanic cavity (Spielberg, 1927) and on an average 1·5 cm from the posterior pharyngeal wall (Mangiaracina, 1942).

The cartilaginous portion of the tube is hook-shaped in cross section and its junction to the bony portion represents the narrowest portion of the tube – the isthmus. The bony portion of the tube lies in the petrous temporal bone in a shallow canal and extends to the anterior wall of the tympanic cavity. In infants the tube is half the length of the adult, it is straighter and wider than in the adult and its pharyngeal orifice lies at a lower level. These anatomical factors may contribute to the frequency of tubal occlusion and middle ear infection in infants. Failure of development of the tympanic portion of the temporal bone results in defective development of the bony Eustachian tube (Greig, 1927).

Mucous glands and mastoid air cells (tubal cells) may open directly into the bony tube. Lindsay (1940) found that 21% of skulls showed pneumatisation of the petrous apex and two thirds of these cells opened into the tympanum and Eustachian tube. These peritubal cells cannot be demonstrated by radiography (Lindsay, 1940) and, according to the same author, because of their free drainage are seldom the site of disease.

Functionally, the Eustachian tube equalises the pressure between the middle ear and pharynx and also acts as a drainage tube for normal and pathological exudates from the middle ear. At rest the approximation of the cartilaginous walls effectively seals the tube and it only opens during swallowing, yawning, deep breathing, coughing and sneezing. Recurring equalising of the external and intra-tympanic pressure is necessary as the air in the tympanum is constantly resorbed and this equalisation is effected by repeated opening of the Eustachian tube. The tube is actively opened by its muscles chiefly the levator palatine but also the tensor tympani.

Radiological appearances. The bony portion of the Eustachian tube can be most clearly visualised in the submento-vertical position and less clearly in the Towne's and transorbital projections. The cartilaginous portion of the tube can be seen in the submento-vertical position when it is distended with air ("Tubenknorpel"), (Corning, 1923). If the Valsalva manoeuvre is performed in the submento-vertical or Towne's position the cartilaginous portion of the tube may be seen.

The Eustachian orifice can frequently be seen in routine views as a dark slit on the lateral wall of the nasopharynx (Larkin, 1944).

Contrast visualisation of the Eustachian tube was first employed by Spielberg (1927) who used iodised oil injected through a Eustachian catheter. Rees-Jones & McGibbon (1941) substituted "pyelectan" as a contrast medium as in their hands iodised oil had proved too viscid. In a series of 34 cases of aviation deafness investigated by this method it was shown that in 90% of cases the obstruction was in the mid-cartilaginous portion whilst 7% were at the isthmus and 3% at the pharyngeal orifice. Films are taken in the postero-anterior and submento-vertical position to visualise the whole length of the Eustachian tube. Because of the difficulty of obtaining a water-tight seal at the pharyngeal orifice the method has not gained widespread use.

Wittenborg & Neuhauser (1963) have demonstrated that contrast demonstration of the Eustachian tube in infancy can be more simply obtained by filling the nasopharynx with oily contrast medium with the head held in a submento-vertical position. During crying and swallowing the oily medium will run along the Eustachian tube to the middle ear (nasopharyngogram). The same method can be used in the adult with forced inspiration and Valsalva's manoeuvre and the tube can be filled in a proportion of cases. In the adult however, it is seldom possible to demonstrate the tube beyond the isthmus (fig. 268).

Compere (1960) has injected watery contrast medium into the middle ear and has used this means to determine patency of the Eustachian tube. In patients with perforated ear drum it has been shown that the instillation of watery contrast medium into the external auditory meatus with a gravity feed will enable the Eustachian tube to be clearly shown. In 30 cases of clinical infection it was shown that in 22% some obstruction of the Eustachian tube in the bony part was present.

Stylomastoid process

The styloid process arises from the under-surface of the petrous bone surrounded in its proximal portion by a sheath of bone. The stylohyoid and stylomandibular ligaments are attached to its distal portion.

In the occipito-frontal views the process can be clearly seen between the mandibular ramus and lateral wall of the antrum whilst in the submento-vertical view it appears as a rounded oval shadow (viewed end-on).

A developmental failure of fusion of the tympano-hyal and stylo-hyal process can be seen in the lateral views and may mimic a fracture. The average length of the styloid process is 2·5 cm but it is subject to considerable variation. Marked elongation or angulation of the process may cause irritation of the tonsillar bed giving rise to glosso-pharyngeal neuralgia. Excision of such a process may relieve symptoms (Wilson & McAlpine, 1946).

Petrous bone

The petrous portion of the temporal bone is a three-sided pyramidal bone inclined at an angle of 45° to the sagittal plane. It forms the bony structure housing the labyrinth, Eustachian tube and part of the tympanic cavity. At the outer extremity of its posterior surface where it joins the mastoid process it is deeply grooved by the sigmoid sinus. This groove varies in depth and is closely related to the mastoid air cells and, according to some embryologists, influences the extent of pneumatisation of that structure.

ANATOMICAL VARIATIONS. An anteriorly placed lateral sinus may deeply subdivide the mastoid air cells into a superficial and deep group relative to the sinus. Detection of an anteriorly placed sinus may prove invaluable pre-operative knowledge in preventing the deeper group of cells being overlooked and diminishing the risk of possible surgical damage to the lateral sinus (fig. 180).

The anterior wall of the lateral sinus is readily seen in the lateral view (the sinus plate) and when the sinus is deep two parallel curved lines can be seen, the posterior and less dense representing the medial overhanging lip of petrous bone and the deeper and more anterior representing the groove on the posterior wall of the petrous bone (sinus plate) (Selander, 1946).

Medially placed on the posterior surface of the petrous bone is the funnel-shaped opening of the internal auditory meatus transmitting the 7th and 8th cranial nerves and the internal auditory vessels. Mostly the walls of the internal meatus are formed by dense compact bone but in some cases extensive pneumatisation of the petrous bone may surround the meatus. A bony ridge (crista falciformis) which separates the upper and anterior part of the external auditory meatus (containing the 7th cranial nerve) from a larger and posterior and lower portion containing the 8th cranial nerve, is an important radiological landmark as its displacement or disappearance may be the earliest radiological evidence of an acoustic neuroma (Valvassori, 1972). There is considerable radiological variation in the size of the internal auditory meatus varying from 2·5 to 8 mm in diameter (Valvassori, 1972).

Midway along the superior surface of the petrous bone is the eminentia arcuata, a bony prominence caused by the cortical bone covering the superior semicircular canal. It can readily be identified in the transorbital and Stenvers' projections of the petrous bone.

The styloid process arises from the postero-lateral portion of the under-surface of the petrous bone and the stylomastoid foramen for the exit of the facial nerve from the skull lies posterior to it. This foramen is only visible in the submento-vertical projection.

The petrous segment of the intracranial portion of the internal carotid artery enters on the inferior surface of the petrous bone anterior to the middle ear. Only a thin plate of bone separates the carotid vessel from the middle ear and in some cases this is defective. The carotid canal then passes forward and medially over the foramen lacerum to its true intracranial portion. In the submento-vertical projection particularly in tomographs in this plane, the carotid canal can be seen as a parallel area of decreased density anterior to the tip of the petrous bone and on the outer side and slightly posterior is the larger opening of the jugular foramen. Agenesis of the carotid canal is readily identified in tomograms and, more important, an ectopic course leading to the presence of the carotid artery in the middle ear can be seen (Potter & Graham, 1974).

The jugular foramen is really a short canal housing the jugular bulb. Anteriorly the overhang of the posterior surface of the petrous temporal bone creates a sloping anterior wall which gives a less well-defined margin than the posterior rim. The jugular process projects into the jugular foramen and gives rise to fibrous septa which subdivide the canal into compartments, medially for the 9th cranial nerve, separated by the inferior petrosal sinus from the 10th and 11th cranial nerves which lie more laterally, and in the postero-lateral compartment and occupying most of the foramen is the internal jugular vein (fig. 179).

Khoo (1946) has drawn attention to the enlargement of the jugular foramen which may occur as a normal variant (giant jugular foramen). The giant jugular foramen can be differentiated from pathological enlargement due to a glomus tumour by the sharp well-defined walls and the jugular process present in the normal variant (fig. 180).

In the majority of petrous bones the degree of cellular development is such that some cells lie both in front and behind the labyrinth. Such cells although numerous may be quite small in size and the individual cell walls are not recognised with the same clarity as cells in the squama. Indeed an appreciation of the extent of cellularity may only be obvious when the increased density of the whole petrous bone is seen when infection has occurred.

Venous markings

The termination of the horizontal sinus in the sigmoid sinus grooving and forming a well-developed 'S'-shaped curve on the postero-lateral angle of the sigmoid has already been mentioned.

The foramen of the mastoid emissary vein is a frequent finding and can be seen in the lateral projection (fig. 178). Considerable variations in the development of the venous sinuses around the petrous bones have been described by Waltner (1944). These veins are developed from venous plexuses which lie on either side of the primitive brain tube (Streeter, 1918). The anterior and mid-venous plexuses drain into the external jugular vein

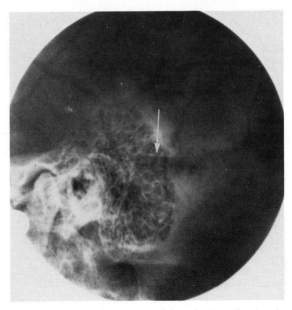

Fig. 177. Abnormal position of lateral sinus showing its relatively low position.

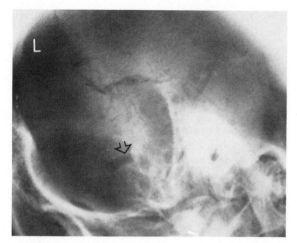

Fig. 178. Large mastoid emissary vein opening into lateral sinus.

the internal jugular vein. The persistence of the spinous jugular foramen accounts for many abnormalities of venous drainage noted.

The variations which are of importance to the radiologist are (Waltner, 1944):

(1) A contracted jugular foramen. Linser (1900) noted 30 out of 1,022 cases examined.
(2) Absence of the lateral sinus; a rare anomaly and usually occurring in the left side (Furstenberg, 1937).
(3) A small transverse sinus leaving the endocranium through the mastoid foramen (Knott, 1881).
(4) Normal lateral sinus leaving the skull through an enlarged mastoid foramen.
(5) The sigmoid sinus absent, the lateral sinus thread-like and a large superior petrosal sinus passing through the mastoid foramen (Williams & Hallberg, 1941).
(6) A sigmoid sinus ending in a blind pouch and draining through a large mastoid foramen (Furstenberg, 1937).
(7) Complete absence of the sigmoid sinus with a large inferior petrosal and narrow lateral sinus (Waltner, 1944).

through a spinous jugular foramen whilst the posterior drains into the internal jugular vein which later forms the sigmoid sinus (figs. 179, 180).

In most mammals the brain is drained through a spinous jugular foramen into the external jugular vein – being phylogenetically an older system than

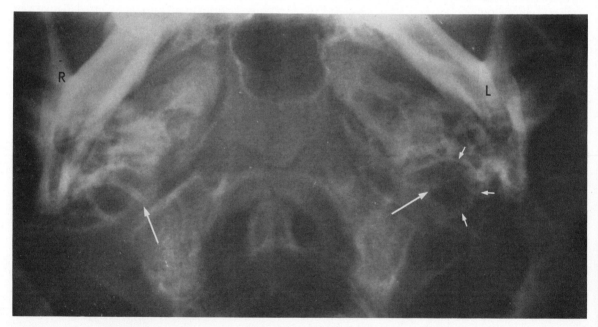

Fig. 179. Jugular foramen. S.M.V. view showing anatomical details of process. Normal jugular foramen on the left side with a well marked processus jugularis (large arrow) which separates the venous from the neurological compartment of the jugular fossa. On the right side the ligament extending from the processus jugularis is calcified (arrow).

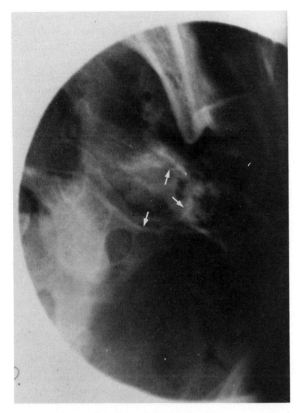

Fig. 180. A normal variant of the jugular foramen associated with a large jugular bulb. It can be differentiated from expansion of the foramen such as from a glomus tumour by the well corticated outline.

(8) Duplication of the lateral sinus is a more frequent anomaly. Streit (1903) and Brown (1921) each reported one case of duplicated sigmoid sinus. Duplication is due to the persistence of two foetal veins.

(9) Hernia-like bulging of the outer wall of the sinus, especially in the region of the upper part of the genu, occurs with relative frequency.

(10) A persistent petro-squamous sinus draining the lateral sinus is a more frequent anomaly. This sinus leaves the skull through the spinous jugular foramen or with the middle meningeal vein through the foramen spinosum.

(11) The sinus may be directly under the periostium, or the cortical layer may be thinned and rendered paper-like by an enlarged sigmoid sinus (Bezold, 1873).

Inner ear

The inner ear is composed of a series of membranous sacs forming the essential organ of hearing, and lying protected in a dense bony capsule (bony labyrinth). Only the bony labyrinth of the inner ear can be visualised by radiological methods.

Three portions of the bony capsule surrounding the inner ear can be recognised radiologically, (a) the vestibule (b) the semi-circular canals, and (c) the cochlea.

The vestibule. The vestibule forms the central portion of the membranous labyrinth and its bony covering forms part of the medial wall of the middle ear. It is ovoid in shape and it is recognised on the radiograph as a small central oval cavity situated near the base of the semi-circular canals.

On its lateral wall is the oval window whilst in the anterior portion of its medial wall is a small depression (Recessus Sphaericus) which lodges the saccule. This portion of the medial wall is perforated by several small holes for the passage of branches of the acoustic nerve. These cannot be recognised on the radiograph.

The Crista Vestibuli is an oblique ridge running across the middle ear which separates the Recessus Ellipticus (containing the utricle) from the Recessus Sphaericus. This wall is also perforated by a small branch of the acoustic nerve proceeding to the utricle. Below the Recessus Ellipticus is the orifice of the vestibular aqueduct.

Facial canal. The facial nerve traverses the petrous bone and because of its importance in microsurgery and diseases of the ear it merits special consideration. The nerve extends from the internal acoustic meatus to the stylo-mastoid foramen. From their attachments to the brain, the two roots of the facial nerve pass into the internal auditory meatus. In the meatus the motor root lies in a groove on the upper and anterior surface of the vestibulo-cochlear nerve, the sensory root being placed between them. At the lateral end of the internal auditory meatus the facial nerve passes through the lamina cribrosa to enter the facial canal. This is divided into three parts: the first or labyrinthine section; the second or tympanic, and the third, mastoid, part. In its first part the nerve runs laterally and then turns anteriorly adjacent to the cochlea and contains the geniculate ganglion. The second part of the facial nerve passes

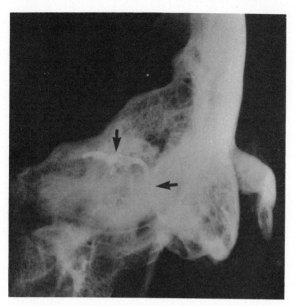

Fig. 181. Facial canal – anatomical specimen of the mastoid process radiographed in the antero-posterior position after the facial canal has been filled with radio-opaque material.

backwards and horizontally beneath the semicircular canal. Finally, the third part descends vertically posterior to the middle ear and external auditory meatus and emerges at the stylo-mastoid foramen (fig. 181).

The first part of the facial canal can be seen on coronal petrous bone tomograms taken anteriorly at the plane of the cochlea and represented in cross section immediately above and lateral to the cochlea. The second part can also be seen in cross section on more posterior cuts where the canal may be identified as a rounded groove or notch below the lateral semicircular canal. In this view however, the facial canal lies obliquely to the tomographic plane (Wilbrand & Bergstrom, 1975), and in most patients is better demonstrated in the half-axial projection. The horizontal and vertical portions of the facial canal are best seen on lateral tomograms, when its outline simulates a walking stick (Guinto & Himadi, 1974), the handle of the stick representing the horizontal section of the canal and its shaft the vertical section.

The semicircular canals. The semi-circular canals form the part of the internal ear concerned with balance. These are three in number, the superior, posterior and lateral and they are situated above and behind the vestibule. Their bony capsules are easily recognisable and form important landmarks in the radiological anatomy of this region.

The superior semicircular canal is vertical in direction and is situated in the petrous bone in a plane transverse to its long axis. Its highest point produces an elevation of the anterior surface of the petrous bone known as the eminentia arcuata. Its anterior end forms the ampulla whilst its posterior end joins with the upper end of the posterior semicircular canal to form the crus commune.

Radiologically, the superior semicircular canal can be easily recognised. It is best demonstrated in Stenvers' position when it appears as a canal 1–1·5 mm wide, surrounded by the dense bony capsule. On the radiograph the upper end of the posterior semicircular canal crosses the superior semicircular canal and the markings produced by this canal on the bony capsule may simulate a labyrinthine fistula. The differentiation can be made by the clear-cut nature of the marking with the absence of any decalcification of the surrounding membrane bone, a feature always noted around a true fistula.

The posterior semicircular canal is placed in a vertical plane and runs roughly parallel to the posterior surface of the petrous bone. It is less easily seen in the Stenvers' position but can be visualised in the Towne's, transorbital, or Chaussé position.

The lateral or horizontal semicircular canal is directed horizontally backwards and laterally. It can be readily visualised in Stenvers' position, Towne's, Chausse and transorbital positions. It forms an important landmark as its most lateral point forms the medial bony wall of the aditus and is of vital importance in the accurate localisation of the exact radiographic position of the aditus ad antrum.

Cochlea. The cochlea, named from its resemblance to a snail's shell, forms the third component of the inner ear. Its apex is directed anteriorly and laterally. The bony canal makes two and three-quarter turns around a central axis (the modiolus). Of the immensely complicated structures of the cochlea, only the modiolus and the bony capsule surrounding the basal turn are visualised by the radiologist. The bony modiolus may be formed of extremely dense bone and may form a confusing dense shadow on the radiograph.

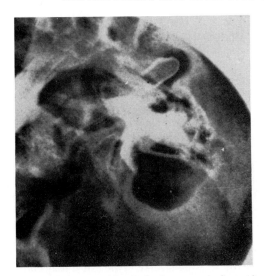

Fig. 182. Aberrant mastoid cell development. Radiograph to illustrate a complete replacement of the mastoid cell system by a giant cell. The appearances are due to a congenital variation in the cell development.

In infants before full development of the mastoid has occurred, the cochlea can be visualised with ease. This is especially true when infection or other cause has produced a relative opacification of the mastoid cells. It may also be unusually prominent in Paget's disease when decalcification of the surrounding petrous bone has occurred in the lytic phase (fig. 254).

The cochlea can be best seen in Stenvers' position, in the modified Towne's position, in Chausse III or transorbital projection but tomography is needed for a comprehensive examination.

The tip of the petrous bone forms an important part of the temporal bone. It may contain diploe or cells of varying size. The tip of the petrous bone may be the site of a giant mastoid air cell (see figs. 182, 183). Apical petrositis depends on a pneumatised tip (Lindsay, 1944) as infection spreads continuously along the pneumatised cells. The petrous pyramid is pneumatised in the perilabyrinthine region in 35% and in the apex in 20% of temporal bones. There are two main routes

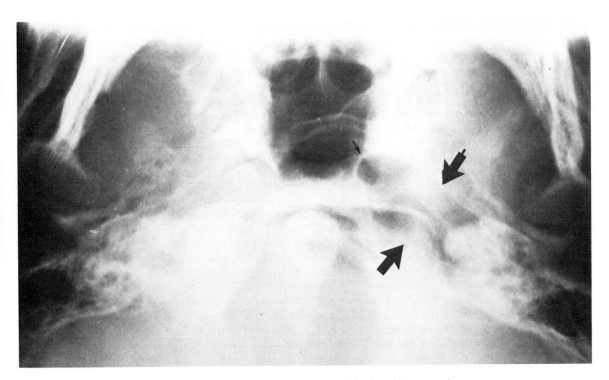

Fig. 183. S.M.V. view of case shown in Fig. 182 showing the extensive pneumatisation of the petrous bone.

of pneumatisation of the petrous pyramid, either anterior or posterior to the labyrinth. Infection tends to follow one or other of these routes and the demonstration of cellular development extending along one or other route is of importance as it enables the surgical approach to be planned. Surgical drainage proceeding along the posterior route may enable the auditory ossicles to be preserved. Perilabyrinthine cells (posterior group) develop from the attic. The anterior group of cells may be pneumatised to a varying extent from the anterior part of the middle ear near the origin of the Eustachian tube. These cells occur in 15% of cases.

Internal auditory meatus is the bony channel transmitting the acoustic and facial nerves through the temporal bone and it forms a valuable radiological landmark.

It can be clearly seen in Stenvers', Towne's and in the postero-anterior projection of the petrous temporal bones particularly so if tomographic cuts are used in the latter position.

Radiologically it appears as a parallel channel with well defined walls. It is smaller than the external meatus and in the lateral views can be visualised as a small oval area of increased translucency lying within the shadow of the external meatus.

The variations in the normal size and shape of the internal auditory meatus are of considerable significance in view of the deformities which may be produced by eighth nerve tumours. In postero-anterior tomographs it can be seen that the outer end of the meatus is slightly bulbous to accommodate the fibres of the auditory nerve as they enter the labyrinth. This must not be mistaken for a pathological enlargement. Postero-anterior tomograms also show a bony ridge to which the septum which divides the internal meatus into a smaller anterior compartment containing the 7th cranial nerve and a larger compartment containing the 8th cranial nerve, is attached (Crista falci-formis). Erosion of this bony ridge has especial significance in detecting 8th nerve tumours.

Considerable variation in the size of the internal auditory canal on both sides may occur in the same individual. Ebenius (1934) found that the meati were identical in 41% to 67% of cases, the difference being related to the projections in which the canals were examined. Camp and Cilley (1939) in an extensive investigation of 250 cases found that the

meati were identical in 41% of cases when examined in the postero-anterior position.

Camp and Cilley (1939) and Valvassori, Naunton and Lindsay (1969) also investigated the average length of the internal auditory canal and the average measurements were 7·9 mm on the right side and 7·8 mm on the left side. The range varied between 3 mm and 16 mm. The greatest variation in width of the internal meatus, of 5 mm, was only noticed in one case.

The mastoid process. Opening out of the posterior aspect of the epitympanic recess is the aditus ad antrum, a short, broad, irregular bony opening leading into the mastoid antrum. The mastoid process may be of the infantile or adult type. The infantile type is poorly pneumatised. It may consist partly of diploic bone and some small cells, the so-called 'mixed type', or it may consist of entirely diploic bone, the true infantile type. Occasionally, the whole mastoid process may be made up of very dense sclerotic bone, the sclerotic mastoid.

The adult type of mastoid shows large well-developed cells throughout the entire mastoid process covered with a relatively thin cortex. These cells usually extend behind the sigmoid sulcus and into the squamous portion of the temporal bone. They may extend forwards into the root of the zygoma and into the petrous bone. Normally, the mastoid processes are symmetrical but asymmetry may occur as a result of unilateral disturbances of cell formation during growth, the mastoid showing deficient cell formation being smaller than the opposite fellow. It has been shown that the degree of pneumatisation of the mastoid process has a very important influence on the natural history of infection of the mastoid and middle ear. The degree of pneumatisation of the mastoid process and its adnexa is therefore a matter of paramount importance.

Several theories have been put forward to account for the great variation in the pneumatisation of the mastoid process, but the most generally accepted view is that of Wittmaack (1912). According to Wittmaack the normal antral mucosa buds out into the surrounding bone, forming air cells and this process continues until the whole mastoid process and part of the squamous and petrous bones are completely pneumatised. This process commences in early infancy. At four months the mastoid antrum is visible on the radiogram as a cavity about a quarter of an inch (6 mm) in diameter situated adjacent to the apex of the lateral semicircular canal. Small peri-antral cells then commence to appear and the process continues until the bone adjacent to the mastoid antrum and the entire mastoid process are occupied by cells. Concurrently, the cells enlarge and expand the bony walls and mastoid process which itself is also enlarged by the pull of the attached cervical muscles. The cells are apt to be of unequal size and not all of them fill with air, those near the mastoid tip being apt to contain a marrow-like substance. This is the sequence of events in a normal mastoid process, where cell formation is unimpeded and results in the adult type of mastoid. In those cases where the middle ear undergoes inflammatory changes in early childhood, disturbances in the normal process of pneumatisation of the mastoid occur. Again, there may be other non-bacterial irritative processes, such as the entrance of sterile amniotic fluid into the middle ear of the foetus, which may inhibit development of the mastoid. This causes a slowly developing inflammatory non-bacterial change which leads to hyperplasia of the mucosa and impedes cell formation. New bone production may be stimulated and a sclerotic mastoid result.

Bacterial infection of the mucosa of the cells may cause fibrosis. If fibrosis occurs early in infancy a complete failure of cellular development with a diploic mastoid results. Fibrosis occurring somewhat later results in an arrest of cell formation and the already formed cells remain small. As cell development primarily occurs around the mastoid antrum the cells remain as small cells grouped around the peri-antral regions.

Other theories have been put forward based on the hereditary factor, but Wittmaack's (1912) theory appears to be the most logical and in accordance with the known facts is the most generally accepted. As will be explained later, there is a very close connection between pneumatisation and the clinical course of infection in the middle ear.

The external meatus. The external auditory meatus extends from the tragus to the membrana tympani. It is about 1 in (2·5 cm) in length, its outer third being cartilaginous and its inner two-thirds bony. The bony portion, with which radiology is primarily concerned, is directed inwards and slightly forwards. It is tapered towards its medial end, which is closed by the membrana tympani, which is firmly attached at its periphery to a bony sulcus (the tympanic ring). The tympanic membrane slopes inwards and downwards at an angle of 55° as mentioned before, and this slope should be borne in mind by the radiologist to enable him to distinguish the upper and lower ellipses of the ring in the radiograms. This slope of the tympanic membrane is demonstrated by filling the external ear with Lipiodol, draining out the surplus and then radiographing in the submento-vertical position. The remains of the Lipiodol will be seen sticking to the outer surfaces of the drum. Because of the slope of the drum, the shadow of the malleus situated on the inner surface of the drum is projected outside the middle ear on to the inner portion of the external meatus in the submento-vertical projection.

The mastoid antrum is separated by only a small thickness of bone from the upper and posterior wall of the auditory canal and cholesteatoma of the antrum not infrequently perforates it. The external auditory meatus is sometimes stenosed by bony exostosis.

Cholesteatoma of the external meatus occurs in rare instances as a result of chronic otitis externa. They can only be recognised on the radiograph when they cause an erosion of the bony walls of the meatus, usually of its upper and posterior wall.

REFERENCES

BEZOLD, F. (1873) Mschr. Ohrenheilk. Lar.-Rhinol., **7**, 130.

BROWN, J. M. (1921) A Double Sigmoid Portion of the Lateral Sinus. Trans. Amer. Lar. rhinol. otol. Soc., **27**, 302.

BRUNNER, S. & PEDERSEN, T. (1970) Roentgen Examination of Facial Canal. Acta radiol. Diag., **10**, 545.

CAMP, J. D. & CILLEY, E. I. L. (1939) The Significance of Asymmetry of the Pori Acustici as an Aid in Diagnosis of Eighth Nerve Tumours. Am. J. Roentg., **41**, 713.

COMPERE, W. E. (1960) The Radiologic Evaluation of Eustachian Tube Function. Archs Otolar., **71**, 386–389.

CORNING, H. K. (1923) Lehrluch der topographischen Anatomie. Munchen: J. F. Bergmann. p. 166.

DAHLBERG, G. & DIAMANT, M. (1945) Hereditary Character of the Cellular System in the Mastoid Process. Acta otolaryng., **33**, 378.

EBENIUS, B. (1934) Results of Examination of Petrous Bone in Auditory Nerve Tumours. Acta radiol., **15**, 284.

FRAZER, J. E. (1914) Second Visceral Arch and Groove in the Tubo-tympanic Region. J. Anat. Physiol., Lond., **48**, 391.

FUCHS, A. W. (1943) Roentgenography of the External Ear. *Am. J. Roentg.*, **49,** 420.

FURSTENBURG, A. G. (1937) Routes of Infection of Sinus. *Trans. Am. Acad. Ophthal. Oto-Lar.,* **42,** 424.

GEJROT, T. & LAUREN, T. (1964) Retrograde Jugularography in the Diagnosis of Abnormalities of the Superior Bulb of the Internal Jugular Vein. *Acta Otolar.,* **57,** 177.

GRAY, H. (1973) *Gray's Anatomy,* 35th Ed. London: Longmans.

GREIG, D. M. (1927) Congenital Absence of the Tympanic Element of Both Temporal Bones. *J. Lar. Otol.,* **42,** 309.

GUINTO, F. C. & HIMADI, G. M. (1974) Tomographic Anatomy of the Ear. *Radiol. Clin. N. Am.,* **7/3,** 405.

HARRISON, J. A. S. & BURROWS, E. H. (1969) Tomography of the Facial Canal, an Experimental Study. *Proc. R. Soc. Med.,* **55,** 166.

KHOO, F. Y. (1946) Giant Jugular Fossae. *Am. J. Roentg.,* **55,** 333.

KNOTT, J. E. (1881) *J. Anat. Physiol.,* **16,** 27.

KOIRANSKY, H. G., ETTMAN, L. K. & WHITE, E. L. (1949) Radiologic Study of Mastoid Bone in Infants. *N.Y. St. J. Med.,* **48,** 1291.

LARKIN, J. C. (1944) Aerotitis Media. *Am. J. Roentg.,* **51,** 178.

LINDSAY, J. R. (1940) Petrous Pyramid of Temporal Bone. *Archs Otolar.,* **31.**

LINDSAY, J. R. (1944) Recent Progress in Management of Acute Suppuration of the Middle Ear. *Archs Otolar.,* **39,** 492.

LINSER, J. (1900) *Beitr. klin. Chir.,* **28,** 642.

MANGIARACINA, A. (1942) The Eustachian Orifice. *Archs Otolar.,* **35,** 6†9.

OVERTON, S. B. & RITTER, F. N. (1973) A High-placed Jugular Bulb in the Middle Ear. A Clinical and Temporal Bone Study. *Laryngoscope,* **83,** 1986.

POPE, T. H. (1969) Bell's Palsy in Pregnancy., **89,** 830.

POTTER, G. D. & GRAHAM, M. D. (1974) The Carotid Canal. *Radiol. Clin. N. Am.,* **7,** 484.

REES-JONES, G. F. & McGIBBON, J. E. G. (1941) Radiological Visualisation of Eustachian Tube. *Lancet,* **ii,** 660.

SELANDER, E. (1946) The Roentgen Appearance of the Anterior Wall of the Sulcus Sigmoideus. *Acta radiol.,* **27,** 60.

SPIELBERG, W. (1927) Visualisation of the Eustachian Tube by the Roentgen Ray. *Archs Otolar.,* **5,** 334.

STREETER, G. L. (1918) The Development Alterations in the Vascular System of the Brain of the Human Embryo. *Contr. Embryol.* (Carnegie Institute, Wash.), **8,** 5.

STREIT, H. (1903) Uber otologisch wichtige anomalien der Himsinus, uber accessorische sinus und bedeutendere veneverbeindugen. *Arch. Ohrenheilk,* **58,** 161.

THERON, C. & SAMUEL, E. (1952) The Radiology of the Auditory Ossicles. *Br. J. Radiol.,* **25,** 245.

TREMBLE, G. E. (1934) Pneumatisation of the Temporal Bone. *Archs Otolar.,* **19,** 172.

VALVASSORI, G. E., NAUNTON, R. F. & LINDSAY, J. R. (1969) Inner Ear Anomalies. Clinical and Histopathological Considerations. *Ann. Otol. Rhinol. Lar.,* **78,** 929.

VALVASSORI, G. E. (1972) Myelography of the Internal Auditory Canal. *Am. J. Roentg.,* **115,** 578.

WALTNER, J. G. (1944) Anatomic Variations of the Lateral and Sigmoid Sinuses. *Archs Otolar.,* **39,** 307.

WELIN, S. (1948) The Roentgen Ray Examination of the Paranasal Sinuses. *Br. J. Radiol.,* **21,** 431.

WILBRAND, H. F. & BERGSTROM, G. (1975) Multidirectional Tomography of Defects in Facial Canal. *Acta radiol., Diag.,* **16,** 436.

WILLIAMS, H. L. & HALLBERG, O. E. (1941) Congenital Absence of the Cranial Venous Sinuses on the Right. *Archs Otolar.,* **33,** 78.

WILSON, C. P. & McALPINE, D. (1946) Glossopharyngeal Neuralgia Treated by Trans-Tonsillar Section of the Nerve. *Proc. R. Soc. Med.,* **40,** 82.

WITTENBORG, M. H. & NEUHAUSER, E. B. D. (1963) Simple Roentgenographic Demonstration of Eustachian Tubes and Abnormalities. *Am. J. Roentg.,* **89,** 1194.

WITTMAACK, K. (1912) *Uber die normale und die pathologische pneumatisation des Schlafenbeines einschliesslich ihrer Beziehungen zu der Mittelohrerkrangkungen. Jena.*

CHAPTER 9

Diseases of the external and middle ear

Congenital lesions

Atresia of the external auditory canal is an uncommon condition and when it occurs it is generally associated with deformities of the pinna (fig. 184). The deformities are not necessarily associated and atresia of the external meatus may occur without any deformity of the pinna (Dean & Gittins, 1917).

Richards (1933) has shown that atresia of the external auditory meatus results either from a failure of the ectodermal invagination from the first gill-cleft to link up with epidermal plate derived from its deeper part, or more commonly, a failure of this plate to split to form the inner end of the external auditory meatus and the tympanic membrane. As the inner ear is derived from a structure (otocyst) developed at an earlier date, congenital abnormalities of the external ear are seldom associated with developmental defects of the internal ear.

Atresia of the external auditory meatus by a skin-like diaphragm has been described by Beck (1930) although this form is questioned by other authors (Richards, 1933). More frequently atresia is caused by a plate of bone in the region of the drum which had been thought to be derived from the proximal part of the hyoid bone (Politzer & Mayer, 1925; Alexander, 1908; Fraser, 1931). Richards (1933) has named this abnormal bony plate – the latero-hyale bone (fig. 185). This is now considered to be developed from the upper part of the cartilage of the second branchial arch (Reichert's cartilage). The malformed ossicles are frequently fused to this abnormal bone (figs. 185, 187).

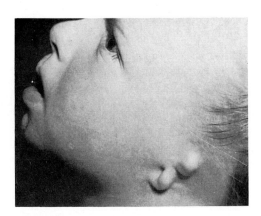

Fig. 184. Microtia associated with congenital atresia of the external auditory meatus. The abnormal external auricle can be seen. The orifice of the external meatus is completely obliterated.

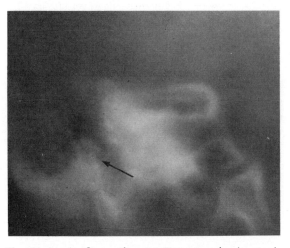

Fig. 185. Atresia of external meatus. Tomogram showing atresia of external meatus with a bony plate and fusion of the malleus to the bony plate obstructing the inner end of the meatus.

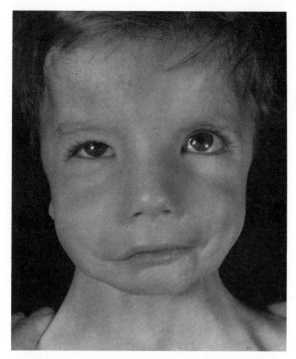

Fig. 186. Möbius syndrome. Clinical photograph showing the cranial nerve palsies, 3rd, 6th and 11th cranial nerves and the congenital deformities of the auricles and the meatus.

The middle ear is generally present in cases of atresia of the external auditory canal, although it may be considerably encroached upon and decreased in size. Frequently, however, it may be filled with bands of scar tissue and be completely airless. In such cases the incus and malleus are fused together into an irregular bony mass,

although the stapes is usually normal. The position of the temporo-mandibular joint may also be abnormal being situated more posteriorly and at a higher level. Atresia of the external meatus may be associated with other congenital deformities as shown in figs. 191, 192.

Frey (1965) has classified abnormalities of the middle ear into five groups:

Group I   Solitary malformation of the ossicles.

Group II   Diminished or atretic external meatus, small atresia plate, a tympanic cavity of normal size, often associated with malformed ossicles.

Group III   Diminished or atretic external meatus, moderate atresia plate, partial atresia of the tympanic cavity, malformed ossicles.

Group IV   Complete atresia of the external meatus, large atresia plate, partial or complete atresia of the tympanic cavity, as a rule no visible ossicles.

Group V   Atypical malformations not included in other first groups.

Anomalies of the carotid canal and jugular bulb may cause serious problems particularly if inadvertent exploration is undertaken. Arteriography may demonstrate the presence of the internal carotid artery bulging into the middle ear when the bony septum separating that structure from the middle ear is congenitally absent (Lapayowker, Liebman & Ronis, 1971).

Aplasia of the malleus and incus may be recognized — fusions of the long process of the malleus to the atretic plate is a frequent finding. Less commonly the malleus and incus may be fused

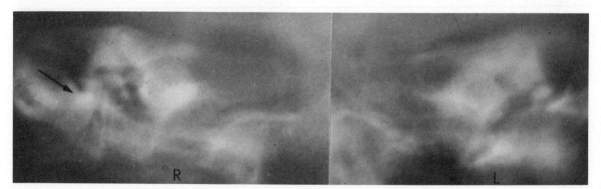

Fig. 187. Atresia of right external meatus. Zonogram showing bony block across the malformed meatus with upward displacement of ossicles.

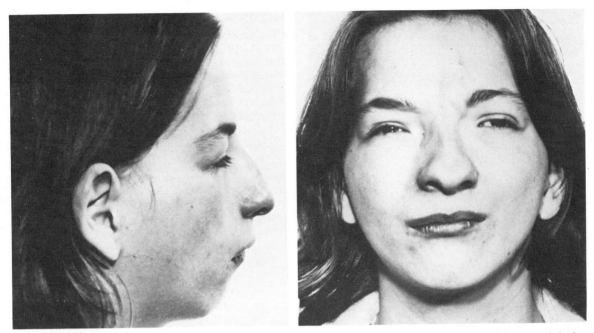

Fig. 188. Treacher-Collins Syndrome with atresia of external meatus. Note the hypertelorism, the high cheek bones and the low position of the auricles.

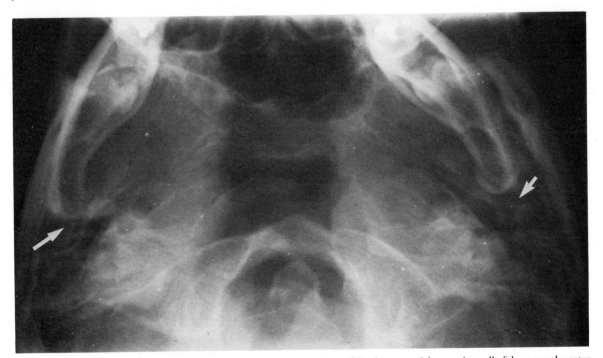

Fig. 189. Submentovertical view; the atresia of the right middle ear with loss of development of the anterior wall of the external meatus with narrowing of the meatus is seen.

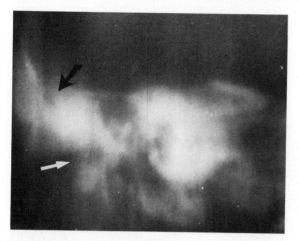

Fig. 190. Tomograph showing narrowing of the external meatus. The middle ear is normally developed and the ossicles are normal. The downward displacement of the floor of the middle cranial fossa is also evident.

to form a single columella – the single ossicle normally present in birds.

The inner ear and middle ears being developed from different germ layers and at different times, congenital deformities are thus not necessarily associated (fig. 192). Thalidomide-induced deformities are exceptions and deformities of both structures are usually present.

Deformities of the semicircular canals usually consist in an underdevelopment with the semicircular canal merely forming a bud from the vestibule. The lateral semicircular canal is most frequently involved, the superior canal the next, and the posterior semicircular canal least commonly affected. Fifty per cent of aplasias of the lateral semicircular canal may be associated with aplasia of the oval window (Terrahe, 1972).

Cochlea malformations usually consist in aplasia of the coils but alterations in size of the coils may be

TABLE I

SYNDROMES WITH ASSOCIATED TEMPORAL BONE ABNORMALITIES

Syndrome	Affected part
Apert's syndrome	Ossicles: inner ear
Crouzon's disease	Ossicles: hyperostosis of petrous bone
First and second branchial arch syndrome (lateral facial dysplasia)	External, middle, or inner ear
Forney, Robinson and Pascoe's syndrome (mitral insufficency, joint fusion and hearing loss)	Fixation of stapes
Fraser's syndrome	External auditory canal
Goldenhar's syndrome	External, middle or inner ear
Klippel-Feil syndrome	Ossicles
Long-arm 18-deletion syndrome	External canal
Mengel's syndrome	Ossicles
Mohr's syndrome	Ossicles
Osteogenesis imperfecta	Otosclerosis-like stapes abnormality
Osteopetrosis	Ossicles
Oto-palato-digital syndrome (Taybi's syndrome)	Ossicles
Pendred's syndrome	Cochlea
Rubella syndrome	Cochlea
Thalidomide syndrome	External, middle and inner ear
Treacher-Collin's syndrome	External ear
Waardenburg's syndrome	Inner ear
Wildervanck-McLaurin syndrome (malformation and conductive hearing loss)	Atresia of the external auditory canal; Inner ear
Winter's syndrome	Ossicles

Reproduced from "Radiologic Clinics of North America", with permission, from article by Fitz & Harwood-Nash.

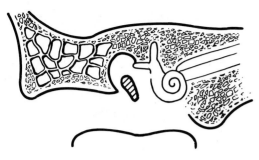

A. Normal ear.

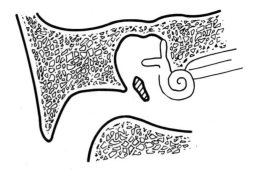

B. Curved external auditory meatus.

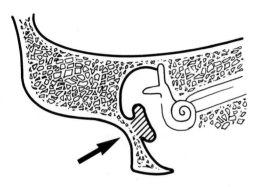

C. Thin atretic plate (arrow) and fused ossicular mass.

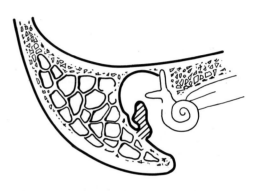

D. Thick pneumatised atretic plate.

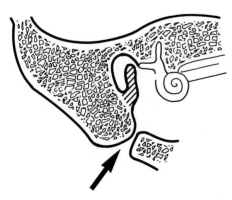

E. Slit attic with "fused" ossicles. The facial nerve (arrow) passes out laterally through floor of the middle ear.

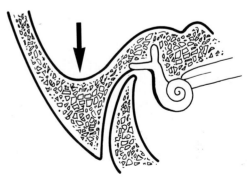

F. Descent of tegmen (arrow). Slit middle ear cavity, no ossicles or oval window and an anteriorly situated facial nerve canal.

Fig. 191. Six line drawings to illustrate typical congenital deformities of the middle and external auditory meatus.

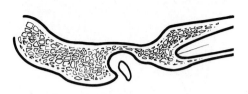

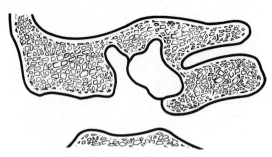

A. Total aplasia of labyrinth.

B. Michel deformity with sac like structure and narrow internal auditory meatus.

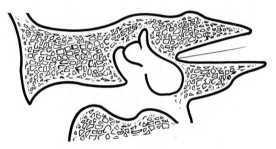

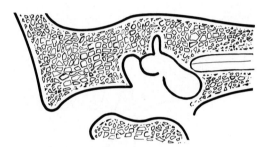

C. Dilated cochlea and vestibule with tapering internal auditory meatus.

D. Mundini deformity.

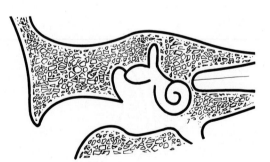

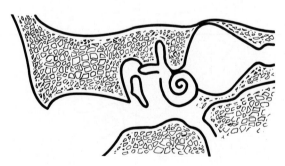

E. Isolated dilatation of lateral semicircular canal.

F. Giant internal meatus.

Fig. 192. Congenital deformities of the inner ear.

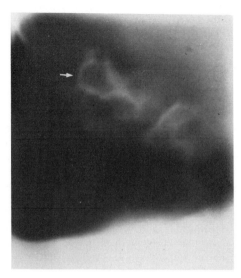

Fig. 193. P.A. tomographic film showing the cochlear spiral deficient in the normal number of turns. Mundini deformity, a congenital deformity of the cochlea. This may occur as an isolated deformity.

a normal variation. The Mundini deformity consists in one-and-a-half turns of the cochlea as opposed to the normal two-and-a-half and radiologically the demonstration of a distinct cavity situated above the normal basal coil is essential. Tomography in the axial or P.A. plane is necessary to demonstrate this deformity (fig. 193). Aplasia of the cochlea occurs without any form of the organ developing and this is usually associated with an underdeveloped internal meatus.

The third type of deformity is one in which a bony labyrinth surrounds a cyst-like space without any suggestion of any cochlear development (fig. 192B).

Aplasia of the internal auditory meatus is not necessarily associated with maldevelopment of the cochlea. Enlargement of the internal auditory meatus has been described in association with retinitis pigmentosa (Jensen, 1974).

Fitz & Harwood-Nash (1974) have summarised the syndromes which may be associated with the deformities and the portions of the temporal bone which may be involved (Table I).

Enlargement of the internal auditory meatus may occur as a normal variant and must not be mistaken for enlargement associated with an acoustic neuroma (fig. 246).

Acquired stenosis. Acquired stenosis of the external auditory canal varies considerably in aetiology and degree. It may be complete or partial. Partial stenosis of the external auditory meatus usually follows chronic inflammation, *e.g.* furunculosis and chronic suppurative otitis media. Atresia of the external auditory meatus may also follow trauma (Palmer & Reifsneider, 1933). Such trauma to the meatal wall may follow attempted removal of wax. Stenosis of the external meatus may also follow a radical mastoidectomy where the skin flaps have become adherent or occur following the development of inflammatory granulations.

Osseous or cartilaginous stenosis generally follows the development of exostosis or chondral thickening of the cartilaginous external meatus. Atresia of the external auditory meatus may also occur as a sequel to gunshot wounds (Conley, 1946).

Radiological features. Radiology can be of considerable assistance in evaluating the type and extent of the atresia and also in determining the presence of a middle ear. An exhaustive radiological examination including tomographs should be undertaken in every case, but especially to enable plastic corrective operations to be performed (Siirala, 1947; Camp & Allen, 1940). The radiological features are:

(1) An *absence of the external meatus* in the routine views when there is a total loss of the bony walls of the external meatus. The anterior wall is particularly defective and this is especially noticeable in cases of partial atresia of the external meatus. These features may be seen in the lateral, submento-vertical and postero-anterior views of the mastoid process.

(2) *Posterior displacement of the condyle* of the mandible. As a result of the lack of development of the bony anterior wall of the external auditory meatus, the temporo-mandibular condyle is seen to be placed more posteriorly than normal. This feature can be well appreciated in the lateral and submento-vertical view.

(3) *Presence of a bony plate.* The demonstration of a bony septum in the external meatus is invaluable information pre-operatively. Tomography in the antero-posterior plane or submento-vertical position will show an extension of the posterior meatal spur forwards

to form a bony plaque. The malleus is usually fused to this bony plaque. More rarely a complete bony block may be seen in the external meatus with no margins visible.

(4) *Tomography is essential for complete radiological examination* of the congenital atresia, and should be carried out in both postero-anterior and lateral planes (Camp & Allen, 1940).

The development of tomographic machines capable of hypocycloidal and ellipsoid movement has provided a means of obtaining more detailed information about the middle ear and labyrinth.

Postero-anterior thin tomographic sections using a small cone taken at 2 mm apart enable the whole of the middle and inner ear to be covered. If the first section is taken at the plane of the anterior wall of the external meatus and six subsequent sections at 2 mm intervals posteriorly the whole middle and inner ear are surveyed. In congenital atresia when the external meatus is absent a guide to the point of commencement of the plane of tomographic section can be gained from reference to the opposite ear.

The information that the radiological study should provide should be as follows (Valvassori, 1963):

(1) Degree and type of abnormality of the tympanic bone.
(2) The structure of the bony septum closing the external meatus (complete or incomplete, thick or thin) (figs. 192c,e).
(3) Degree of development of the tympanic cavity.
(4) Condition of the ossicular chain.
(5) Degree and localisation of the pneumatisation of the mastoid antrum and mastoid cells.
(6) Route of the facial canal.
(7) The status of the labyrinthine windows.

The use of thalidomide as an anti-emetic drug in pregnancy produced a large number of congenital deformities of the ear. It is estimated that 4,000 such cases are present in Germany and many have occurred in other European countries. These auricular deformities may be associated with varying degrees of phocomelia. Reparative surgery may considerably help with hearing loss in these subjects and as it is difficult to differentiate between neurosensory deafness and conductive deafness in the young a careful radiological study at as early an age as possible is essential. Heavy basal narcosis or

even light general anaesthesia is necessary in these young subjects to allow immobilisation of the head to obtain good tomographic films.

The radiological appearances of congenital ear anomalies may be summarised as follows.

External auditory meatus

The external auditory meatus may be shown to be narrow, short or completely atretic. It may run in an abnormal direction, sloping upwards towards the middle ear, and sometimes curved in two planes, the horizontal section being at its medial end. In external meatal atresias, both soft tissue and bone are involved, and the tympanic ring may be absent, deformed or hypoplastic. Complete atresia is associated with a posteriorly situated temporo-mandibular joint. Atresia plates may be due to a deformed tympanic bone or to extension of the squamous temporal bone downwards. Both processes occur, and in the latter circumstance the atresia plate may be pneumatised by extension of the mastoid air cells (fig. 191e).

Middle ear cavity

In isolated unilateral atresias the middle ear cavity is usually of relatively normal shape and even in the most severe deformities there is rarely complete absence of the middle ear and usually at least a slit like hypo-tympanum. The middle ear cavity may be reduced in size by encroachment of the atresia plate, a high jugular bulb, or by descent of the tegmen tympani. The latter is typical of a mandibulo-facial dysostosis (Treacher Collins syndrome) and the attic and antrum are absent or slit-like. The middle ear cavity may contain thin bony septa dividing it into two or more compartments.

Ossicles

In most instances of atresia of the external ear there is an associated abnormality of the ossicular chain. The most usual deformity is a fusion of the bodies of the malleus and incus. The fusion may be bony or fibrous and the ossicular mass may be fixed to the walls of the middle ear cavity by bosses of bone. Because of the replacement of the tympanic membrane by a bony plate the handle of the malleus is the part of the ossicular chain which is most commonly abnormal. Often the handle of the malleus is bent towards the atresia plate to which it may be fixed. Deformities of the stapes super-structure cannot be recognised radiologically but fixations of the footplate may be associated with a massive stapes and the stapes is then more clearly demonstrated on tomography than in the normal patient.

Facial nerve

Congenital deformities of the first part of the facial nerve are rare, but congenital abnormalities of the middle ear and external meatus may be associated with an abnormal course of the second and third parts of the facial nerve. The nerve is more anteriorly placed than normal and follows a direct course out of the temporal bone. These changes are often associated with an abnormal oval window.

The facial nerve may cross the middle ear cavity without being in a bony canal. This cannot be shown radiologically but usually the exit foramen through the floor of the middle ear cavity can be identified.

The facial canal may divide into two or more branches before leaving the mastoid but narrowing or widening of the canal is of no significance.

Inner ear abnormalities

Congenital labyrinthine abnormalities vary from total aplasia of the labyrinth to minor anomalies of the semicircular canals (fig. 192). A solitary sac-like deformity of the labyrinth was first described by Michel (1863) in which both cochlea, vestibule and semicircular canals are replaced by an amorphous sac. In some patients barely recognisable differentiation may occur, usually with one or more semicircular canals appearing to arise from the sac. The Michel deformity is usually associated with an absent or narrow internal auditory meatus, and a total absence of hearing.

In moderate deformities of the labyrinth some cochlea function may be retained (Phelps, Lloyd & Sheldon, 1975). The most important lesion in this group is that in which the modiolus or central bony spiral of the cochlea is deficient, and the distal one and a half coils are replaced by a sac (Mundini, 1791). The typical tomographic appearance is that of an "empty" cochlea due to the deficient modiolus. There may be some associated dilatation of the semicircular canals in the Mundini defect but

the anomaly is usually present with a normal internal auditory meatus.

A congenital deformity of the internal auditory meatus and labyrinth sometimes associated with a cerebrospinal fluid fistula has been described by Phelps & Lloyd (1976). Typically these patients show a tapering internal auditory meatus, which narrows at its lateral end and is associated with a generalised dilatation and dysplasia of the labyrinth, with the cochlea represented as an amorphous sac completely lacking a modiolus.

Congenital dilatations of the semicircular canals are the commonest inner ear abnormalities to be shown radiologically. When confined to the lateral semicircular canal there is not as a rule any loss of hearing. Radiologically the finding of a short, wide, lateral semicircular canal is therefore without significance as an isolated phenomenon (fig. 192c).

Congenital dilatation of the internal meatus may be mistaken for pathological enlargement caused by an acoustic neuroma. The well defined bony walls and a nipple-like projection of the inner end of the enlarged meatus help to differentiate the two conditions (fig. 246).

FOREIGN BODIES

External auditory meatus

The exposed nature and easy accessibility of the external auditory canal makes it a frequent site for the lodgement of foreign bodies. Young infants and mental defectives are especially prone to insert foreign bodies into the external auditory meatus.

Foreign bodies which have been removed from the external ear vary greatly in size and nature, only those which are radio-opaque are of interest to the radiologist. Radiology can, however, offer considerable assistance in diagnosis as, although the vast majority of foreign bodies can be readily seen through a speculum, the oedema of the walls of the external meatus may obscure an underlying foreign body.

Glass beads are the commonest of foreign bodies found in the external auditory meatus and are generally composed of lead glass of sufficient density to cast a radio-opaque shadow. Some beads, notably plastic ones, are of such a low radio-opacity as to cast no shadow (Longaker, 1929). It should be remembered that most plastic buttons cast no shadow.

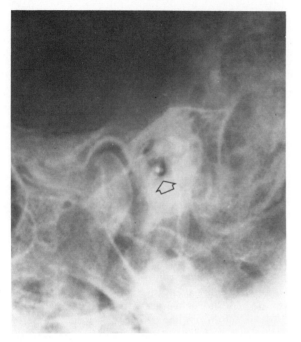

Fig. 194. Lateral oblique view showing the clouding of the mastoid cells, with the dense metallic foreign body lying in the middle ear.

Middle ear

Foreign bodies in the middle ear almost invariably reach that site through the external auditory canal after perforation of the drum. This may follow attempted removal of the foreign body from the external auditory meatus when the whole or a fragment of the foreign body may be displaced into the middle ear. Such foreign bodies become lodged in the attic giving rise to persistent discharge and may subsequently lead to the development of a mastoid infection.

The use of acetylene welding has resulted in foreign bodies in the middle ear becoming an industrial hazard. Otitis media may result from a perforation of the eardrum by molten metal (Britton & Walsh, 1940) and partial or complete deafness may be a serious aftermath of burning of the tympanic membrane by "slag", the byproduct of the welding process (Lund, 1929).

In virtue of its high radio-opacity the presence of such slag in the mastoid process may be readily demonstrated radiologically and may prove of considerable help in elucidating the aetiology of a chronic otitis media or a chronic mastoiditis (figs. 194, 195, 196).

Eustachian tube

Foreign bodies in the Eustachian tube are an exceedingly rare occurrence. Hastings (1937) has recorded a piece of gold bougie and Mangiaracina (1940) a piece of twisted wire removed from the Eustachian tube (fig. 197).

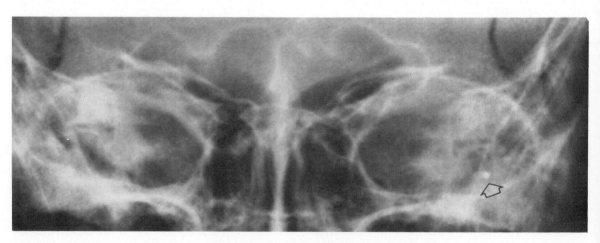

Fig. 195. Transorbital view demonstrating metallic fragment lying in middle ear (same case as Fig. 194).

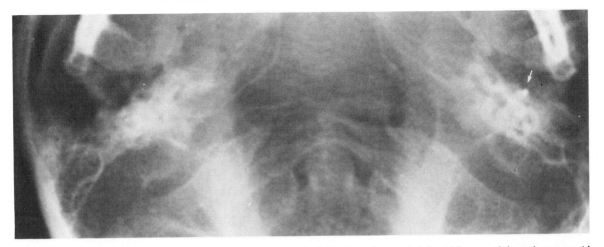

Fig. 196. Submentovertical view of same case as Fig. 194 showing diminished translucency in left middle ear and throughout mastoid air cells on the left side.

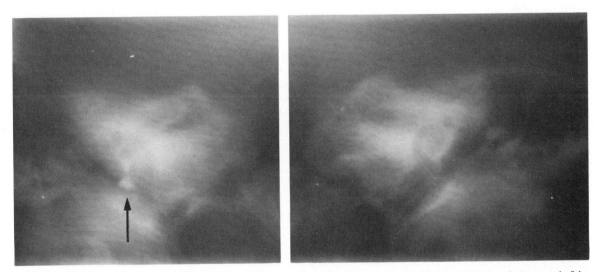

Fig. 197. Foreign body in Eustachian tube. Antero-posterior tomogram showing a metallic foreign body lodged in the inner end of the right Eustachian tube.

INFLAMMATORY AND DEGENERATIVE CHANGES

Auricle

Inflammatory conditions involving the auricle seldom call for radiological examination owing to the ease of clinical examination.

Certain degenerative conditions of the auricular cartilage, however, are best demonstrated by radiology. Calcification in the auricular cartilages is a rare occurrence but when it occurs it can readily be demonstrated. Scherrer (1932) was able to find only 40 such cases reported in the literature between 1866 and 1931. Childrey (1932), however, recorded a series of eight cases and in a later article collected 61 cases reported in the literature and added a further seven cases.

The aetiological factors concerned in the development of calcification in the auricular cartilage are numerous. Frostbite appears to be the most constant whilst senile keratosis, syphilis, Addison's disease (Jarvis *et al.,* 1954), acromegaly (Nathanson & Losner, 1947), ochronosis (Pomeranz, Friedman & Tunick, 1941), and perichondritis have all been mentioned as predisposing factors.

Haug (1939) reported a male aged 60 years where the ossification was confined to the helix and antihelix. The ear had previously been the site of frostbite which was probably the cause of the subsequent calcification. This author considered three possibilities as regards the formation of the calcification: destruction of the cartilage followed by the deposition of calcium salts (dystrophic calcification); metaplasia of cartilage to bone; a combination of partial calcification with islets of bone formation.

The radiological appearances are those of calcification closely following the anatomical markings of the auricular cartilages. Other radio-opaque deposits such as the tophi noted in gout generally do not contain sufficient calcium to throw a significant shadow on the radiograph.

The easiest position for the radiographic demonstration of the auricle is by placing an occlusal film end-on against the side of the head, and directing the ray perpendicularly through the centre of the ear and tangentially to the lateral aspect of the head (Fuchs, 1943).

INFECTIONS OF THE MIDDLE EAR

Aetiology

In most cases of otitis media infection spreads by way of the Eustachian tube from the nasopharynx, vigorous blowing of a congested nose often aiding the spread of infection. In infants the Eustachian tube is short and straight and as they spend a considerable period lying supine secretions from the nose readily gravitate into the Eustachian tube. In children the lymphoid tissue forming the pharyngeal cushion at the orifice of the Eustachian tube may become hypertrophied and by occluding the Eustachian tube, predispose to an otitis media. Diving and swimming, by increasing the pressure in the nasopharyngeal air space, may cause infected water or secretions to be forced or sucked up the Eustachian tube.

Infection of the middle ear may also occur through direct spread from the outside through a perforated eardrum. Fractures of the skull may pass through the middle ear producing haematoma (haemo-tympanum) in the middle ear which later becomes secondarily infected.

Blows on the ear, loud explosions or rapid alterations in atmospheric pressure, *e.g.* Caisson's disease, flying, gun-fire *etc.,* may occasionally rupture the eardrum with a subsequent development of a middle ear infection. Infection of the middle ear may also arise from the bloodstream; tuberculous infection of the middle ear almost certainly occurs by this route.

The mucosa of the middle ear, being continuous with that of the nasopharynx, is subject to the same allergic disturbance as the nasal mucosa. During an attack of hay fever the tympanic mucosa usually reacts in much the same way as the nasal mucosa and in this way allergic mucosal swelling may give rise to an otitis media.

It has been established that mastoid infections in diabetes are associated with relatively early and extensive bone destruction and are particularly liable to intracranial complications. This finding was challenged by Kecht & Dibold (1936), Dibold & Huber (1938), and Mayer (1939) but the later investigations of Druss & Allen (1942) of 49 patients with diabetes associated with acute mastoiditis confirmed the original observations. These latter authors found that 41% of such cases showed intracranial complications.

Lymphatic leukaemia sometimes shows infiltration of the tympanic mucosa producing a purulent discharge loaded with the same type of cells found in the blood (Fowler & Swenson, 1939).

The organisms responsible for an otitis media are extremely varied, among the commonest being the streptococcus pyogenes, the pneumococcus, staphylococcus albus and aureus, the diphtheroids, and haemophilus influenzae (Friedman, 1957). Klebsiella pneumoniae is one of the most destructive of these organisms invading the middle ear – often being asymptomatic and insidious. Rarely, tuberculosis and fungal organisms such as actinomycosis (Brown, 1942) may affect the middle ear. The correct diagnosis in reported cases was only made at autopsy and there were no specific radiographic signs.

Infection of the middle ear differs from infection in the other nasal spaces in that there is no

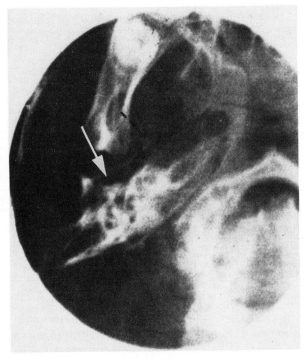 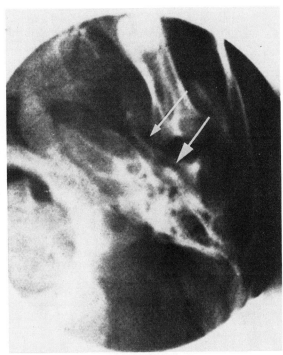

Fig. 198. Acute suppurative otitis media. Submentovertical view of a male child aged 10 who had complained of pain in the left ear for one week's duration. On examination the left eardrum was red and pulsating. The radiograph demonstrates a loss of translucency of the left middle ear associated with diminished translucency of the aeration of the left Eustachian tube (indicated by arrows). The normal appearances can be seen on the right side.

concomitant enlargement of the lymphatic glands. No lymphatics have been identified in the temporal bone (Fowler & Swenson, 1939). The mucosa of the middle ear becomes oedematous and swollen and the inflamed tissues infiltrated with leucocytes. The Eustachian tube becomes occluded, the air in the middle ear absorbs, and an exudate fills the middle ear which later becomes purulent. The drum then becomes reddened and bulges outwards and unless paracentesis is performed, spontaneous rupture occurs. Perforation usually occurs in the postero-superior quadrant, less often in the anterior quadrant. If exudate accumulating in the niche of the round or oval windows or in the attic around the malleus and incus becomes organised, the scar tissue formed interferes with the movements of the ossicles and causes conductive (adhesive) deafness. Severe infection may spread through the membranous and bony capsule causing a labyrinthitis.

In every case of otitis media there is to a greater or lesser degree an associated infection of the mastoid antrum and the immediate mastoid cells opening from it (fig. 198).

Infection of the middle ear may involve the ossicles causing a destruction and absorption of these bones – the incus as a consequence of its precarious blood supply is especially prone to be involved. Occasionally, particularly if there is a dehiscence of the covering bone, infection may spread into the facial canal causing facial paralysis (figs. 199, 200). Facial palsy is especially liable to occur in those cases where there is a congenital absence of the roof of the facial nerve. If the cells in the apex of the petrous temporal bone are affected the 6th nerve may be involved, producing paralysis of the external rectus muscle (Gradenigo's syndrome).

The natural history of the infection following otitis media is largely dependent on the degree of pneumatisation of the petrous bone. It has long been recognised that approximately 93% of cases of

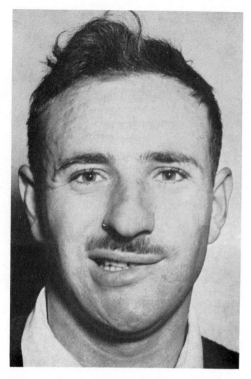

Fig. 199. Left facial palsy associated with acute middle ear infection. This feature is especially liable to develop when there is a dehiscence of the bony covering of the facial canal.

chronic otitis media occur in patients with diploic or poorly pneumatised mastoids ("infantile" type of mastoid). Acute otitis media may occur with either the "infantile" or "adult" type of mastoid

process but a consequential acute mastoiditis is more prone to occur in the cellular type as diploic bone is more resistant to infection.

Diamant (1940) investigated the mastoid process in approximately a thousand persons all over the age of 10 years. Approximately 40% had no symptoms of ear disease; the remaining 60% were suffering from acute or chronic otitis media. Radiographs of the mastoid processes of these patients (lateral oblique projection) were taken and the cell system measured by means of a planimeter. This investigation showed that the cell system in adults normally varies from 0 to 30 sq. cm. The examination of patients with chronic otitis media showed an average cell system which is only one-fourth of the normal. In practically every case of Diamant's series suffering from chronic otitis media, the size of the cell system fell far short of the average normal value. Diamant (1940) states that "if a cell system is found to exceed 15 sq. cm. one may assert that otitis media, if it should occur, will not give rise to a permanent change in the tympanic membrane". According to him this means that such a person will never suffer from chronic otitis media irrespective of the type of treatment, or lack of treatment, which he may receive. This far-reaching statement, if correct, is of important prognostic value. Diamant emphasises that this conception of chronic otitis media is in accordance with Brock's definition (1926) and refers to the state of the tympanic membrane and not to the type of infection. The following table is reproduced from Diamant's article.

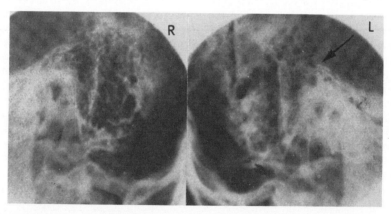

Fig. 200. Lateral oblique radiograph of patient shown in fig. 199 showing both mastoid processes. Both mastoid processes are cellular, the cells in the periantral region of the left mastoid processes are opaque but the inter-sinus cell walls are visible.

SUMMARY OF DATA

Diagnosis	Ears examined	Age group (years)	Average value of cell system (sq. cm.)	Highest value of cell system (sq. cm.)
Normal mastoid	356	10–30	12·27	27·6
Chronic otitis	138	10–30	2·89	15·1
Marginal perforation	101	10 & over	1·68	9·2
Central perforation	136	10 & over	3·54	16·1
Atrophic scar	89	10 & over	4·94	16·4
Acute otitis	91	10 & over	9·6	20·5

If the cell system is asymmetrical in the petrous bones and the patient contracts a unilateral otitis media which becomes chronic, it is the ear with the smaller cell system that is most commonly affected.

Diamant, however, states that the persons with the largest cell systems exceeding 23 sq. cm. in practically no instances develop otitis media but experience is at variance with this statement as acute infections of mastoids with such cell systems can occur.

Later work by Dahlberg & Diamant (1945) has shown that hereditary factors play an important part in the evolution of the cell pattern of the mastoid process. Schwartz (1951) investigating the influence of heredity on pneumatisation, found that uniovular twins showed similar mastoid pneumatisation, whereas binovular twins did not. Diamant (1952) concurs that heredity is the determining factor in the type of mastoid pneumatisation that occurs.

The freely communicating cells of a pneumatised mastoid are prone to the rapid spread of an acute infection. The cortex of the cells is thin and signs of acute inflammation appear earlier and are more obvious both clinically and radiographically than they are in a small cell or diploic type of mastoid. In such cases a conservative approach would preferably be the line of choice and if operation is eventually performed, it would probably be a conservative mastoidectomy. Radiology can be of great value in determining the topography of the mastoid cells and in indicating groups of cells which extend beyond the limits of normal and are likely to be overlooked during operation. On the other hand, the diploic or sclerotic type of mastoid is more resistant to spread of infection from the middle ear, but if infection occurs the course of events may differ considerably from that seen in a cellular mastoid. Both the clinical and radiological signs are much less apparent. Normally there is a considerable thickness of bone between the mastoid antrum and the cortex, but only a thin layer of bone divides the antrum and middle ear from the meninges; infection consequently may spread inwards and lead to dangerous intracranial complications in a diploic mastoid.

Studies in a working class general practice (Lowe, Bamforth & Pracy, 1963) have confirmed previous findings that malnutrition and poor domestic hygiene greatly contribute to the persistence of infection. A cure failure rate of 29% was noted by these authors, and 25% of this group showed significant deafness six months later. The radiologic anatomical information is of equal importance to the pathological findings in acute otitis media and may be summarised as follows:

Anatomical

(1) Is the cellular development of mastoid process symmetrical or asymmetrical? Is it of adult or infantile type?
(2) If cellular, what is the distribution of the cells? Do they extend into the zygoma, squamous, temporal or the petrous bone beyond the labyrinth? What is their relationship to the lateral sinus?
(3) If of infantile type, is the mastoid process diploic, sclerotic or diploic with a few small cells (mixed type)?

Pathological

(1) Is the middle ear of normal transradiancy?
(2) Are the ossicles visible?
(3) Is the Eustachian tube outlined by air and consequently visible or is it de-aerated and, therefore, faint or invisible?

(4) If there are any cells in the petrosa anterior to the labyrinth are they clear-cut and transradient or are they ill-defined and cloudy? Is the bone of the petrosa of normal texture?

(5) If the mastoid process is of adult type, are the cells clear-cut and transradiant or are they hazy, opaque, sclerosed or blurred in outline? Is there any evidence of cell wall destruction and abscess formation?

(6) If the mastoid is of infantile type are the mastoid antrum and any small peri-antral cells clear or cloudy. Is the bone of normal x-ray texture and density or is it rarefied, cloudy in texture, destroyed or does it show sclerosing osteitis?

If there is any bone destruction present is it adjacent to or does it involve the walls of the mastoid antrum, tympanum or the posterior wall of the external auditory meatus?

Otitis media

Pathologically otitis media may be:

(a) Acute catarrhal and suppurative otitis media.
(b) Chronic otitis media.
(c) Healed (quiescent) otitis media.

Acute catarrhal otitis media usually follows a nasopharyngeal infection. A catarrhal oedema of the mucosa of the middle ear and of some or all of the mastoid cells takes place. The drum may be reddened and hearing be impaired but no suppuration occurs. Usually, the condition subsides after a few days, but in unfavourable cases it may go on to a suppurative otitis media. It is probable that some cases of catarrhal otitis media are not infective but are allergic in origin. Both benign and malignant tumours of the nasopharynx by obstructing the Eustachian tube may cause a catarrhal otitis media. Catarrhal otitis media may occur in xanthomatosis or may follow radiation therapy applied to any structure in the vicinity of the nasopharynx or mastoid process.

In acute non-suppurative otitis media, the mucosa of the middle ear, mastoid antrum, and peri-antral cells becomes oedematous and appears hazy on the radiograph. This haziness may be very slight, the affected areas having a ground glass appearance. Because of the minimal nature of these changes they may escape detection in the antrum of diploic mastoid, but they can usually be observed in the cellular mastoid (fig. 218). In a diploic or cellular type of mastoid the cell walls are not appreciably obliterated though the cells themselves are cloudy.

A post-auricular adenopathy or cellulitis may show an apparent loss of translucency of the peri-antral cells but in such cases the middle ear and Eustachian tube are unaffected and in the submento-vertical projection the opacity may be seen to extend beyond the limits of the cell system.

Acute suppurative otitis media. In acute suppurative otitis media the inflammatory process proceeds to suppuration with reddening and bulging of the drum and severe clinical symptoms. Loss of air conduction occurs and mastoid tenderness may be present and the mastoid lymph gland may be enlarged. The subsequent course depends on the treatment and unless a paracentesis is performed, spontaneous rupture of the drum usually occurs. The discharge varies in character and infection may spread from the middle ear into the mastoid process. The mucous membrane of the mastoid air cells then becomes thickened and the cells filled with pus. The cell walls become decalcified and an osteomyelitis may occur with breakdown of the cell walls and with the coalescence of two or more cells an abscess forms, usually situated in the peri-antral cells. If the apical cells are involved, and especially if the cortex of the mastoid process is thin, perforation may occur with a resulting abscess formation in the soft tissues of the neck (Von Bezold's abscess) (cf. Chap. X, fig. 217). If there is a congenital dehiscence of the facial canal facial palsy may occur (fig. 200).

If the posterior group of cells around the sigmoid sinus become infected, a lateral sinus thrombosis may occur. There is sometimes considerable difficulty in distinguishing clinically between a case of acute suppurative otitis media and one of acute external otitis. In both there may be acute pain and a purulent discharge, although with simple acute external otitis there is usually a history of itching and eczema of the auricle. X-ray examination will assist in the diagnosis as in external otitis the mastoid cells are comparatively unaffected, whilst in an otitis media there is a loss of translucency of the middle ear generally associated with a clouding of the peri-antral cells and a de-aeration of the Eustachian tube (fig. 198).

Radiological findings. Initially the radiological features in an acute catarrhal and suppurative otitis media are similar and, as spread of infection into the mastoid process occurs, the signs of mastoiditis are superimposed.

(1) *Loss of the normal translucency of the middle ear and Eustachian tube.* The haziness first seen in the Eustachian tube, middle ear and the peri-antral cells rapidly spreads through the cell system. This haziness rapidly changes to a definite cloudiness and is more readily seen in the submento-vertical projection (fig. 198).

(2) *Increase in the prominence of normal markings.* As a result of a loss of translucency in the cells, normal structures such as the sinus plate and tegmen tympani become more apparent because of an enhancement effect of the opaque cells.

(3) *Loss of shadow of the ossicles.* The shadow of the ossicles becomes hazy and blurred by the thickened mucosa and exudate and as the translucency of the middle ear diminishes the shadows of the ossicles become lost. The upper and lower parts of the tympanic ring become difficult to distinguish. The Eustachian tube on the affected side becomes faint or completely invisible owing to a loss of its air content.

(4) *General increase in density of petrous bone.* In addition to the radiological change mentioned it will be found that in the majority of cases a generalised increase in opacity takes place in the affected petrous bone. This opacity which may be quite noticeable is obviously not due to bone change in the acute phase and must therefore be due to pathological changes in the cells in the body of that bone. These cells, as previously mentioned are contiguous with the mastoid cells, but owing to their small size and the density of the surrounding bone are invisible in the normal. When infected, however, they cause a generalised increase in density of the petrous bone which is best seen in the submento-vertical view and transorbital view.

(5) *Loss of outline of cell walls.* As infection progresses the opacity of the mastoid cells increases and the cell walls become more and more indistinct until they may become completely invisible. This is due to two factors, the pus or thickened mucosa in the cells obscures the walls and secondary decalcification of the cell walls takes place due to hyperaemia. Though actual rupture of the cell walls due to erosion and pressure of contained pus may occur, it is often impossible to appreciate this destruction radiologically as previous decalcification may have already made the cell walls invisible on the radiograph. Where, however, the case can be followed by serial radiographs gradual and progressive thinning and destruction of the cell walls may be observed and the resulting abscess noted.

Acute suppurative otitis media in sclerotic mastoids. With good radiographs and a well-pneumatised process and especially if the infection is unilateral, the x-ray diagnosis of acute otitis media is usually easy but an x-ray diagnosis in a diploic or sclerotic mastoid is often a matter of very great difficulty. No peri-antral cells may be present and the sclerotic bone may completely conceal the mastoid antrum. In such a case polycycloidal tomograms taken in the true antero-posterior position may be helpful. Naturally, if virulent infection of the peri-antral cell wall persists, ultimately the resulting bone destruction will become radiologically visible. This destruction will usually be in the direction of the tegmen tympani with possible perforation into the cranial cavity. Once it has been shown that the mastoid is diploic or sclerotic in a case of acute otitis, it should be appreciated that no further x-ray evidence can be expected until actual bone destruction has taken place. X-ray evidence of infection in the middle ear and Eustachian tube may be evident and there may be a generalised abnormal opacity of the petrous bone and mastoid antrum. Generally speaking, the otologist should ignore negative x-ray evidence in cases with sclerotic mastoids and rely on his clinical findings.

Otitis media and chemotherapy. The administration of chemotherapeutic agents has considerably modified the course of the acute otitis media. Resolution of the inflammatory process is the rule (Falbe-Hansen & Becker-Christiansen, 1944) with antibiotics (Weinstein & Atherton, 1945) but unless they are used with correct dosage they may mask the infection without effecting a proper cure. In such cases, the symptoms may be masked but the failure of x-ray appearances to return to normal in "clinically recovered" patients should be viewed with the gravest suspicion. Serial radiography may

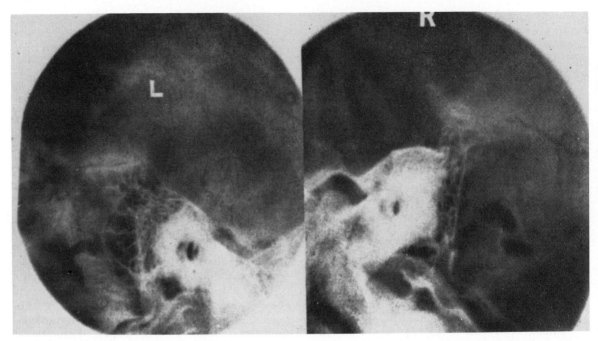

Fig. 201. Mastoiditis and chemotherapy. Lateral views of the mastoid process in a female child aged 10 showing an infected right mastoid but with no obvious breakdown of the cell walls. Pain in the right mastoid was the presenting feature (see also p. 173).

be of utmost importance in assessing re-aeration of the middle ear and mastoid cells which is one of the indices of complete resolution of infection (figs. 201, 202).

Complications. The complications of acute suppurative otitis media are as follows:

(1) *Mastoiditis.* Spread of infection to the mastoid antrum and air cells is almost an invariable complication of acute suppurative otitis media to some degree. The infection may be acute or chronic. The radiological features are discussed later.

(2) *Intracranial spread of infection.* This complication generally follows as a direct sequel of spread of infection through the mastoid process. Meningitis, cerebral abscess or lateral sinus thrombosis all may follow intracranial spread of infection. The radiological features of these conditions are discussed in Chapter 10.

(3) *Infection of the temporo-mandibular joint.* Spread of infection anteriorly may result in an infective arthritis involving the temporo-mandibular joint. Such a sequel is uncommon but Shambaugh (1941) was able to collect three cases showing this complication. The diagnostic criteria are swelling over the temporo-mandibular joint without displacement of the auricle, pain on mastication, limitation of movement, fever and leucocytosis. Radiologically, evidence of involvement of the joint can be seen by widening of the joint space. According to Shambaugh (1941), in cases where the diagnosis is in doubt, diagnostic aspiration of the joint should be undertaken.

Chronic otitis media

Chronic suppurative otitis media is usually the result of persisting infection or of repeated recurrence of the acute attacks. In some cases with a low-grade infection occurring in a diploic or sclerotic mastoid, the condition may be chronic from the outset. The drum usually shows a large perforation and is thickened and retracted. The ossicles may be wholly or partially destroyed. In advanced cases there is often granulation tissue or

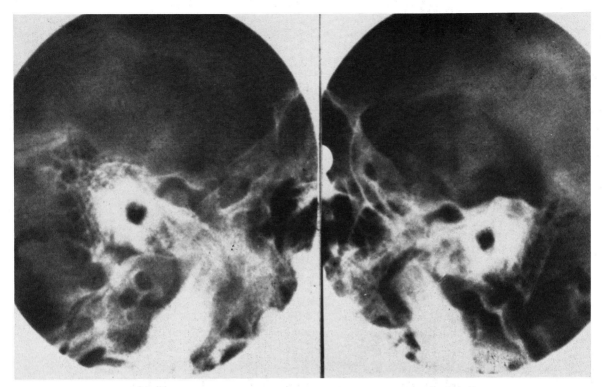

Fig. 202. Same case as fig. 201 seven months later after two further attacks of temperature and pain. Radiological appearances are those of an infected right mastoid showing obliteration of the cell walls with thickening of the walls and general sclerosis. In view of the failure of response to chemotherapy operation was performed and disclosed a chronic suppurative mastoiditis.

polypoid mucosa which may push through the perforated drum and fill the external meatus.

Diploic bone offers a high degree of resistance to infection but once invaded the infection is very persistent. The result is virtually a chronic osteomyelitis of the mastoid process. If the organisms are of low virulence and the patient's resistance good, a cholesteatoma may form. The condition is often associated with a continued foul smelling discharge and a marginal perforation of the drum. The other symptoms of infection such as deafness, vertigo and headache may be prominent. As cholesteatoma forms on the chronic infection it gradually increases in size, completely filling the bony cavity in which it lies, causing erosion of the surrounding bone. Owing to the slow nature of its progress a thin partial or complete reactive ring of sclerosed bone surrounds the cholesteatoma which can be seen in the radiographs. If this process of erosion continues unchecked, eventually per-

foration of the surrounding bony walls occurs. This may be inwards through the tegmen tympani into the cranial cavity, or in other instances perforation may occur into the external auditory meatus, usually in the upper part of its posterior wall. Perforation may also take place into the external semicircular canal resulting in a labyrinthine fistula.

Healed otitis media

Clinically the drum in these cases is often milky and less transparent than normal and the light reflex is lost. It is usually retracted and there are frequently scar areas where previous perforations have occurred. The patient gives no history of ear pain or discharge but complains of deafness. If the deafness is bilateral it may be difficult to distinguish clinically between those cases that give no history of past ear infection and otosclerosis. In this connection, radiology can be of great assistance by demonstrating the signs of past inflammation in the mastoid and the middle ear. It must be borne in mind, however, that a patient suffering from otosclerosis is also liable to otitis media.

Otitis media due to specific organisms

Risch (1939) collected 29 reports of actinomycosis of the ear – of these only 12 affected the middle ear. The condition is uncommon. The vast majority of these cases were fatal, deaths being due to meningitis. Infection of the middle ear is thought to spread up *via* the Eustachian tube. Tuberculous infection of the middle ear may be associated with extensive bone destruction, but there may be no specific radiological features. Successful treatment with streptomycin and surgical treatment has been recorded (Banham & Ransome, 1951).

Secretory otitis media (hydrops of the middle ear)

This is associated with a sterile effusion into the middle ear associated with a blocked Eustachian tube. It may be due to an infection which has been sterilised by antibiotics or an infection of low virulence (Hopple, 1950). Allergy and autonomic imbalance have been also suggested (Hartman, 1952) and lymphoid remnants may cause the Eustachian block. It may present as an acute, subacute or recurrent clinical condition and usually responds to myringotomy or repeated aspiration. Compere (1958) has shown that the rate of clearing of contrast medium injected into the middle ear may be a useful means of differentiating it from infective conditions.

Radiologically the middle ear shows loss of translucency associated with blurring of the shadow of the ossicles. No change is visible in the mastoid cells and the cellular development is normal.

TRAUMATIC LESIONS OF THE MIDDLE EAR

The most frequent result of violence of the middle ear is a rupture of the external fibro-membranous wall – the tympanic membrane. Radiologically, the mishap is not as a rule demonstrable unless the middle ear becomes the seat of a haematoma when loss of translucency may readily be seen.

Fractures involving the middle ear are generally an extension of the fractures of the base of the skull and of the temporal bone – their radiological features will be considered with fractures of the petrous temporal bone. There is, however, one form of trauma that the middle ear is particularly susceptible to, namely, barotrauma. The effects of rapid alteration in barometric pressure on the paranasal sinuses are discussed in Chapter 5. The changes in the middle ear are due to the same mechanism but are probably of greater importance.

Aero-otitis media or barotrauma

One of the main purposes of the Eustachian tube is to equalise between the middle ear and the atmospheric pressure. If the air pressure in the external auditory meatus rises above that in the nasopharynx, there is a sensation of fullness and pain. This inequality of pressure results in invagination of the drum into the cavity of the middle ear and a forcible shift or possible subluxation of the ossicles. Rupture of the drum may occur if the difference in air pressure is sufficient. This may be caused by exposure to factors to which the human ear is structurally unfitted, such as deep sea diving (Schilling, 1945), submersion in caissons, and proximity to violent displacement of the air by loud explosions. By far the commonest cause of this disability, however, has been the rapid alterations in atmospheric pressure produced by flying (Armstrong & Heim, 1937). Aero-otitis media may be best defined as a traumatic inflammation of the middle ear caused by a difference in pressure on the two sides of the drum (Whaley, 1942; Stewart, Warwick & Bateman, 1945). During ascent, air spills from the Eustachian tube into the nasopharynx and this as a rule causes no symptoms. The reverse conditions hold during descent, when air is forced into the middle ear along the Eustachian tube. If the Eustachian tube is blocked aero-otitis occurs. Any infection of the nose or nasopharynx by virtue of its tendency to block the Eustachian tube will, of course, increase the risk of aero-otitis media.

Kelly & Langheinz (1946) have reported cases in which they believe that dental malocclusion had been partly responsible for the development of aero-otitis media. These and other authors believe that free drainage of the middle ear *via* Eustachian tube is interfered with by muscular tensions due to abnormal jaw movements. They believe that restoration of normal mandibular movements relieves the mucosal congestion of the Eustachian tube. Radiographs of the temporo-mandibular joint are made in both the open and closed positions and the range of movement is then compared with the normal.

Larkin (1944) of the United States Naval Medical Services made an extensive roentgenological study of aero-otitis media. He demonstrated radiologically the shift of the ossicles due to retraction of the drum. In aero-otitis media, as a result of a change in the osmotic pressure a resulting exudation of lymph causes the middle ear to fill with fluid and become opaque.

REFERENCES

ALEXANDER, G. (1908) Die Ohrenkrankheiten im Kindesalter. F. C. W. Vogel, Leipzig 1912. Z. Ohrenheilk., 55, 144.

ARMSTRONG, H.G. & HEIM, J. W. (1937) Effect of Flight on the Middle Ear. J. Am. med. Ass., 109, 417.

BANHAM, T. M. & RANSOME, J. (1951) Tuberculous Mastoiditis Treated with Streptomycin. J. Lar. Otol., 65, 102.

BECK, O. (1930) Quoted by JACKSON, C. & COATES, G. M. The Nose, Throat and Ear and their Diseases. Philadelphia: W. B. Saunders Co.

BRITTON, J. A. & WALSH, E. L. (1940) Health Hazards of Electric and Gas Welding. J. ind. Hyg. Toxicol., 22, 125.

BROCK, W. (1926) Trommelfellbild und pneumatisation des Warzenteils; eine röntgenologische Studie. Z. Hals-Nasen-u.-Ohrenheilk., 15.

BROWN, J. M. (1942) Actinomycosis of Temporal Bone. Laryngoscope, 52, 507.

CAMP, J. D. & ALLEN, E. P. (1940) Microtia and Congenital Atresia of the External Auditory Canal. Am. J. Roent., 43, 201.

CHILDREY, J. H. (1932) Calcigerous Metaplasia in the Auricle. Archs Otolar., 15, 883.

COMPERE, W. E. (1958) Tympanic Cavity Clearance Studies. Trans. Am. Acad. Ophthal. Oto-lar., May–June, p. 444.

CONLEY, J. J. (1946) Atresia of External Auditory Canal Occurring in Military Service. Report on Correction of this Condition in 10 Cases. Archs Otol., 43, 613.

DAHLBERG, G. & DIAMANT, M. (1945) Hereditary Character of the Cellular System in the Mastoid Patient. Acta otolar., 33, 378.

DEAN, L.W. & GITTINS, T. R. (1917) Congenital Osseous Atresia of External Auditory Canal. Laryngoscope, 27, 461.

DIAMANT, M. (1940) Otitis and Size of the Air Cell System. Acta radiol., 21, 543.

DIAMANT, M. (1940) Otitis and Pneumatisation of Mastoid Bone. Acta otol. (Suppl.), 41, 1.

DIAMANT, M. (1952) Chronic otitis: a Critical Analysis. Pract. Oto-Rhino-Laryng., 14/1 (Suppl.).

DIBOLD, H. & HUBER, K. (1938) Wundheilung bei diabetes. Fortschr. Ther., 14, 113.

DRUSS, J. G. & ALLEN, B. (1942) Acute Mastoiditis in Diabetes Mellitus. Archs Otolar., 36, 12.

FALBE-HANSEN, & BECKER-CHRISTIANSEN, D. (1944) On Sulfonamide Therapy in Acute Suppurative Otitis Media with Special Reference to Otitis in Children. Acta Otolar., 32, 209.

FITZ, C. R. & HARWOOD-NASH, D. C. F. (1974) Radiology of the Ear in Children. Radiol. Clin. N. Am., 12, 553.

FOWLER, E. P. & SWENSON, P. C. (1939) Petrositis. Am. J. Roentg., 41, 317.

FRASER, J. S. (1931) Maldevelopment of the Auricle, External Acoustic Meatus and Middle Ear. Archs Otolar., 13, 1.

FREY, K. W. (1965) Die Tomographe der Labyrinthmissbildungen. Fortschr. Geb. RöntgStrahl., 102, 1.

FRIEDMAN, J. (1957) Bacteriology of Acute Otitis Media. Proc. R. Soc. Med., 50, 406.

FUCHS, A. W. (1943) Roentgenography of the External Ear. Am. J. Roent., 49, 420.

HARTMAN, O. (1952) Secretory Otitis Media. Classification Based on Amenability. Bull. N.Y. Acad. Med., 28, 817.

HASTINGS, H. (1937) A piece of Gold Bougie (20 Years in situ) Removed from Distal Half of Eustachian Tube During a Radical Mastoid Operation. Ann. Otol. Rhinol Lar., 44, 213.

HAUG, R. (1939) Ein fall von Verknöcherung der Ohrmuschel. Mschr. Ohrenheilk. Lar.-Rhinol., 73, 287.

HOPPLE, G. D. (1950) Otitis Media with Effusion – a Challenge to Otorhinolaryngology. Laryngoscope, 60, 315.

JARVIS, J. L., JENKINS, D., SOSMAN, M. C. & THORN, G. W. (1954) Roentgenological Observations in Addison's Disease. Radiology, 62, 16.

JENSEN, J. (1974) Congenital Anomalies of the Inner Ear. Radiol. Clin. N. Am., 12, 473.

KECHT, B. & DIBOLD, H. (1936) Diabetes und Eiterungen im Mittelohr, Nasennebenholen und Rachen. Z. Hals-Nasen-u-Ohrenheilk., 39, 288.

KELLY, W. J. & LANGHEINZ, H. W. (1946). Dental Treatment for Prevention of Aerotitis Media. Ann. Otol. Rhinol. Lar., 55, 13.

LAPAYOWKER, M. S., LIEBMAN, E. P. & RONIS, M. L. (1971) Presentation of the Internal Carotid Artery as a Tumour of the Middle Ear. Radiology, 98, 293.

LARKIN, J. C. (1944) Aero-otitis Media. Am. J. Roentg., 51, 178.

LONGAKER, E. P. (1929) Two Interesting Foreign Body Cases of the Mastoid and the Nose. *Ann. Otol. Rhinol. Lar.*, **38**, 1158.

LOWE, J. R., BAMFORTH, J. S. & PRACY, R. (1963) Acute Otitis Media. *Lancet*, **ii**, 1129.

LUND, H. (1929) *Arch. Ohr.-Nas.-u. KehlkHeilk.*, **122**, 195.

MANGIARACINA, A. (1940) Foreign Bodies in the Eustachian Tube. *Archs Otolar.*, **32**, 517.

MAYER, E. H. (1939). Outis bei diabetes. *Mschr. Ohrenheilk. Lar.-Rhinol.*, **73**, 305.

MICHEL, E. M. (1863) Memoire sur les anomalies congenitales de l'oreille interne. *Gaz. méd. Strasb.*, *1*, *ser.*, *23 anee*, **55**: (14).

MUNDINI, C. (1791) Anatomici surdi nati sectro Bononiensi scientarium et artium instituto atque academia commentarii VII, 419.

NATHANSON, L. & LOSNER, S. (1947) Ossification of auricles of the External Ears Associated with Acromegaly. *Radiology*, **48**, 66.

PALMER, F. E. & REIFSNEIDER, J. S. (1933) Plastic Reconstruction of the External Meatus. *Laryngoscope*, **43**, 618.

PHELPS, P. D., LLOYD, G. A. S. & SHELDON, P. W. E. (1975) Deformity of the Labyrinth and Internal Auditory Meatus in Congenital Deafness. *Br. J. Radiol.*, **48**, 973.

PHELPS, P. D. & LLOYD, G. A. S. (1976) Congenital Deformity of the Internal Auditory Meatus and Labyrinth associated with Liquor Fistula. *VII International Congress of Radiology in O.R.L., Copenhagen, 1976*.

POLITZER, G. & MAYER, E. G. (1925) Uber Angeborenen Verschluss und Verengening des aussfen Gehörgangs und ihre formale genese. *Virchow's Arch. path. Anat. Physiol.*, **258**, 206.

POMERANZ, M. M., FRIEDMAN, L. J. & TUNICK, I. S. (1941) Roentgenological Findings in Alkaptonuric Ochronosis. *Radiology*, **37**, 295.

RICHARDS, L. (1933) Congenital Atresia of the External Auditory Meatus. *Ann. Otol. Rhinol. Lar.*, **42**, 692.

RISCH, O. C. (1939) Actinomycosis of Ear. *Archs Otolar.*, **29**, 235.

SCHERRER, F. W. (1932) Calcification of the External Ear. *Ann. Otol. Rhinol. Lar.*, **41**, 867.

SCHILLING, C. W. (1945) Aero-otitis Media and Loss of Auditory Acuity in Submarine Escape Training. *Archs Otolar.*, **42**, 169.

SCHWARTZ, H. W. (1951) The Influence of Heredity on the Pneumatisation of the Temporal Bone. *J. Lar. Otol.*, **65**, 317.

SHAMBAUGH, G. E. (1941) Involvement of the Jaw Joint in Acute Suppurative Otitis Media. *Archs Otolar.*, **33**, 975.

SIIRALA, U. (1947) Influence of Sulphonamides on Infectious Otitis Interna. *Acta otolar.*, **35**, 77.

STEWART, C. B., WARWICK, O. H. & BATEMAN, G. L. (1945) Acute Otitic Barotrauma Resulting from Low Pressure Chamber Tests. *J. Aviat. Med.*, **16**, 385.

TERRAHE, K. (1972) Diagnostik der Missbildungen des Ohres und des Ohrschädels. *Arch. klin. exp. Ohr.-Nas.-u.-KehlkHeilk.*, **202**, 85.

TERRAHE, K. (1965) Malformation of the Inner Ear due to Thalidomide Embryopathy. Results of Tomography of the Ear. *Fortschr. Geb. RöntgStrahl.*, **102**, 14.

VALVASSORI, G. E. (1963) Laminagraphy of the Ears. *Am. J. Roentg.*, **89**, 1168, also p. 1158.

WEINSTEIN, L. & ATHERTON, H. B. (1945) The Treatment of Acute Suppurative Otitis Media with Penicillin. *J. Am. med. Ass.*, **129**, 503.

WHALEY, J. B. (1942) Problems of Aviation Medicine Relating to Ear, Nose and Throat. *Archs Otolar.*, **26**, 438.

CHAPTER 10

Traumatic and other lesions of the Temporal bone

TRAUMA

(a) Rupture of the drum

Rupture of the tympanic membrane is the commonest result of injury to the ear. It usually follows a blow on the ear or less frequently is the result of a sudden alteration in atmospheric pressure (*e.g.* in aircraft decompression or in deep sea diving). Blasts from gunfire or explosions can also rupture the drum.

Clinical inspection is the surest and most rapid means of diagnosis but submento-vertical views will frequently reveal blurring and haziness of the middle ear due to haemorrhage into the tympanic cavity.

(b) Ossicular chain

Damage to the auditory ossicles may complicate rupture of the tympanic membrane or may occur with an intact drum. These injuries result in conductive deafness but as they are frequently associated with multiple injuries, as in motor car accidents, the hearing defect may be initially overlooked.

The incus because of its relative instability is particularly prone to dislocation and displacement. Complete displacements can usually be readily seen in lateral tomographs when the "molar tooth" appearance of the ossicles is lost. Postero-anterior tomographs will reveal the incus lying in an abnormal position. Dislocations of the incudo-stapedial joint are more difficult to see and demand a high technical standard (Hough, 1959). Dislocations and displacement of the incus may also be associated with longitudinal fractures of the petrous bone. Submento-vertical tomographs are superior to lateral tomograms in demonstrating

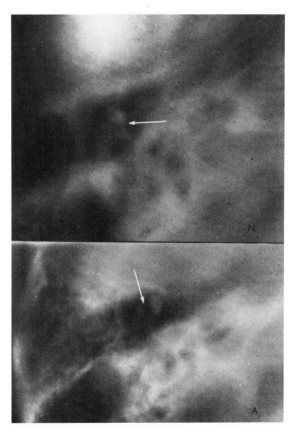

Fig. 203. Dislocation of the ossicles.
N—zonogram in submento-vertical position showing the normal inco-malleal joint.
A—the displacement and disruption of this joint is seen.

minor displacements of the incudo-mallear joint (fig. 203).

The malleus, because of its attachment to the drum, is less liable to displacement whilst fractures of the crura – or footplate of the stapes – usually occur in association with fractures of the petrous bone. Hough & Stuart (1968) found that in approximately 38·5% of cases of conductive deafness occurring after injury the following changes were found in the ossicular chain. In the remainder no changes were shown.

TABLE I

SURGICAL FINDINGS IN 31 EARS

1. Posterior bony canal wall fracture	66·66%
2. Incudostapedial joint separation	82·3%
3. Massive dislocation of the incus	57·1%
4. Fracture of the stapedial arch	30·0%
5. Fracture of the malleus	11·0%
6. Fixation of the upper ossicular chain	25·0%
7. Multiple concomitant middle ear pathology	34·5%

(Table reproduced with kind permission of Drs Hough and Stuart)

Full radiological examination for possible middle ear damage frequently has to be delayed until the patient has recovered sufficiently from associated injuries to allow full cooperation during the examination.

(c) Fractures

Fracture of the petrous bones is usually an extension from fractures of the vertex or base of the skull (Grove, 1939). Fractures may be seen often with some difficulty in 80–90% of conventional views. Pleuridirectional tomography is a much more rewarding investigation (Wright, 1974). Valvassori (1964) has classified the radiological appearances of fractures as follows (fig. 204):

(i) *Extra-labyrinthine fractures* – these are the commonest fractures and are usually an extension of a fracture from the squamous temporal and extend through the epitympanic recess into the thin roof of the tegmen tympani.

(ii) *Labyrinthine fractures (transverse, vertical)* – these fractures extend through the petrous bone and are often known as transverse or vertical fractures. They commence in the region of the jugular foramen and extend forward either laterally through the vestibule, cochlea or semicircular canal, or medially through the internal auditory meatus to the region of the foramen rotundum. These fractures invariably produce inner ear deafness. As the petrous bone is

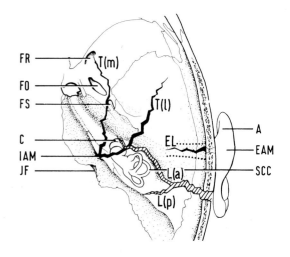

T=Transverse   L=Longitudinal   EL=Extra labyrinthine

Fig. 204. Fractures of petrous bone. Schematic drawing to illustrate the course of the three types of fracture lines involving the mastoid process. Note that the course of both transverse and longitudinal may be in two directions, in the case of the transverse fracture in a medial (Tm) and lateral route (Tl), and in an anterior (La) and posterior (Lp) in the case of the longitudinal fracture.
FR and FO—foramen rotundum and ovale
FS—foramen spinosum
IAM and EAM—internal and external meatus
C—cochlea.

enchondral in origin these fractures fail to unite and can be seen years after the injury (figs. 205, 206).

(iii) *Tympano-labyrinth (Longitudinal – Druss, 1951)* – These fractures extend obliquely across the petrous bone starting as an extension of the squamous fracture in the region of the lateral sinus or external auditory canal, through the tympanic cavity into the labyrinth. The fracture line may proceed anteriorly into the middle cranial fossa or may veer behind to the posterior surface of the petrous bone. These fractures as they frequently cross the medial wall of the tympanic cavity may involve the facial canal or ossicular chain (Hough & Stuart, 1968) (fig. 204).

Radiological features

Estimation of the full extent of fractures of the petrous bone can only be made by accurate tomo-

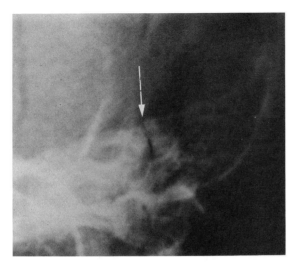

Fig. 205. Transverse fracture through petrous bone, the fracture line passes through the bony labyrinth. Such fractures are almost invariably associated with deafness.

Barrois, 1959) but Du Boulay & Bostick (1969) claim that oblique linear tomography may be as good, and in some cases, even better than the more complex tomographic movements.

When the fracture extends from the vertex the mastoid cells through which it traverses usually give a clue to the involvement of the petrous bone as the cells surrounding the fracture line become blurred and hazy due to extravasated blood and oedema. If however, the cell walls in the affected area become lost this indicates that infection has supervened although Whittaker (1944) found that superadded infection was not a frequent complication when the only associated injury was a ruptured tympanic membrane.

Determination of the site and extent of fracture of the petrous bone is most frequently required in cases developing facial paralysis after a head injury. In those cases lateral tomography to outline the facial canal is of utmost importance to indicate the exact site and extent of injury. The tympano-labyrinthine fracture is particularly liable to involve the facial nerve below the genu, and then effective decompression of the facial canal (if necessary associated with a nerve graft) may be of the utmost value in securing complete healing (fig. 207).

Compression of the facial nerve by depressed

graphy in both antero-posterior and lateral planes and even then the length of fracture is usually considerably greater than demonstrated. Tomography using ellipsoid or hypocycloidal movement is superior to linear tomography (Francois &

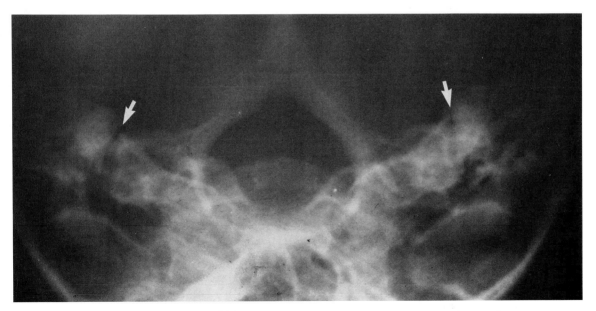

Fig. 206. Bilateral fractures of the petrous temporal bone in a young child of 12 after a motor car accident. Deafness was present on both sides.

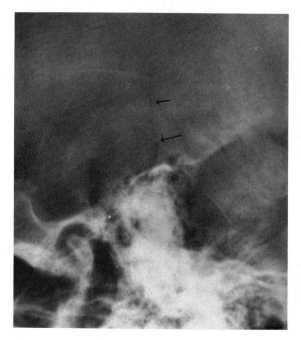

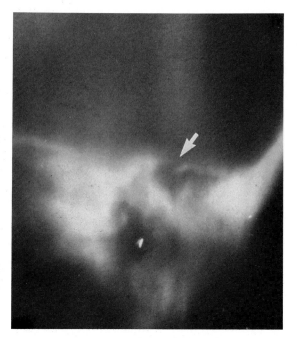

Fig. 207. Fracture of Petrous Bone.

Motor car accident Head injury. One week later developed facial palsy. Lateral oblique view showing downward spread of parietal fracture into the mastoid process and involving the facial canal. Involvement of the descending portion of the facial canal indicates a site of possible success with surgical interference. Fracture lines involving the horizontal portion are not amenable to surgical treatment.

Fig. 208. Fracture of petrous bone. Tomograph in postero-anterior view demonstrating fracture line extending through petrous bone into region of mastoid antrum.

bone spicules from the walls can be seen on the lateral tomograms and is an indication for early **decompression (Wright, 1974)** (figs. 208, 209, 210 and 211).

Fractures of the external auditory meatus usually involve the anterior wall and may follow blows on the angle of the jaw. They can be seen in lateral tomographs but the normal fissure (petro-mastoid fissure) must not be confused with a fracture line. Bleeding from the external meatus may occur infrequently as a result of this type of fracture but haemorrhage from the external meatus is far more likely to be due to a ruptured drum.

FOREIGN BODIES

Industrial accidents concerned with the welding process result in fragments of molten metal (slag) entering the middle ear. As the result of the

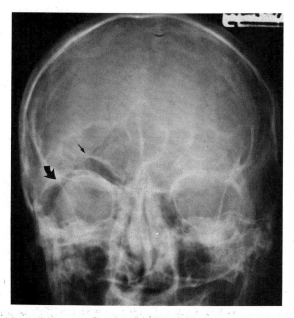

Fig. 209. Fracture of vertex of skull extending into petrous bone (longitudinal type) with wide separation of fractured fragments.

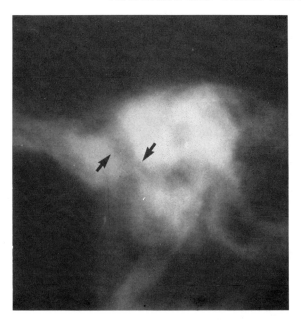

Fig. 210. Lateral tomograph of case shown in fig. 209 showing wide separation of fracture line.

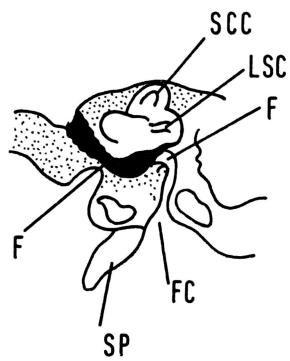

Fig. 211. Line drawing of fig. 210.
SSC—superior semicircular canal   F—fracture
LSC—lateral semicircular canal   SP—stylomastoid process.
FC—facial canal

presence of a foreign body infection and trauma almost invariably occur with the development of an acute or subacute middle ear infection with a mastoiditis (see Chapter 9, figs. 194 and 195).

An elongated stylo-mastoid process may present as an unexplained cause of pain in the tonsillar bed acting as a foreign body involving the tonsillar bed.

Radiographic examination of these cases reveals an elongated styloid process directed forwards or a normal sized process angled more medially than normal. Lateral films determine the length of the process and lateral or medial deviation of the process or curvature of the tip are seen in the antero-posterior view.

The exact amount of the styloid process to be excised at operation to relieve symptoms can be estimated from the radiograph and excision is generally associated with complete relief of symptoms (Wilson & McAlpine, 1946).

INFLAMMATORY DISEASE OF THE MASTOID PROCESS

As already stated, in the vast majority of instances, infection spreads to the mastoid *via* the middle ear. Only on rare occasions with a specific type of infection, *e.g.* tuberculosis, is the infection borne by the blood stream. Inflammatory diseases of the mastoid process may be classified as follows:

Acute mastoiditis

— catarrhal or suppurative
— with abscess formation

Chronic mastoiditis

— with abscess formation
— cholesteatoma
— acute on chronic mastoiditis

MASTOIDITIS

Acute mastoiditis

The mucosal changes in catarrhal mastoiditis are represented by oedema and swelling of the mucosa of the cells but without pus formation. These

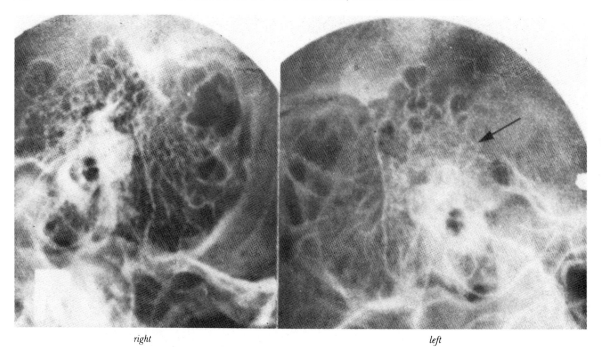

right   *left*

Fig. 212. Acute left mastoiditis – early changes visible in a cellular mastoid with clouding and loss of translucency of the cells particularly in the peri-antral region but no breakdown of cell walls.

changes are especially well seen in the peri-antral mastoid cells when the middle ear is the site of an acute otitis media. The appearance of clouding in these cases should not necessarily be taken to imply a developing mastoiditis as oedema of the cell mucosa alone will produce demonstrable clouding on the radiograph. The differentiation of catarrhal mastoiditis from a developing suppurative mastoiditis may be impossible on radiographic grounds.

Shadows in the subcutaneous tissue overlying the mastoid process may also give the appearance of clouding of the mastoid cells. Thus with an external otitis the swelling of the post-auricular gland may cast a shadow over the mastoid process suggesting early infection of the mastoid cells.

Opacities of the mastoid cells may also be caused by physical agents. Thus, as a sequel of radium or x-ray treatment to skin lesions, *e.g.* rodent ulcer in the region of the auricle, clouding of the mastoid cells may develop.

Trauma to the external ear may also produce oedema and haemorrhage into the mastoid cells, giving an appearance similar to that seen in catarrhal mastoiditis. If there is any degree of swelling of the pinna it may overlie the mastoid process and mimic a catarrhal change in the underlying mastoid cells.

In acute suppurative mastoiditis the mastoid cells become filled with pus and as the inflammatory process proceeds the cell walls become decalcified and destroyed. Radiologically demonstrable destruction of the cell walls usually appears some 10–12 days after the onset of infection.

Radiological appearances

(i) The earliest change is a *loss of translucency of the cells particularly around the mastoid antrum*. These changes rapidly spread throughout all the mastoid air cells (fig. 212).

(ii) As a result of the diminished translucency of the whole of the mastoid process, *certain bony structures which are not normally visible become prominent*. The sinus plate becomes accentuated and for the same reason the tegmen tympani can be more clearly visualised (figs. 213, 214).

(iii) *The bony cell walls as a result of infection decalcify*

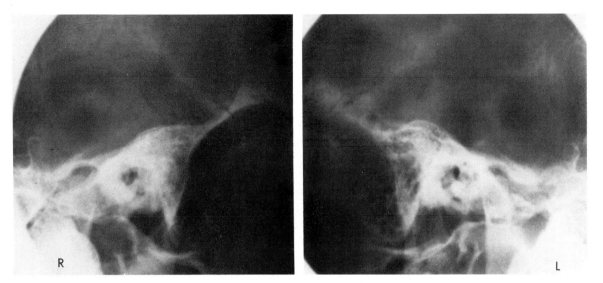

Fig. 213. Acute mastoiditis. Lateral oblique views of right mastoid shows blurring of all cell outlines and loss of translucency throughout the mastoid cells. Left mastoid process shows normal cell translucency.

and disappear (fig. 215). The interpretation of such changes in the bony walls calls for considerable experience and care. In the acute stage some cell walls can apparently be clearly seen whilst operative findings indicate that breakdown of these cell walls has clearly occurred. In such cases the explanation proposed (Pancoast, 1940) is that the portion of the cell wall remaining is sufficiently dense to cast a shadow indistinguishable from normal cell walls.

Likewise, in many radiographs the cell walls have apparently disappeared whilst at operation distinct cells walls can be seen. In these cases the radiographic appearances have been produced by a decalcification of the cell wall rather than an actual bony destruction.

The radiographic determination of destruction as opposed to decalcification of cell walls can only definitely be made by serial x-ray examination. In cases

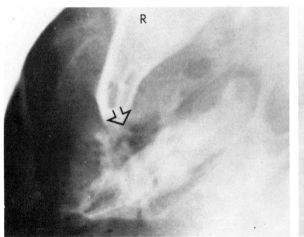

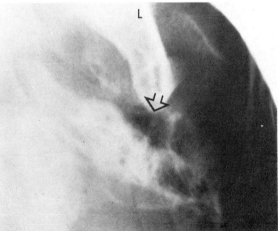

Fig. 214. Submentovertical view of case shown in fig. 213. The right middle ear shows loss of translucency and blurring of the ossicular shadows due to the exudate present in the middle ear.

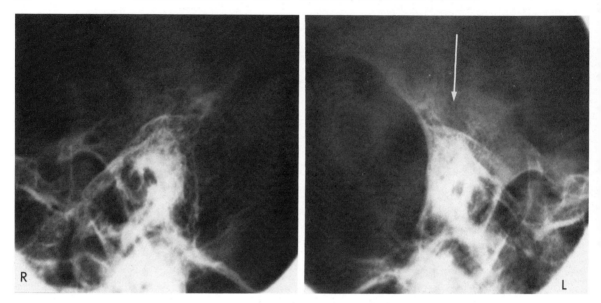

Fig. 215. Acute mastoiditis. The left mastoid process shows a diffuse loss of translucency affecting the whole of the left mastoid cell system. In the peri-antral region (arrow), however, there is a breakdown of the cell walls with the development of abscess formation. The sinus plate in the left mastoid process is clearly seen.

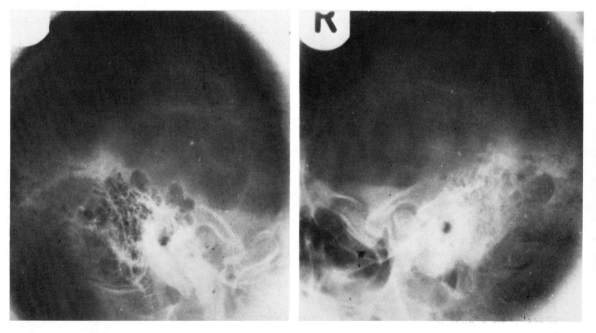

Fig. 216. Acute mastoiditis in a cellular mastoid, clouding of the cells with some disappearance of cell walls in the perisinus region of the right mastoid process.

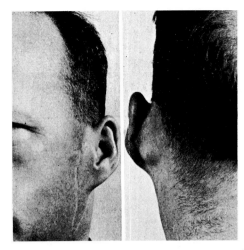

Fig. 217. – Von Bezold's abscess. Abscess formation presenting in the soft tissues near the tip of the mastoid process. Von Bezold's abscess usually presents at a considerably lower level. The scar in front of the auricle is from the removal of a parotid tumour. A left mastoidectomy had been performed in infancy and had no symptoms until a few weeks previously he developed pain in the left ear. On examination a fluctuant swelling was present behind and below the left ear.

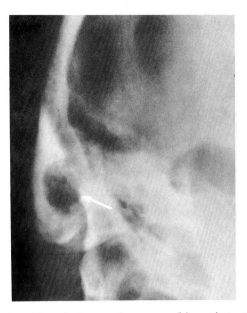

Fig. 218. Mastoid abscess – large area of bone destruction present in the mastoid cavity with sclerosis and irregularity of outlines of the cavity.

where serial films are impracticable the following features assist in the diagnosis of destruction of the cell walls (fig. 215).

(a) The outline of the cell wall becomes blurred and hazy.
(b) The wall may become "spotty". Variation in the density of the cell wall at any point is strong evidence of actual necrosis of the cell wall (fig. 216).
(c) The cavities of the cells themselves become widened.

Abscess formation. As infection spreads the cell walls may necrose and disappear. Coalescence of the pus-filled cells gives rise to abscess formation. As infection spreads from the mastoid antrum destruction is most marked in the cells around the mastoid antrum and it follows that the first signs of bone absorption are seen in this region. The location of the abscess cavity is of considerable importance to the otologist and the radiologist can furnish valuable assistance by indicating the site and the extent of the abscess. The abscess cavity may originate in the region of the sinus plate and its development should be suspected when the clarity with which the sinus plate was previously visualised

in a clouded mastoid becomes lost. In other instances the abscess may track upwards towards the tegmen tympani and a radiographic demonstration of a loss of the normal clear-cut outline of this structure indicates the possibility of an intracranial spread with the formation of an extradural abscess.

If the abscess involves the tip of the mastoid process, a site where a large solitary cell (tip cell) is often located, the abscess may erode the cortex of the bone and spread into the soft tissues of the neck (Bezold's abscess) (figs. 217, 218).

In more fortunate circumstances the abscess tracks in a more superficial direction and may perforate the posterior meatal wall with spontaneous discharge of the abscess. The detection of erosion of the posterior meatal wall is difficult to visualise radiologically and erosion may be overlooked.

In the diagnosis of an abscess care must be taken not to mistake normal cell markings for bone destruction. A normal marking frequently mistaken for a large antrum or abscess cavity is an anteriorly placed lateral sinus or an unusually prominent genu in the sinus. In the Towne's projection the genu of the sinus overlies the mastoid antrum and

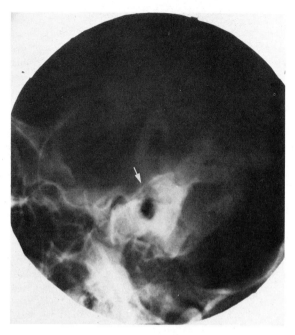

Fig. 219. Chronic mastoiditis. The cells in the mastoid process are absent and the process is composed of dense sclerotic bone. Some erosion of bone is, however, present in the attic region (arrow).

may be mistaken for an abscess cavity. In the lateral views the true nature of the marking can be quickly appreciated.

One fallacy in the interpretation of an abscess formation is the appearance of a giant mastoid cell (Law, 1920). In such cases a careful examination will reveal a well defined bony cortex usually paper-thin, a feature practically never seen in an acute abscess.

Acute mastoiditis occurring in a diploic or mixed type of mastoid process is a disappointing field for the radiologist. The radiological signs in such cases may be absent and reliance on clinical judgment is essential. In the mixed type of mastoid the small cells with thick bony walls seldom give rise to sufficient changes to allow an accurate radiological diagnosis unless bony destruction is pronounced.

Chronic mastoiditis

Chronic infection of any bone is characterised by new bone formation and sclerosis and in this the mastoid process is no exception. The presenting radiological feature in chronic mastoiditis is thus sclerosis. The extent of sclerosis is dependent on the infecting organism, the duration of the disease and the adequacy of treatment. The role played by infection on the degree of pneumatisation in the mastoid process has already been considered. Thus mastoid processes which have been subjected to infection during their development are usually poorly pneumatised and the cell walls are sclerosed and dense (fig. 219). The number of cells present in the mastoid process largely depends on the extent of pneumatisation which had already occurred when infection supervened and arrested the process of pneumatisation, but obliteration of the mastoid air cells may occur directly as the result of sclerosing osteitis associated with infection.

The few cells visible in the peri-antral region in chronic mastoid infection generally show such thick walls as to make the interpretation of changes in the translucency of the cells extremely difficult.

Chronic mastoiditis is usually a sequel of acute or subacute mastoiditis but in some cases it may be due to a specific organism, *e.g.* tuberculosis or actinomycosis. These organisms, however, differ in their radiological appearances from the usual type of chronic mastoiditis in that they produce destruction rather than sclerosis. Proctor & Lindsay (1942) reported on the clinical and pathological aspects of eight cases of tuberculosis involving the temporal bone. Adams (1942) noted that a tuberculous infection of the middle ear frequently followed thoracoplasty, material presumably being aspirated through the Eustachian tube. Actinomycotic infection of the temporal bone is excessively rare, only 14 cases involving the temporal bone were reported between 1890 and 1939 (Brown, 1943). This infection spreads by direct continuity and intracranial complications may develop without warning. The lesion is entirely destructive – sclerosis being unusual and in this feature resembling tuberculosis.

Chronic mastoiditis with abscess formation. Owing to the bony density of the mastoid process, abscess formation in a chronic mastoid is often overlooked radiologically until the abscess is quite large. In the early stages the radiological changes are those of small mottled areas of increased translucency. At this stage there may be considerable difficulty in differentiating these translucent areas from residual small cells. The presence of a white pencil-line bony wall will assist in the recognition of a cell. Ultimately coalescence of the areas of translucency may occur with the formation of a single translucent area representing the abscess cavity.

The abscess cavity may extend throughout the mastoid process burrowing along the sinus plate and beneath the tegmen tympani. The condition has to be differentiated from a destruction due to other causes such as a cholesteatoma of an operation cavity. The differentiation from a cholesteatoma can usually be made on the blurred outline of the abscess cavity contrasting with the well defined outline of a cholesteatoma. The detection of a residual or abscess cavity in a mastoid containing an operation cavity presents an extremely difficult radiological problem. In such cases an irregular extension with ill-defined, blurred walls extending from a clear-cut operation cavity points to abscess formation.

Cholesteatoma, defined by Young (1950) is a "smooth-walled silvery cyst" lying in a bony cavity and easily detached from its bed. The cyst wall consists of concentric layers of epithelium, the parietal surface actively growing and shedding squames so that the wall is a series of successive layers. Friedman (1974) has suggested the term "epidermoid cholesteatoma" to emphasise the origin from squamous epithelium. Two types of cholesteatoma are recognised by most authors:

(i) The epidermoid (cholesteatoma) tumour which is undoubtedly derived from a congenital epithelial rest (Jefferson & Smalley, 1938). Such tumours are frequently intradural and confusion with the second type only really arises when the latter occurs in the temporal bone. Mahoney (1936) adding five personal cases, was able to find 142 examples of intradural epidermoid recorded in the literature.

(ii) Cholesteatoma associated with chronic suppuration. There is considerable controversy as to the origin of the squamous epithelium forming a cholesteatoma. The majority of otologists subscribe to Habermann's and Von Bezold's original hypothesis that the epithelium is derived from the external auditory canal or middle ear and is the sequel of metaplasia of the epithelium. Polvogt (1929) considered that the epithelium of the external auditory canal grew into the middle ear and attic through a perforation in the tympanic membrane. Cellular metaplasia of the mucosa of the middle ear is also considered by the same author to be a possible source of cholesteatoma. Tumarkin (1954) however, produced evidence which suggests that the attic was lined by specific epithelium which became hyperplastic, giving origin to the cholesteatoma. The researches of Hallpike (1950) have greatly illuminated the possible origins of cholesteatoma. He subscribes to the opinion that cholesteatomas are of two types – the true congenital (embryonal) type and a more common type, a sequel of chronic suppuration. These considerations are based on Hallpike's routine sections of temporal bones which showed isolated masses of epithelial cell rests in the attic without any evidence of previous infection or perforation of the drum. He and others (Cawthorne & Pickard, 1965) claim that the cholesteatoma is produced by irritation of these cell rests leading to proliferation and pseudo-tumour development.

On rare occasions cholesteatoma may develop as foreign body reaction and they have been noted to develop after the use of sulphonamide powder (Jongkees, 1948). This author does not record any radiological appearances but from the description of the operative findings it would appear that these appearances would not differ from other types of cholesteatoma.

Radiological appearances. The vast majority of cholesteatomas arise in the middle ear or attic and it has been stated that 20% of cholesteatomas remain entirely attic in site (Becker & Woloshin, 1962). Cholesteatoma itself casts no shadow and its presence can only be inferred from the bone erosion it produces. Consequently those cholesteatomas which do not produce bone erosion cannot be diagnosed radiologically (Waltner, 1949).

Considerable discussion has occurred as to the number of cholesteatoma which cannot be shown by radiology. Figures showing the extreme rarity of normal cell development in cases of cholesteatoma have been collected by Nilsson (1948), Gaben (1936) 0·3%; Steurer (1937) 0·25%; Wustman (1942) 0·2% – (an average figure of 0·2% to 0·3%. Welin, 1941). Winderen & Zimmer (1954) are not in agreement with these figures and they found that the percentage of pneumatisation was considerably higher. This is of importance as the complications of cholesteatoma were far higher in a cellular than in a sclerotic mastoid. Cholesteatoma occurring in

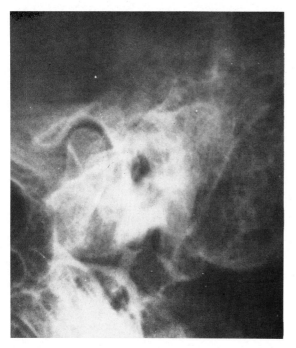

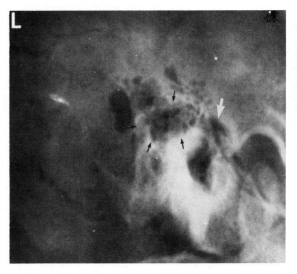

Fig. 221. Cholesteatoma occurring in cellular mastoid. The attic is expanded (white arrow) and the extension posteriorly into the mastoid antral cavity is shown (black arrows).

Fig. 220. Cholesteatoma occurring in a cellular mastoid. Some breakdown of cell walls and loss of translucency is present. The development of a cholesteatoma in a cellular mastoid is exceptional.

cellular mastoids particularly in children may be a **cholesterol granuloma** (black cellular cholesteatoma, Birrell, 1956) and fundamentally consists of granulation tissue with cholesterol crystals (figs. 220, 221).

Winderen & Zimmer (1954) claim an accuracy of 91% in the radiological diagnosis of cholesteatoma. These figures must be qualified in that in cases of chronic otitis media negative radiological findings were far less accurate, and in almost one-third of cases of chronic otitis media cholesteatoma was diagnosed when in fact it was not present. The accuracy of radiological examination undoubtedly depends on the extent of bone destruction, but also on the meticulousness of radiological technique and on the experience of the examiner.

Bone erosion. The cause of bone erosion in cholesteatoma is due to enzymal or chemical factors rather than to pressure erosion (Friedman, 1974). As the majority of cholesteatoma arise in the attic the bone erosion depends on the pathway of spread if upwards, to involve the tegmen tympani, anteriorly into the Eustachian tube, more com-

monly backwards through the aditus ad antrum into the mastoid antrum.

More difficult to appreciate radiologically is erosion of the medial or lateral wall of the attic or middle ear. Spread of the cholesteatoma with erosion of the walls of the external auditory meatus may be very difficult to recognise although polycycloidal tomography is of immense help.

It is important to appreciate that cholesteatoma can occur without any radiological changes and that other causes of bone erosion, indistinguishable from cholesteatoma, may be abscess formation or granulation tissue.

The area of bone erosion has a clear-cut outline with a marginal sclerosis surrounding the bone defect. The larger and more evenly contoured the area of bone destruction the more easy the diagnosis, but the recognition of the bone erosion with a thin marginal sclerotic line is the key in early diagnosis.

Detection of early erosive changes is easier in the sclerotic than in a cellular mastoid. If a small area of bone erosion is overlaid by many cells it may be impossible to detect.

Active infection may considerably alter the radiological picture and the sharply defined cavity walls may become blurred and indistinguishable from an osteitis associated with chronic infection. Equally important is the fact that the cholesteatoma cavity

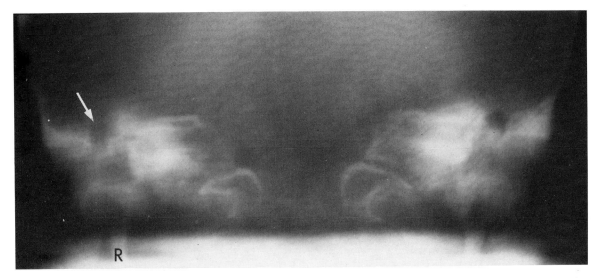

Fig. 222. Attic cholesteatoma. P.A. zonogram (thick section tomograph). The erosion and expansion of the attic is clearly seen on the right side as compared with the normal left.

demonstrated on the radiograph may not actually contain cholesteatomatous material, this having been liquefied or discharged and the cavity being empty.

The demonstration of the sites of maximum bone erosion enables the type of cholesteatoma to be recognised.

Buckingham & Valvassori (1970, 1973) have classified cholesteatoma on a radiological basis into four groups.

Group 1. Involving the middle ear and attic only.
Group 2. Involving the middle ear and attic and the adjacent mastoid, the adjacent mastoid antrum and air cells being infected and filled with granulation tissue.
Group 3. The cholesteatoma sac extends into the mastoid antrum.
Group 4. The cholesteatoma sac extends beyond the antrum into the mastoid process.

Attic cholesteatoma. Enlargement of the attic can be seen in the lateral oblique projection (Brunner & Sandberg, 1970) and the thinning of the bony walls of the attic can be recognised by the ease with which the detail of the internal ear can be seen in the lateral oblique projection on an otherwise dense mastoid. The upward spread of the bone erosion is

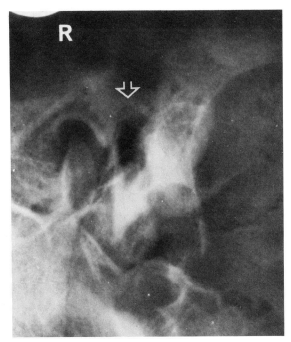

Fig. 223. Right attic cholesteatoma. Lateral oblique view demonstrating erosion of roof of attic by attic cholesteatoma in a 14-year-old girl who presented with aural discharge and vertigo.

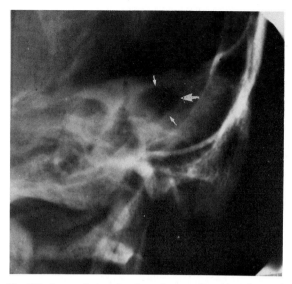

Fig. 224. Stenvers' view showing a large cavity with a clear-cut outline in the region of the mastoid process. The well-defined and sharp outline of the cavity favours the diagnosis of cholesteatoma rather than an abscess. Cholesteatoma may, however, occur without such a clear-cut outline.

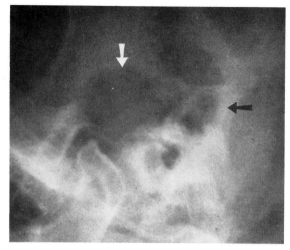

Fig. 225. Large cholesteatoma. Lateral oblique view of mastoid process showing extensive destruction extending forwards into the zygomatic process. The mastoid is sclerotic.

also easily seen in the transorbital and tomographic views (figs. 222, 223).

Antral cholesteatoma. Antral cholesteatoma usually show an enlargement of the mastoid antrum and as they are usually a backward extension from attic cholesteatoma some widening of the aditus ad antrum with erosion of its walls occurs as an early feature of the disease. Antral cholesteatoma can best be seen in lateral oblique, Towne's, Chaussé IV, transorbital and Stenvers' views (figs. 224, 225, 226).

Rarer varieties such as *Eustachian Tube Cholesteatoma* and extension of the cholesteatoma along the tympanic tube are best recognised in the submento-vertical view by widening and thinning of the bony walls of this tube (see Chapter 12). Lateral extension into the *external auditory meatus* is seen in the lateral oblique view by erosion of the floor and posterior wall of that structure.

If the middle ear itself is involved general enlargement of the middle ear may be associated with loss of the shadows of the incus and malleus, seen in the submento-vertical, transorbital or Chaussé III views if these bones are involved by the cholesteatoma.

The older radiological projections used to demonstrate cholesteatoma have been largely superseded by polytomography. Detection of early bone erosion so vital in the diagnosis of cholesteatoma is best recognised on the polytome sections. The value of polytome sections in the diagnosis of cholesteatoma (Buckingham & Valvassori, 1970) are as follows:

(i) The size and extent of the cholesteatomatous mass can be defined.

(ii) Erosion of the lateral attic wall, particularly erosion of the posterior meatal spine (tympanic spine) is an important diagnostic sign. Likewise erosion of the bony walls *e.g.* the dural plates, the mastoid process, the posterior meatal wall and the ossicles can be recognised.

(iii) Demonstration of erosion of the facial nerve canal.

(iv) Visualisation of fistula formation into the semicircular canals (figs. 227, 228).

(v) The integrity of the ossicular chain can be delineated.

Differential diagnosis

(a) *Normal mastoid antrum.* MacMillan (1936) showed that in the antero-posterior plane the average height of the mastoid antrum was 10 mm and its breadth 6 mm. Large antra may occasionally exceed these measurements and may cause confusion. In the Meyer's projection the overlap shadow of the external ear may mimic a

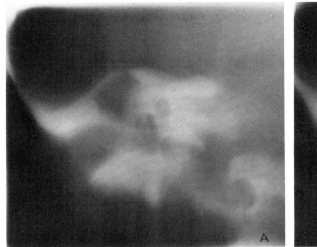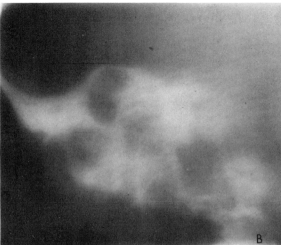

Fig. 226. Attico-antral cholesteatoma. Tomograms showing extension of bone destruction from the attic region (A), and posteriorly into the mastoid antrum (B).

large antrum, but Stenvers' or Chaussé views will enable the true nature of the translucency to be appreciated.

(b) *Granuloma or abscess formation.* The bone destruction produced by granulation tissue or chronic abscess formation does not differ from that

produced by cholesteatoma unless the outline of the latter is clear cut with a thin marginal sclerosis. As has been stated, superadded infection may modify the radiological appearances.

(c) *Histocytosis X.* Histocytosis X of the temporal

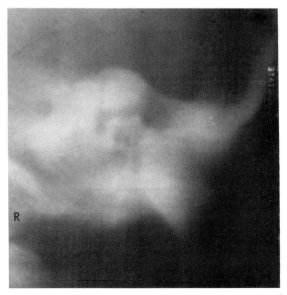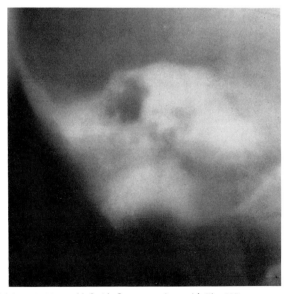

Fig. 227. Fistula into the right lateral semicircular canal caused by bone erosion from a cholesteatoma. The normal thinning of the bony wall of the lateral semicircular canal in this region must not be confused with a fistula.

Fig. 228. Normal left side for comparison with Fig. 227.

bone has to be distinguished from choles-teatoma. The features of both these conditions are extremely similar and radiological differen-tiation may only be possible by the detection of other deposits in bones, skin, or lung fields. The demonstration of radiological signs of infection is not of diagnostic value as a xanthoma may become secondarily infected.

(d) *Glomus jugulare tumour.* The destruction produced by a small glomus jugulare tumour may be extremely similar although in the latter the clinical syndrome and usually the extensive nature of the bone destruction should enable accurate diagnosis to be made.

Complications of mastoiditis

Otitic hydrocephalus. Although this complication may follow an otitis it also may arise de novo (McAlpine, 1937). Cairns (1930) however, main-tained that acute otitis with labyrinthitis is the basic aetiological factor in the origin of the disease. The majority of authors believe that the condition is the result of increased secretion from the choroid plexus or of diminished absorption of cerebro-spinal fluid.

Davidoff & Dyke (1937) have introduced the term "hypertensive meningeal hydrops" to indicate that the syndrome is not dependent on an infectious intracranial disease.

The plain radiograph apart from the signs of mastoid infection shows no signs. Ventriculo-graphy or computerised axial tomography show:

 (i) A normal ventricular system in relation to size and shape.
(ii) Difficulty in filling the ventricular system by encephalographic measures owing to the ease with which air escapes into the subarachnoid space (Hamberger, 1946).

Apical petrositis. Fowler & Swenson (1939) define apical petrositis as inflammation of the petrous bone anterior and medial to the arcuate eminence. According to these authors pneumatisation of the petrous apex is present to a greater or lesser degree in most mastoid processes and consequently possible involvement of this portion of the temporal bone must always be anticipated in all cases of middle ear infection.

The association of an apical petrositis associated with paralysis of the homolateral sixth cranial nerve constitutes "Gradenigo's syndrome".

Despite the probable frequency of apical petro-sitis in mastoiditis the occurrence of Gradenigo's syndrome is relatively rare. Gradenigo's syndrome occurs most frequently in patients who have had a previous mastoidectomy.

The value of radiological examination in cases of apical petrositis is directly proportional to the care and patience expended in making the examination. Negative findings on x-ray examination are not significant (Bateman, 1939).

In the investigation of apical petrositis the trans-orbital views are particularly valuable.

Radiological features. The radiological features of apical petrositis are dependent on the degree of pneumatisation of the petrous bone. In the sclerotic petrous bone radiological changes are not visualised until the changes of osteomyelitis have made their appearance.

In the pneumatised petrous tip the first radio-logical changes are:

 (i) *An increased density of the petrous apex.* In assessing this feature it should be remembered that some degree of loss of translucency of the petrous tip occurs in most cases of acute mastoiditis.
 (ii) *Decreased density of the petrous apex with a loss of bony detail.* As the infection develops, destruction and decalcification of the bone and of the bony cortex of the apex results in a blurred appearance.
(iii) *Bone destruction.* In more advanced cases actual destruction of the bony walls occurs and the break through the bony cortex may be recognised. This is associated with the formation of an extradural abscess.
(iv) *Bone sclerosis.* If the infection is more chronic, actual sclerosis develops with a marked increase in density of the apex of the petrous bone. Thornval (1946) noted changes consisting of loss of outline of the cells in the apex of the petrous bone associated with an increased density in this area while the remainder of the mastoid process appeared normal.

Sinus thrombosis. Involvement of the lateral sinus with the complication of sinus thrombosis occurs in a small percentage of acute mastoid infection. Lateral sinus involvement may also occur less frequently in a chronic mastoid infection. Regules & Canbarrere (1944) believe that there are radiological signs to indicate involvement of the lateral sinus. These authors describe what they refer to as two gutters (visible in the lateral projection) running along the entire course of the sinus. They believe that changes in the anterior wall of the gutter herald the involvement of the lateral sinus. They found the sign positive in 19 out of 24 cases.

Intracranial complications. Intracranial abscesses may follow sinus infection or be of otitic origin (Davis, 1945). Intracranial abscess is now best recognised by technetium isotope scans or by the more sophisticated computerised axial tomography which conclusively demonstrates the presence of an intracranial abscess.

Mastoiditis and chemotherapy

Christie & Wyatt (1946) have summarised the modifications in the radiological appearances of various diseases following chemotherapy treatment. Altemeier & Helmsworth (1945) showed that, in osteomyelitis in other sites such as long bones, the radiological appearances lagged behind or even deteriorated despite the apparent improvement in the clinical condition. This delay in the appearances of bone changes has a considerable bearing on the interpretation of the radiological appearances in the mastoid process as some degree of osteomyelitis of cell septa is present in most cases of acute suppurative mastoiditis.

There has been general agreement amongst otologists that the familiar clinical signs and symptoms of mastoiditis are frequently masked after the administration of antibiotics (Fenton, 1943; Maybaum, Snyder & Coleman, 1939; Maxwell, 1942; Converse, 1939; Bowers, 1940; Lillie, 1940; Babcock, 1940; Watkyn-Thomas, 1945; Dingley, 1944; Livingston, 1941; Fenton, 1939; Florey & Florey, 1943).

Law & Taylor (1939) state that sulphanilamides also change the radiological picture. The bony septa appear thinner and the cell contents more translucent. The same appearances may be noted after the use of antibiotics.

Johnson, Weinstein & Spence (1945) report a series of 23 acute mastoid cases which were treated by mastoidectomy plus instillation of penicillin into the mastoid cavity. In these authors' opinion when surgical drainage was combined with chemotherapy the results were greatly improved. Whether, however, antibiotics alone have reduced the development of chronic mastoiditis is still a matter of doubt.

Radiological appearances. The modern chemotherapeutic measures produce the following modifications in the radiological picture:

(i) *There is considerable delay in the appearance of the radiological changes.* Normally radiological changes in the mastoid process can be demonstrated within 24 hours following the onset of a mastoid infection. With a mastoid infection under treatment with chemotherapeutic drugs, radiological signs may not appear until four or five days after the onset of symptoms.

(ii) *There is a general diminution in the severity of the radiological signs.* The cloudiness and the opacification of the mastoid process are not nearly as marked as in the untreated case. This corresponds to the features described by Law (1940) and is explained by the fact that the secretions formed in the mastoid cells are thinner and consequently less dense than with an untreated case and fewer cells are involved.

(iii) *The radiological changes frequently progress after the clinical signs have subsided* and indicate that chemotherapy should be continued until the radiological appearances have returned to normal. The presence of radiological signs (cloudiness of the cells and loss of the cell walls) indicates persisting infection. In those cases which fail to return to normal after the clinical signs have completely subsided, surgical drainage will probably be necessary if the development of a chronic mastoid is to be avoided. It is probable that, where reliance is placed entirely on the clinical symptomatology without radiological control, many cases of mastoiditis treated by chemotherapy suffer too rapid withdrawal of the antibiotic, resulting in persistence of infection and the development of a chronic mastoiditis. Chronic mastoiditis is also especially prone to develop in those cases where the dosage of the antibiotic has been inadequate. As has already been indicated serial radiological control is especially desirable in those cases where bone destruction has not occurred, as the clinical condition may rapidly become normal and this should be confirmed by a return of the radiological appearances to normal (figs. 201, 202).

Otosclerosis

Otosclerosis is an inherited disease and pathologically consists of otosclerotic foci of bone arising in the endochondral bone of the labyrinth which progressively invade the labyrinthine windows (oval and round) and also involve the bone deep to both these windows. The otosclerotic process leads to fixation of the stapes in the oval window and also to blockage of the round window. These changes lead to progressive deafness and the condition is bilateral in 80% of cases.

Radiological examination in a suspected case of otosclerosis is taken to exclude other conditions which mimic otosclerosis and secondly to look for specific radiological signs of otosclerosis. Polytomography is essential when attempting to delineate changes of otosclerosis and the tomographic cuts are taken first in the axial and half-axial positions (see Chapter 6).

The site of predilection of otosclerosis is around the vestibular window and according to Nylen (1949), 90% of cases of otosclerosis are located around the labyrinthine windows. The normal vestibular window is about 2 × 3 mm and the cochlear window is slightly smaller.

Mild changes consist in a loss of the normal sharpness of the outline of the window; in more advanced cases narrowing of the window to a slit-line opening can be seen. In severe cases there is total obliteration of the vestibular window by dense calcified bone and the spread of the process to the vestibule results in dense opacities being superimposed on the vestibule. Similar changes occur around the cochlear window but they are more difficult to visualise. The pathological process of otosclerosis involves the promontory (normally 1 mm thick) and in the active phase it appears decalcified, thickened and blurred; whilst in the inactive phase it shows as a dense sharply defined thickening with dense bony foci bulging into the tympanic cavity or the fossula of the oval window.

Jensen et al. (1966) reviewing a series of 39 patients with fenestral otosclerosis, described three types of change seen on polytomography:

(1) Narrowing of the oval window.
(2) Total obliteration of the oval window with increased density of the surrounding bone.
(3) Generalised thickening and sclerosis of the bone surrounding the vestibule and semi-circular canals.

Valvassori (1969) has also described two other distinct x-ray signs in fenestral otosclerosis: apparent enlargement of the oval window due to osteolytic changes in its margins, in the early stages of the disease; and central otosclerosis involving only the footplate of the stapes, appearing as a prominent bony structure within the outline of the oval window.

Involvement of other parts of the bony labyrinth (retro-fenestral otosclerosis) occurs (Frey, Kleinman & Michael, 1967) and these changes largely occur around the cochlea. The basal turns of the cochlea become thickened and dense, the lumen narrowed and foci of otosclerosis may protrude into the basal turn. When the whole cochlea is involved in the active stage, the whole of the bony wall is decalcified and the cochlea cannot be clearly seen. In inactive sclerosis the whole of the bony wall is thickened and the bone thickening spreads into the surrounding bone making it difficult to demonstrate the bony outlines.

Valvassori (1969) recognises three degrees of otosclerotic involvement of the cochlea as shown by tomography: changes limited to the capsule of the basal turn of the cochlea; diffuse changes involving other parts of the cochlea; and widespread changes throughout the labyrinthine capsule. The x-ray appearances described consist in the first instance of an osteolytic process followed later by sclerosis; the first stage corresponding to actively enlarging vascular otosclerotic foci, while the sclerotic changes are the result of mature foci. In some patients there is a mixed radiological picture, with both sclerotic and osteolytic changes. In the author's experience these changes in the cochlea are difficult to demonstrate convincingly. However, Britton & Linthicum (1970) have been able to confirm otosclerosis histologically in one case diagnosed by x-ray as cochlear otosclerosis. They record this as the first time the correlation has been made.

Although at the present time the x-ray findings in cochlear otosclerosis are of little practical significance, this may not always remain so. Britton & Linthicum (1970) point out that attempts are being made to treat cochlear otosclerosis. Shambaugh (1969) for example has used fluorides in treatment and surgical attempts have been made to revascularise the cochlea and improve blood supply. If a successful method of treating sensorineural hearing loss due to cochlear otosclerosis is discovered, it will be necessary to establish a baseline as a guide to therapy and radiology should be able to make an important contribution.

Meniere's disease

The syndrome of episodic vertigo, tinnitus, fullness, deafness, and pressure in the ear constitutes a fairly clear clinical entity which allows the diagnosis of this syndrome.

It is now thought that failure of resorption of endolymph in the endolymphatic sac results in an increase in the quantity of endolymph present (endolymphatic hydrops).

Radiological investigation has two special functions in the investigation of Meniere's disease, first the exclusion of other pathological conditions which may mimic the syndrome, e.g. acoustic neuroma and secondly the demonstration of changes in the temporal bone which may be specific for Meniere's syndrome.

Polytome studies of the temporal bone have revealed changes in the vestibular aqueduct. Axial tomographs or tomographs with the sagittal plane turned 40° towards the film (Brunner & Pedersen, 1971) will normally demonstrate the posterior surface of the petrous bone and the vestibular aqueduct.

Scanlan & Graham (1974) have found that in 30% of patients with Meniere's disease the cochlear aqueduct could not be identified, in comparison with 3% of the control group. Narrowing or absence of the vestibular aqueduct was noted in 50% of patients with inner ear disorders (Clemis & Valvassori, 1963) whereas in 200 controls visualisation of the vestibular aqueduct was found in 90%.

In view of the frequency with which bilateral abnormalities are found it is essential to study both temporal bones even in cases of unilateral Meniere's disease.

REFERENCES

ADAMS, J. G. (1942) Tuberculous Otitis Media: a Complication of Thoracoplasty. *Ann. Otol Rhinol. Lar.,* **51,** 209.

ALTEMEIER, W. A. & HELMSWORTH, J. A. (1945) Penicillin Therapy in Acute Osteomyelitis. *Surgery Gynec. Obstet.,* **81,** 138.

BABCOCK, J. W. (1940) Role of Sulfanilamide in the Treatment of Acute Otitis Media. *Archs Otolar.,* **32,** 246.

BATEMAN, G. H. (1939) Petrositis. *J. Lar. Otol.,* **54,** 476.

BECKER, J. A. & WOLOSHIN, H. J. (1962) Mastoiditis and Cholesteatoma – a Roentgen Approach. *Am. J. Roentg.,* **87,** 1019.

BIRRELL, F. (1956) Black Cholesteatomata in Children. *J. Lar. Otol.,* **70,** 26.

BOWERS, W. C. (1940) Observations on 793 Cases of Acute Purulent Otitis Media with Chemotherapy in 396 Cases. *J. Am. med. Ass.,* **115,** 178.

BRITTON, B. H. & LINTHICUM, F. H. Jr. (1970) Otosclerosis: Histologic Confirmation of Radiologic Findings. *Ann. Otol.,* **79,** 5.

BROWN, J. M. (1943) Actinomycosis of the Temporal Bone. *Archs Otolar.,* **37,** 126.

BRUNNER, S. & SANDBERG, L. E. (1970) Tomography in Cholesteatoma and Chronic Otitis Media. *Archs Otolar.,* **91,** 560.

BRUNNER, S. & PEDERSEN, C. B. (1971) Experimental Roentgen Examination of the Vestibular Aqueduct. *Acta radiol.,* **11,** 443.

BUCKINGHAM, R. A. & VALVASSORI, G. E. (1970) Tomographic Evaluation of Cholesteatoma. *Archs Otolar.,* **91,** 464.

BUCKINGHAM, R. A. & VALVASSORI, G. E. (1973) Tomographic Evaluation of Cholesteatoma of Middle Ear. *Otol. Laryng. Clinics N. America,* **6,** 363.

CAIRNS, H. (1930) Abscess of the Brain. *J. Lar. Otol.,* **45,** 385.

CAWTHORNE, T. & PICKARD, B. (1965) Pathology and Treatment of Cholesteatoma Auris. *J. Lar. Otol.,* **79,** 945.

CHRISTIE, A. C. & WYATT, G. M. (1946) Roentgen Diagnosis. *J. Am. med. Ass.,* **132,** 895.

CLEMIS, J. W. & VALVASSORI, G. E. (1963) Recent Radiological and Clinical Observations on the Vestibular Aqueduct. *Otol. Clin. N. America,* **1,** 339–346.

CONVERSE, J. M. (1939) Recurrence of Otitic Infections due to Beta-haemolytic Streptococcus following Inadequate Sulfanilamide Therapy. *J. Am. med. Ass.,* **113,** 1383.

DAVIDOFF, L. M. & DYKE, E. G. (1937) Hypertensive Meningeal Hydrops. *Am. J. Ophthal.,* **20,** 908.

DAVIS, E. D. D. (1945) Treatment of Abscess of the Temporo-sphenoidal Lobe of the Brain arising from the Ear. *J. Lar. Otol.,* **60,** 129.

DINGLEY, A. R. (1944) Some Dangers of Sulphonamides in Ear Infections. *Br. med. J.,* **i,** 747.

DRUSS, J. G. (1951) Fractures of the Petrous Pyramid. *Archs Otolar.,* **53,** 541.

DU BOULAY, G. & BOSTICK, T. (1969) Linear Tomography in Congenital Abnormalities of the Ear. *Br. J. Radiol.,* **42,** 495.

FENTON, R. A. (1939) Sulfanilamides in Otolaryngology. *Ann. Otol. Rhinol. Lar.,* **48,** 17.

FENTON, R. A. (1943) Local Use of Sulfathiazole in Otolaryngologic Practice. *Archs Otolar.,* **37,** 491.

FLOREY, M. E. & FLOREY, H. W. (1943) General and Local Administration of Penicillin. *Lancet*, **i**, 387.

FOWLER, E. P. & SWENSON, P. C. (1939) Petrositis. *Am. J. Roentg.*, **41**, 317.

FRANCOIS, J. & BARROIS, J. (1959) Anatomie tomographique de l'os temporal normale. *Ann. Radiol.*, **11**, 71.

FREY, K. W., KLEINMAN, J. & MICHAEL, M. (1967) Tomographie der Otosklerose. *Fortschr. Rontgenstr.*, **106**, 428.

FRIEDMAN, I. (1974) *Pathology of the Ear*. Oxford: Blackwell, p. 84.

GABEN (1936) *Quoted by Nilsson.*

GROVE, W. G. (1939) Skull Fractures Involving the Ear. *J. Lar., Otol.*, **49**, 678.

HALLPIKE, C. S. (1950) Discussion in Section of Otology. *Proc. R. Soc. Med.*, **43**, 81.

HAMBERGER, C. A. (1946) On Otitic Hydrocephalus. *Acta otolar.*, **34**, 11.

HOUGH, J. V. D. (1959) Incudo-stapedial Joint Separation. *Laryngoscope*, **69**, 644.

HOUGH, J. V. D. & STUART, W. D. (1968) Middle Ear Injuries in Skull Trauma. *Laryngoscope*, **78**, 899.

JEFFERSON, G. & SMALLEY, A. (1938) Progressive Facial Palsy Produced by Intra-temporal Epidermoids. *J. Lar. Otol.*, **53**, 417.

JENSEN, J., ROVSING, H. & BRUNNER, S. (1966) Tomography of the Inner Ear in Otosclerosis. *Br. J. Radiol.*, **39**, 669.

JOHNSON, L. F., WEINSTEIN, L. & SPENCE, P. S. (1945) Penicillin and Primary Suture in Treatment of Acute Surgical Mastoiditis. *Archs Otolar.*, **41**, 408.

JONGKEES, L. B. W. (1948) Formation of Cholesteatoma Around a Deposit of Sulfa-powder. *J. Lar. Otol.*, **62**, 754.

LAW, F. M. (1940) *Quoted by Pancoast, p. 490.*

LAW, F. M. (1920) Mastoids Roentgenologically Considered. *Ann. Roentgen.*, **1**, 000.

LAW & TAYLOR (1939) *Quoted by Scal, J. S., N.Y. St. J. Med.*, **39**, 1790.

LILLIE, H. I. (1940) Treatment of Acute and Chronic Suppurative Otitis Media. *J. Am. med. Ass.*, **115**, 506.

LIVINGSTON, G. S. (1941) Local Sulfonamide Therapy in Acute Mastoiditis. *J. Am. med. Ass.*, **117**, 1081.

MAHONEY, W. (1936) Die Epidermoide des Zentralnervesystems. *Z. ges. Neurol. Physchiat.*, **155**, 416.

MAXWELL, J. H. (1942) The Sulphonamide Drugs in the Treatment of Acute Suppurations in the Middle Ear. *Surgery, Gynec. Obstet.*, **74**, 573.

MAYBAUM, J. L., SNYDER, E. R. & COLEMAN, L. L. (1939) Experiences with Sulfanilamide Therapy for Otogenous Infections. *Archs Otolar.*, **30**, 557.

MACMILLAN, A. S. (1936) Cholesteatoma in Chronic Otitis Media. *Am. J. Roentg.*, **36**, 747.

MCALPINE, D. (1931) Toxic Hydrocephalus. *Brain*, **60**, 180.

MCKENZIE, D. (1931) The pathogeny of Aural Cholesteatoma. *J. Lar. Otol.*, **46**, 163.

NILSSON, G. (1948) Attic Cholesteatoma Following Longitudinal Fracture of Pyramid. *Acta otolar.*, **36**, 85.

NYLEN, B. (1949) Histopathological Investigation on the Localisation, Number, Activity and Extent of Otosclerotic Foci. *Uppsala Läk-För. Förh.*, **54**, 1.

PANCOAST, H. K. (1940) *The Head and Neck in Roentgen Diagnosis*. Springfield: C. C. Thomas.

POLVOGT, L. M. (1929) Pathogenesis of Cholesteatoma. *Archs Otolar.*, **9**, 597.

PROCTOR, B. & LINDSAY, J. R. (1942) Tuberculosis of the Ear. *Archs Otolar.*, **35**, 221.

REGULES, P. & CANBARRERE, N. (1944) *An. Oto-rino-lar. Urug.*, **14**, 26.

SCANLAN, R. L. & GRAHAM, M. (1974) Radiology of Meniere's Syndrome. *Quoted by Rumbaugh et al., Radiologic Clinics of North America*, **12/3**, 517.

SHAMBAUGH, G. E. (1969) Sodium Fluoride for Inactivation of the Otosclerotic Lesion. *Archs Otolar.*, **89**, 381.

STEURER, F. (1937) Uber ozonbehandlung in der hals-nasen-ohren-heilkunda. *Z. Hals-Nasen-v. Ohrenheilk.*, **42**, 404.

THORNVAL, A. (1946) On the Treatment of Apicitis Suppurativa. *Acta Otolar.*, **34**, 546.

TUMARKIN, A. (1954) *Modern Trends in Diseases of the Ear, Nose and Throat*. London: Butterworths. p. 159.

VALVASSORI, G. E. (1964) *Radiographic Atlas of the Temporal Bone*, Book II. American Academy of Ophthalmology and Otolaryngology.

VALVASSORI, G. E. (1969) Tomographic Findings in Cochlear Otosclerosis. *Archs Otolar.*, **89**, 377.

VON BEZOLD, F. (1890) Cholesteatom, Perforation der Membrana flaccida Schrapnelli und Tuben verschluss. *Z. Ohrenheilk.*, **20**, 5.

WALTNER, J. G. (1949) Roentgendiagnosis of Cholesteatoma of Middle Ear. *Am. J. Roentg.*, **62**, 674.

WATKYN-THOMAS, F. W. (1945) Treatment on Endocranial Complications of Otitis Origin. *J. Lar. Otol.*, **60**, 129.

WELIN, S. (1941) Roentgendiagnostik der otitis media acuta. *Acta radiol.*, Suppl. No. 42.

WHITTAKER, H. (1944) Wounds in the Ear and Mastoid Region. *J. Lar. Otol.*, **59**, 205.

WILSON, C. P. & MCALPINE, A. (1946) Glossopharyngeal Neuralgia Treated by Transtonsillar Section of the Nerve. *Proc. R. Soc. Med.*, **40**, 82.

WINDEREN, L. & ZIMMER, J. (1954) Cholesteatoma of Middle Ear. *Acta radiol.*, Suppl. No. 3.

WRIGHT, J. W. (1974) Trauma to the Ear. *Radiologic Clinics N. America*, **12/3**, 527.

WRIGHT, J. W. & TAYLOR, C. L. (1975) *Polytomography of the Temporal Bone*. St. Louis: Warren H. Green. Chap. 6.

WUSTMAN (1942) *Hals-Nas.-u. Ohrenarzt.*, **32**, 406.

YOUNG, G. (1950) Cholesteatoma or Cholesteatosis – a Review. *Proc. R. Soc. Med.*, **43**, 75.

CHAPTER 11

Tumours of the ear, mastoid process and petrous bone

Neoplasms of the middle ear and mastoid processes are rare. In a series of 6,000 cases of pathological conditions involving the middle ear reported by Schall (1935), malignant disease occurred only once.

Tumours involving the auditory apparatus may be classified as follows:

External Auditory Meatus

(a) BENIGN
  (i) Osteoma
  (ii) Haemangioma
  (iii) Adenoma

(b) MALIGNANT
  (i) Carcinoma
  (ii) Rodent ulcer

Middle Ear Cleft

(a) BENIGN
  (i) Osteoma
  (ii) Angioma
  (iii) Tympanic body (glomus jugulare) tumour

(b) MALIGNANT
  (i) Squamous celled carcinoma
  (ii) Adenocarcinoma

Eustachian Tube

(a) BENIGN TUMOURS
(b) MALIGNANT TUMOURS

Petrous – Temporal Bone
Primary Tumours

(a) BENIGN
  (i) Osteoma – localised hyperostosis

  (ii) Histiocytosis X
  (iii) Neurofibroma
  (iv) Acoustic neuroma
  (v) Plasmacytoma
  (vi) Meningioma

(b) MALIGNANT
  (i) Haemangioendothelioma
  (ii) Rhabdomyosarcoma
  (iii) Fibrosarcoma
  (iv) Osteogenic sarcoma
  (v) Chondrosarcoma

Secondary Tumours

  (i) Meningioma
  (ii) Carcinoma
    Direct extension (from carcinoma of nasopharynx, cervical glands)
    Distant spread (from breast, kidney, bronchial tumours)

External auditory meatus

(a) BENIGN
(i) **Osteoma.** Osteomas are the commonest benign tumours to occur in the external auditory meatus. They may arise from any part of the external meatus and produce symptoms by compression and occlusion of the external auditory meatus. Swimming in cold water is an aetiological factor in the production of osteomas of the external auditory meatus. Adams (1951) confirms the views of Field (1873), van Gilse & Belgraver (1938) and Fowler & Osmun (1942) that water entering the external auditory meatus is a major cause of exostoses and maintains that lowering of the temperature of the meatus to 35°C is an important aetiological factor.

  Histologically osteomas arising in the external

177

auditory meatus are generally of the compact variety, cancellous osteomas being rare.

Radiological appearances. Radiology gives considerable assistance in the diagnosis and in assessing the size of the osteoma. Clinical inspection may reveal the site of origin of the tumour but an estimation of its inner extent can only be made by tomography. In other cases the presence of an otitis externa may obscure the osteoma. The lateral film enables the diagnosis to be established and tomographs in the lateral and anteroposterior planes assist in determining the size and degree of narrowing of the meatus.

(ii) **Haemangioma.** Haemangioma of the external ear, middle ear and mastoid process is rare (Miller, 1949). It may occur at any age. The presenting symptom is tinnitus often occurring synchronously with the pulse. Loss of hearing is generally associated with the tinnitus and the presence of a polypoid mass in the external auditory meatus. The radiographic features are those of a destructive tumour often associated with considerable dilatation of the vessels in the bone adjoining the mastoid process. Phleboliths may be seen in the tumour and angiography will demonstrate its vascular nature.

(b) MALIGNANT

Malignant tumours affecting the external auditory meatus are generally extensions of growths arising in the pinna or in the middle ear.

Malignant growths arising from the pinna are either basal celled (rodent ulcer) or squamous celled carcinoma. Rarely melanoma or adenoid cystic carcinoma arising from the ceruminous glands may occur. Unless treated early these tumours may infiltrate widely and the walls of the external auditory meatus may be extensively destroyed. Clinical diagnosis is usually obvious and radiology is mainly required to determine the extent of bone involvement. In such circumstances the radiograph shows destruction with little or no bony reaction of the outer cortex of the squamous temporal bone or the posterior wall of the external auditory meatus. Superadded infection may involve the middle ear and mastoid processes, clouding the mastoid cells. In such cases, unless a careful clinical examination is carried out and biopsy taken the malignant nature may be overlooked (figs. 229, 230, 231).

Malignant tumours of the external meatus have to be differentiated from "malignant external otitis", a condition appearing in elderly patients with long-standing uncontrolled diabetes. Facial nerve involvement is a frequent occurrence and tomography is necessary for the demonstration of bone destruction but differential diagnosis from carcinoma of the external meatus is difficult on

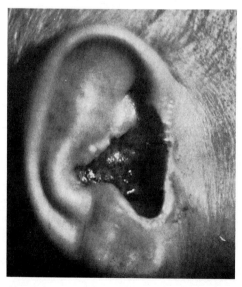

Fig. 229. Carcinoma of external auditory meatus. A male who had noticed a blood-stained discharge from the external auditory meatus with pain in the ear. The growth extending through the external meatus is seen.

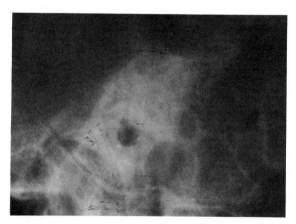

Fig. 230. Lateral view of case shown in Fig. 229 merely shows a sclerotic mastoid and no obvious radiological features to indicate malignancy.

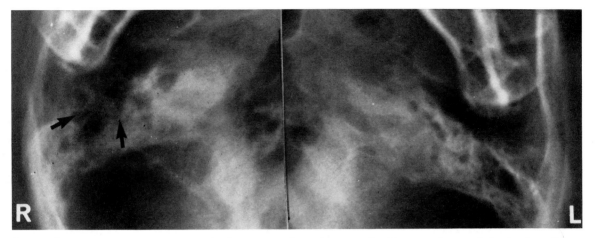

Fig. 231. Submento-vertical view shows extensive destructive change in the bony walls of the external meatus indicating the malignant nature of the process.

radiological grounds (Kim, 1971), and may only be made on biopsy.

Middle ear cleft

(a) BENIGN. Benign neoplasms involving the middle ear are extremely rare. Primary cholesteatoma (Epidermoid) is the commonest tumour to be found in this region but the controversy as to its aetiology and nature has already been discussed, and there is considerable doubt as to whether it should be regarded as a true tumour. Radiologically the inferior margin of the lateral wall of the attic is seen to be intact whilst the lateral wall of the same structure is eroded from within, features which enable congenital cholesteatoma to be differentiated from acquired cholesteatoma (Valvassori, 1974).

(i) **Osteomas** are the most frequently found benign tumours occurring in the mastoid process. Cinelli (1941) found 28 examples recorded in the literature. He found that histologically there were three types:

(1) Osteoma compactum
(2) Osteoma Cancellare
(3) Osteoma cartilagineum

There has been considerable controversy as regards the aetiology of osteoma compactum (fig. 232). Heymann (1919) considered that these tumours started at puberty and their growth was dependent on the growth of cranial bones. Stuart (1940) suggested that pituitary dysfunction might influence their development. Friedberg (1938) on the other hand regarded trauma with a subsequent ossifying periostitis and chronic inflammation as the predisposing agent.

(ii) **Angiomas.** Angiomas of the middle ear have been described and in 1923 Fischer recorded an example and Hampton & Sampson (1939) reported two further cases. The histological features of angiomas of the middle ear do not differ from those of haemangiomas elsewhere.

Radiological appearances. The radiological features are:

(1) Tomographs reveal the middle ear cleft to be filled with a soft tissue mass which occasionally may contain phleboliths.
(2) Widening of the vascular channels in bone adjoining the mastoid process may be present.
(3) Enlargement of the mastoid emissary vein. If the latter two features are especially marked, the diagnosis of an angioma is extremely likely although with any highly vascular tumour such changes may appear. Arteriography may assist but it should be remembered that chemodectoma may be very vascular and may be confused with angiomas.

Chemodectoma. Glomus or tympanic body tumour occurring in the middle ear was first described by Rosenwasser (1945). It may extend

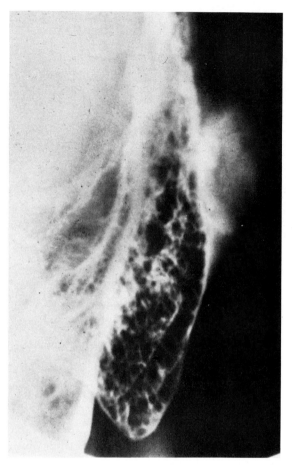

Fig. 232. Ivory osteoma involving mastoid process. Tangential views demonstrate dense exostosis arising from the bony cortex over the mastoid process. The patient was a soldier who complained of pain when wearing his steel helmet.

through the tympanic membrane and be mistaken for an aural polyp. Often, however, the growth may extend posteriorly into the mastoid process destroying the cell system. The tumour does not metastasise but frequently recurs after incomplete removal.

Chemodectomas show marked sex predominance in females, (22 out of a total of 28 cases – Alexander, Bramer & Williams, 1951).

Radiological features. The radiological features are dependent on the exact site of origin and the path along which the tumour extends. With the tumour confined to the middle ear, little or no radiological change may be found. Some clouding of the peri-

antral cells may precede invasion and destruction of the mastoid cell systems. A more common radiological finding is invasion of the petrous bone with extensive destruction (figs. 233a, 233b). The growth of the tumour is extremely slow. Arteriography reveals an extremely vascular tumour often with tumour staining although subtraction films may be necessary to show this feature. Jugular venography is particularly useful in detecting spread of tumours into the jugular vein (fig. 234), a not uncommon finding with large tumours.

(b) MALIGNANT TUMOURS OF THE MIDDLE EAR. Malignant tumours of the middle ear and mastoid process are almost invariably carcinoma. According to Furstenburg (1924), if neoplastic change develops in a chronically infected mastoid the growth is usually a squamous celled carcinoma – otherwise the growth is an adenocarcinoma.

Carcinoma of the middle ear is a rare condition. Rosenwasser (1940) found an incidence of one in 5,000 of tumours seen at the Mount Sinai Hospital. The clinical features are persistent pain, paralysis of the facial nerve and an intractable otitis media. The largest series reported by a single author has been a series of 13 cases reported by Thorell (1935) from the Radiumhemmet, Stockholm. Thorell added another histological type to Furstenburg's classification, namely a basal celled carcinoma, but as his series included tumours which had secondarily invaded the middle ear it is possible that this type of growth had originated from skin.

All authors are agreed that long-standing chronic otorrhoea frequently precedes the development of a neoplasm (Zizmor & Noyek, 1969). Ellis & Bracy (1954) reviewed 120 cases of carcinoma of the middle ear and added five personal cases. Analysis of 27 cases of carcinoma of the middle ear (Adams & Morrison, 1955) showed that an area of sclerosis frequently surrounded the bone destruction. The bone sclerosis is probably an index of the pre-existing infection. Widening of the external meatus was also found frequently. Supervoltage therapy was used by these authors in treatment with some degree of success.

Radiological appearances. The value of radiology in cases of malignant disease of the middle ear is twofold. First, as a diagnostic measure and as a means of assessing whether the growth is primarily derived from the middle ear or from secondary invasion from the pinna, and secondly in evaluating

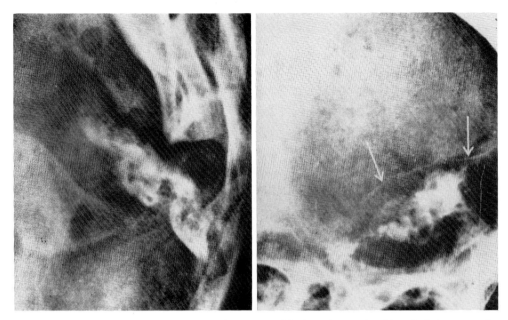

Fig. 233. Glomus tumour. (a) Submentovertical view. (b) The erosion of the bone is extensive although the bony capsule around the internal ear appears intact. A thin rim of bony cortex still remains. On clinical examination a pulsating mass could be seen occupying the whole of the middle ear. Progressive destruction of the temporal bone had occurred since the patient had first come under observation 16 years before. The radiological features of any chemodectoma of the petrous bone may be identical with these appearances.

the extent of the bony infiltration and destruction. The findings of carcinoma originating in the middle ear are as follows:

1. *Destruction of the bone:* malignant invasion of bone results in destruction with little or no reactive change. As growths of the middle ear are associated with infection which in itself also produces bone destruction, the evaluation of this sign may be difficult. A disproportionate amount of bone destruction in an otherwise sclerotic mastoid may suggest that malignant change has supervened. This feature is not diagnostic of malignant disease as in certain types of mastoid infection, notably in those caused by pneumococcal or tuberculous infection, extensive destruction of bone may occur. In Thorell's (1935) series of 25 cases of carcinoma, 32% showed extensive destruction of bone (figs. 236, 237, 238, 239, 240 and 241).

2. *Cloudiness of the mastoid cells:* malignant disease of the middle ear is almost invariably associated with infection and this results in cloudiness of the mastoid cells. A mistaken radiological diagnosis of infection may be made because of these changes. In Thorell's series, 28% of cases showed this sign. Cloudiness of the mastoid cells is usually caused by infection but in some instances it may be due to invasion of the cells by tumour tissue.

3. *Sclerosis of the mastoid process:* the frequency with which malignant change is superimposed on chronic infection has already been emphasised, hence it is not surprising to find that many cases show sclerosis of the mastoid process. In a sclerotic mastoid the recognition of areas of early destruction may be extremely difficult. Extensive tomography is essential for the early diagnosis of bone destruction.

4. *Post-operative defect:* some cases of malignant disease of the middle ear may not be diagnosed

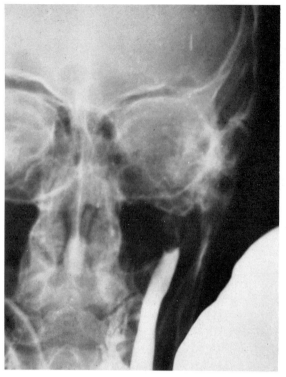

Fig. 234. Jugulogram. Contrast injection of internal jugular vein showing invasion of upper portion of the vein by tumour and complete occlusion of the lumen of the vein.

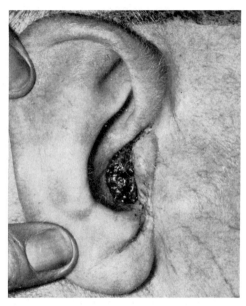

Fig. 235. Carcinoma of the middle ear. A male aged 58 who had been partially deaf following scarlet fever aet. three years. Discharge from the right ear had been present at intervals for ten years. One month prior to examination pain had commenced in the right ear and this had increased in severity. On examination a bleeding polypoid mass projected from the right external auditory meatus.

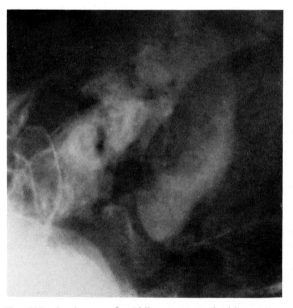

Fig. 236. Carcinoma of middle ear. Lateral oblique view showing destruction of the cells due to a mixture of infection and tumour invasion.

pre-operatively or may be even overlooked at operation. In those cases persistent discharge and a failure of the lesion to heal may suggest the diagnosis. Such cases show a post-operative cavity with an area of bone destruction (16% of Thorell's series).

Carcinoma which secondarily invade the mastoid process arise from the external auditory meatus, pinna or scalp. Radiology is of value in these cases to determine the presence and extent of bone involvement. Bone involvement is indicated by destruction of the cortical bone, in other cases cloudiness of the mastoid cells may be the earliest indication of involvement of the mastoid process.

Sarcoma of the middle ear. Sarcoma of the middle ear is extremely rare. Figi & Hempstead (1943) report that of 38 malignant tumours of the middle ear, only three were sarcomatous, whilst in Scott & Colledge's review (1939) of 70 cases of malignant disease, two only were sarcomas.

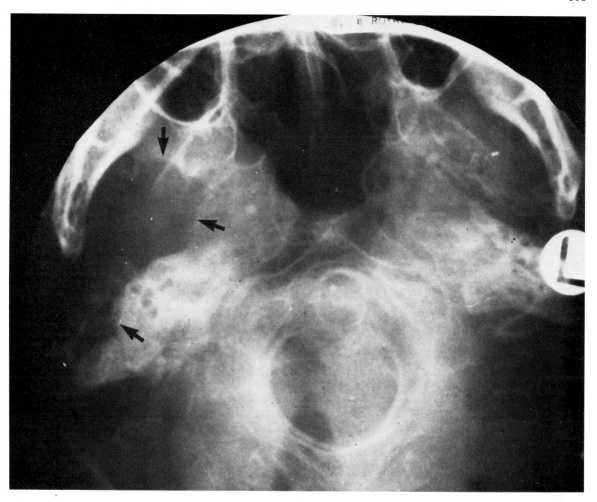

Fig. 237. Carcinoma of right middle ear showing extensive destruction of the middle cranial fossa bone by extension of the growth (case shown in figs. 235, 236).

Zimmerman (1934) reported the only recorded cases of Ewing's sarcoma occurring in the middle ear. Maconie (1944) records a case of a spindle-celled sarcoma involving the middle ear in a young boy aged five years. Embryonal rhabdomyosarcoma may occur in the middle ear in young children under the age of seven years.

The radiological features of sarcoma do not differ from those of carcinoma except in the rate at which they grow. Extensive destructive changes with little or no reactive change dominate the radiological appearances particularly in the case of the embryonal rhabdomyosarcoma.

Eustachian tube

Primary tumours involving the Eustachian tube are exceedingly rare. According to Graves & Edwards (1944) only 30 cases have been recorded since 1888. Proctor in 1912 recorded the first case of a highly malignant carcinoma involving the Eustachian tube. Further reports of primary malignant tumours of the Eustachian tube were recorded by Schumaker (1940) and Lawson (1943).

Radiologically, the presenting features are those of a suppurative otitis media with a secondary involvement of the mastoid process. The true state

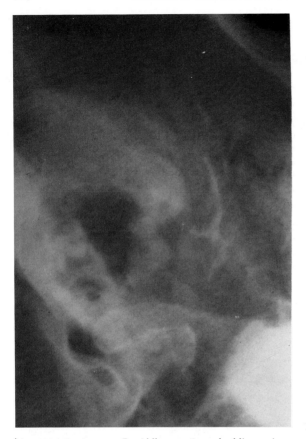

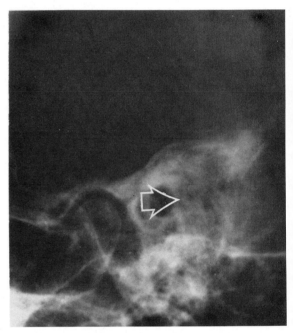

Fig. 238. Carcinoma of middle ear. Lateral oblique views showing extensive area of destruction associated with the malignant growth.

Fig. 239. Carcinoma of middle ear. Lateral oblique view. Relatively little bone destruction is apparent in this view and other views and careful tomography is necessary to search for any evidence of bone destruction.

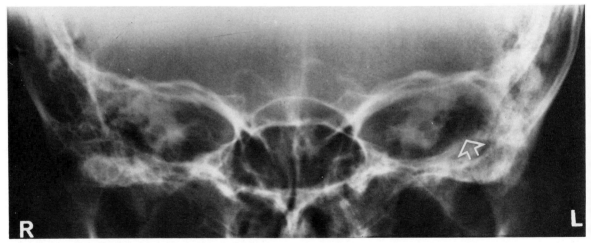

Fig. 240. Transorbital view of case shown in fig. 239 shows that the main extent of destruction has extended downwards.

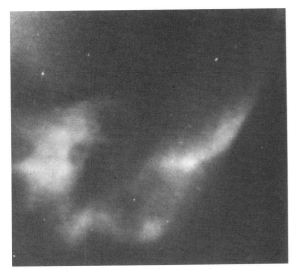

Fig. 241. Tomograph in P.A. position demonstrating the extensive degree of bone destruction caused by a downward spread of the growth (see figs. 239, 240).

of affairs is generally only discovered at operation. The periosteum tends to protect the temporal bone from invasion and limit its spread when the temporal bone is involved (Schuknecht, Allan & Murakami, 1971). Secondary involvement of the Eustachian tube frequently occurs with malignant nasopharyngeal growths involving the lateral wall of the nasopharynx.

Petrous bone

(a) PRIMARY TUMOURS. Primary tumours of the petrous bone are not common. They may arise from the temporal bone itself, *e.g.* dermoid cysts (Waltner & Karatay, 1947) or osteomas, or from structures contained in the temporal bone, *e.g.* neuroma from the facial nerve.

Osteoma. Osteomas occur infrequently in the petrous temporal bone. Radiologically their appearances are identical with those occurring in other parts of the skull. They have to be differentiated from reactive hyperostosis produced by intracranial meningiomas and hyperostosis from generalised bone disease, *e.g.* fibrous dysplasia. Reactive hyperostosis of the petrous bone is, however, not a common finding with meningiomas in the region of the petrous bone, which usually result in destruction rather than sclerosis. Reactive

hyperostosis can be distinguished from an osteoma by the diffuseness of the lesion and by the ill-defined edges of the affected area. A further condition which has to be differentiated is the bony thickening which occurs in fibrous dysplasia and less frequently in Paget's disease. In the latter case the involvement of the vertex of the skull indicates the correct diagnosis. Difficulties may arise with monostotic Paget's disease confined to the temporal bone, but when this occurs it is usually of the decalcifying type (osteoporosis circumscripta).

Generalised thickening of the temporal bone in association with a thickening of the base of the skull may be met with in fibrous dysplasia. The bony changes may occur in the base of the skull without any associated lesion in any other part of the skeleton (Towson, 1950).

Histiocytosis X. Xanthoma of the petrous bone is not uncommon and according to Snapper (1946) generalised xanthomatosis is frequently associated with other deposits in the temporal bone.

Xanthomatosis of bone (Hand-Schüller-Christian syndrome) is classified by Thannhauser & Magendantz (1938) into the group of xanthomatosis unassociated with any alteration in the blood cholesterol level (normocholesteraemic group). It may first present with a deposit in the temporal bone. The xanthoma may involve the middle ear and as a result of infection may give rise to persistent discharge. A mastoidectomy may be performed without the true nature of the condition being recognised. Schuknecht & Perlman (1948) report seven cases of Hand-Schüller-Christian disease where three cases showed an initial destructive lesion in the temporal bone. These authors reported a case in which the lesion involved both mastoid processes six months before the remainder of the skeleton. Greifenstein (1932) found that in a series of 26 cases reported in the literature, 12 cases showed involvement of the temporal bone.

Radiologically xanthomas occurring in the temporal bone appear as:

1. *A clear-cut destructive lesion with little reactive change in the surrounding bone.* The edges of the area of destruction are clear-cut and the destruction may be extensive.

2. As the destructive process extends from the petrous temporal and involves the mastoid process *secondary infection may be superadded and the*

radiological appearances become obscured. A "solitary" xanthoma has been recorded in the external auditory canal (Rosenberger, 1937). As part of a generalised disease xanthomatosis may occur bilaterally.

The destructive nature of the xanthomatous lesion may cause considerable difficulty in diagnosis from a malignant growth. This is especially true when superimposed infection is present.

Neurofibroma. Other benign tumours which give rise to radiological changes in the petrous temporal bone are the neurofibromas. The commonest type is a tumour involving the eighth nerve but rare examples of neurofibromas occurring in the facial nerve have been recorded.

The radiological signs of these tumours are those of pressure atrophy of the petrous bone, the internal auditory meatus may be expanded and the walls thinned. The changes may be identical with those of acoustic neuroma.

Acoustic neuroma. Eighth nerve tumours histologically form a mixed group of tumours occurring in an anatomical space below the tentorium, the "cerebello-pontine angle" (subtentorial angle – Stibbe, 1939). The anatomical boundaries of the

subtentorial angle are, below and laterally the posterior surface of the petrosa, above and medially the inferior surface of the sub-arachnoid space. It is approximately 13 mm in width and 25 mm in depth.

Histologically eighth nerve tumours can be classified into three groups:

(1) *Acoustic neurinoma* (perineural fibroblastoma). This type constitutes 90% of the total of acoustic neuromas.
(2) *Neurofibroma.* This type of cerebello-pontine tumour may be familial and bilateral and may represent a variety of Von Recklinghausen's disease (figs. 242, 243, 244).
(3) *Meningioma.* This is a rather unusual type of eighth nerve tumour which again is generally associated with Von Recklinghausen's disease.

Neuromas may arise from any of the cranial nerves but they have a peculiar tendency to occur in the eighth nerve. Henschen (1915) postulated that these tumours arose from the vestibular division of the eighth nerve. Post-mortem histological investigation of 250 healthy petrous pyramids showed unsuspected small acoustic tumours in six cases (Hardy & Crowe,

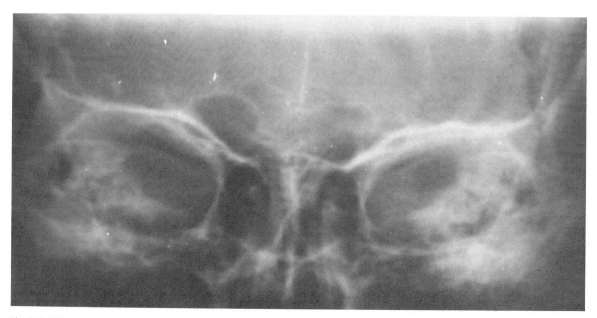

Fig. 242. Bilateral acoustic neurofibroma. Transorbital view showing enlargement of both internal auditory meati with erosion of the tips of the internal meati.

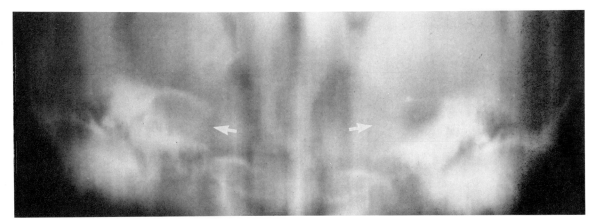

Fig. 243. P.A. tomograph. The enlargement and bone destruction in the apices of both petrous bones is seen.

1936). Neurofibromas tend to be bilateral and often show a familial tendency. This trait is well illustrated by the Gardner-Frazier family (1930) in which bilateral deafness was transmitted as a Mendelian dominant to 217 relations through five generations. Meningiomas also occur in the Von Recklinghausen's group and there is a tendency for

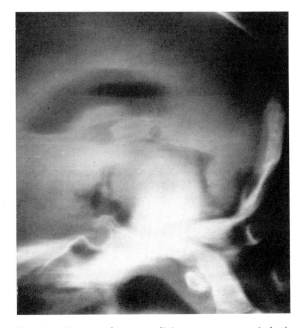

Fig. 244. Air encephalogram outlining tumour masses in both internal meati.

these tumours to be disseminated throughout the brain.

The macroscopic appearance of these three histological types is identical. They are all greyish-yellow in colour, oval in shape, well encapsulated and slow-growing. A small nipple-like projection on one part of the tumour projects into the porus acousticus and indicates the origin from within the internal meatus.

The progress of clinical symptoms falls into three stages: first the symptoms are limited to changes in function of the seventh and eighth nerves; secondly the stage of cerebellar ataxia, and finally all those symptoms associated with intracranial pressure. The vastly different prognosis and the surgical management between small and large intra-canalicular tumours is of utmost importance and emphasises the need for early diagnosis.

The value of the radiographic signs in the diagnosis of eighth nerve tumours was first appreciated in 1926 by Towne. Later in 1928 Lysholm standardised the technique for roentgen examination of the petrous bones. Various authors have shown individual preference for various projections which in their opinion are of greatest value in demonstrating erosion of the tip of the petrous bone. Hodes, Pendergrass & Young (1949) found that in a series of 129 cases, Towne's view gave most information in 40%, the submento-vertical position in 8%, postero-anterior view in 37%, and Stenvers' in 8%. Undoubtedly, no study of the petrous bone should be regarded as complete until the bone has been examined in all views and

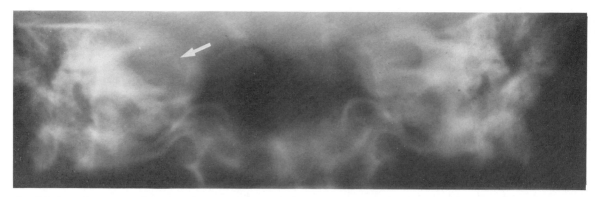

Fig. 245. Acoustic neuroma. Zonogram showing enlargement of the right internal meatus. Bone erosion of the apex of the petrous bone is also present.

confirmation of this is obtained from Hodes *et al.* (1949) series, where 15% of tumours would have been overlooked if all the projections used to show the tip of the petrous bone had not been taken. Tomography demonstrates the bone erosion more clearly and has largely replaced the standard views (Denny, 1955; Elliott & McKissock, 1954) and pleuridirectional tomograms are essential in the detection of acoustic neuromas (Lapayowker, Carter & McGann, 1962).

The radiological features are:

1. *Decalcification or displacement of the crista falciformis and bony walls of the internal auditory meatus.*

This is one of the earliest features of a tumour and one of the most difficult to appraise. The postero-anterior projection with the tips of the petrous projected through the orbit forms the best view to assess this change. Six per cent of a series of 125 internal auditory tumours showed this change (Hodes *et al.*, 1949). Pleuridirectional tomography in the postero-anterior plane is essential in recognising erosion and loss of the crista falciformis, and is an invaluable sign in identifying small intracanalicular types of tumour before marked expansion of bone has occurred.

2. *Expansion of the bony walls of the internal auditory meatus* is a change more readily appreciated (Hodes,

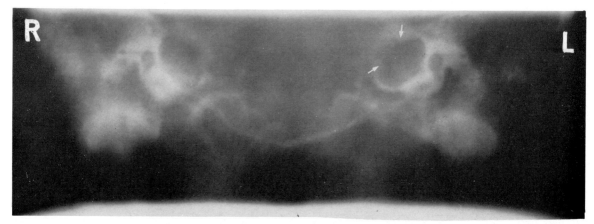

Fig. 246. Giant internal auditory meati. Normal variations which may mimic enlargement from tumour formation. The nipple-like bone projection at the internal end of the meatus representing normal walls is a useful pointer in differentiating the condition from pathological expansion (zonogram).

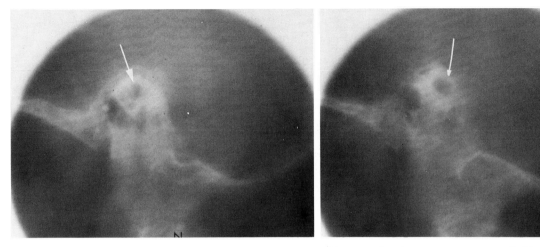

Fig. 247. Lateral tomogram of acoustic neuroma showing enlargement of the internal auditory meatus as compared with the normal (N). Tomography in the lateral plane is especially valuable in estimating enlargement of the internal meatus.

Pendergrass & Dennis, 1951). The expansion of the internal auditory meatus can be clearly demonstrated in the Stenvers', Towne's and postero-anterior transorbital views of the petrous bone. In 26% of cases this consists simply in a widening of the internal auditory canal but in 36% of cases the canal is both shortened and widened (fig. 245).

3. *Erosion of the tip of the petrous bone.* This represents an advanced change and indicates a large extra canalicular component of the tumour. The tip of the petrous bone may be eroded by direct pressure from the tumour (8% of cases). Complete destruction of the internal auditory canal and apex of the petrous bone occurs in 14% of cases. Erosion of the tip of the petrous bone must not be confused with:

(a) Normal variations. The degree of ossification of the tip of the petrous bone is proportional to the size of the venous lake forming the origin of the superior and inferior petrosal sinuses.

(b) Aneurysms of the carotid artery and even atherosclerotic carotid arteries in the elderly may also erode the tip of the petrous bone.

(c) Infection – apical petrositis (Gradenigo's syndrome) seldom causes the same degree of bone destruction as a tumour.

(d) Differentiation of normal variations. The internal auditory meatus may be grossly expanded but shows a normal bony cortex and usually has a nipple-like projection indicating the normal part of the meatus. The variation is frequently bilateral (fig. 246).

4. *Tomography.* Valvassori (1969) gives the following criteria of abnormality in the internal auditory canal, as shown by polytomography:

(a) Erosion of the cortical line surrounding the lumen of the canal seen in the lateral tomograms (fig. 247).

(b) Widening of 2 mm or more by measurement of any portion of the internal auditory canal when compared with the corresponding segment of the opposite canal.

(c) Shortening of the posterior wall of the canal by at least 3 mm in comparison with the opposite side.

(d) Demonstration of the crista falciformis running closer to the inferior than to the superior wall of the internal auditory canal. The crista should normally be located at or above the midpoint of the vertical diameter of the canal.

5. *Raised intracranial pressure.* These consist in a decalcification affecting the posterior clinoid processes, associated with a slight generalised enlargement of the sella turcica. Displacement of a calcified pineal gland seldom occurs and when it does it consists of a lateral shift rather than an upward displacement as would be anticipated.

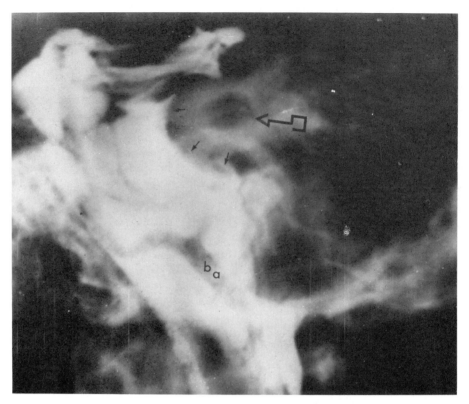

Fig. 248. Contrast myelogram showing filling defect (small arrows) and enlargement of internal auditory meatus (large arrow).
ba—Basilar artery
A 40-year-old hospital porter who had noticed recent giddiness and slight deafness for only three months duration.

6. *Contrast examination.* The successful development of the translabyrinthine operation for the removal of acoustic neuromas has demanded more sophisticated methods to detect early tumours which show little change in the plain films.

Both positive contrast (Myodil) and negative contrast (air) have been used to detect tumours and both have been used in conjunction with tomography. Positive contrast methods appear to be of more value in detecting small tumours (fig. 248).

Valvassori (1972) found that the average width of the internal auditory meatus was 4·5–5 mm with a range of 2 mm to 10 mm. In the smaller internal meatii those of between 2 and 2·5 mm showed no filling with contrast medium, in those between 3 and 3·5 mm only that part above the crista falciformis (containing the facial nerve) filled, whilst in those meati between 3 and 4·5 mm contrast streaks above and below the nerve fibres were seen. In canals of more than 4·5 mm width the filling of the canal was complete with the end of the column of contrast medium being convex.

The development of computerised axial tomography has proved to be of immense value in the early diagnosis of acoustic neuroma. Intravenous injection of 40–60 ml of iodine containing contrast medium will enhance the image and make the tumour far easier to visualise. Even with contrast enhancement some cases of acoustic neuroma have been confused with cerebello-pontine angle arachnoid cysts (fig. 249).

The differential diagnosis is:

(a) Normal variations.

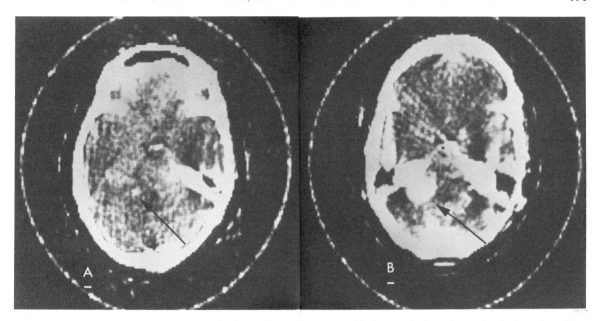

Fig. 249. Computerized transverse axial scan of right sided acoustic neuroma. (a) Showing the bone destruction in the region of the internal meatus, and (b) showing the contrast enhancement of the tumour after the injection of intravenous iodine containing contrast medium.
(Acknowledgement to Dr. N. Lewtas.)

(b) Meningioma (hyperostosis of petrous apex).
(c) Cholesteatoma (primary). Bone erosion occurs in this lesion without real expansion of the canal.
(d) Meningeal adhesions and cysts.

Plasmacytoma. The occurrence of extra-medullary plasmacytoma in the mastoid processes is excessively rare and only three cases have been reported (Cappell & Mathers, 1935). In Gros' case (1945) the plasmacytoma was associated with a Gradenigo's syndrome. Eagleton (1936) believes that plasmacytic mastoiditis is a metaplasia of bone marrow originating in a virulent suppuration in the petrous apex and filling the mastoid process with plasmacytes.

(b) MALIGNANT TUMOURS. Primary malignant tumours occurring in the petrous temporal bone are generally tumours of vascular origin. Spicht & Volker (1929) reported a haemangio-endothelioma affecting the temporal bone and discussed its aetiology in detail. Haemangio-endothelioma occurs at any age and Sullivan (1934) reports a haemangio-endothelioma occurring in a young child aged five years who showed a cauliflower-like mass in the middle ear with a facial paralysis and paralysis of the soft palate. Haemangio-endothelioma, judged from the reports in the literature, frequently gives rise to facial paralysis, although in Goekoop's cases (1934) the paralysis appeared to be due to simple pressure. The familial nature of the tumour in this author's cases was extremely unusual.

Radiological appearances
1. Destruction of bone: this may be extensive and involve the petrous bone.
2. Calcification within the tumour: this seldom is seen but if it occurs it helps considerably in diagnosis.
3. Secondary involvement of other parts of the skeleton.

Meningioma. Occasionally the temporal bone becomes secondarily involved by a meningioma. Such involvement is uncommon but appears to be more common in female subjects.

Radiological appearances
(1) Destruction of the temporal bone, which may be extensive with little or no bone reactive change.

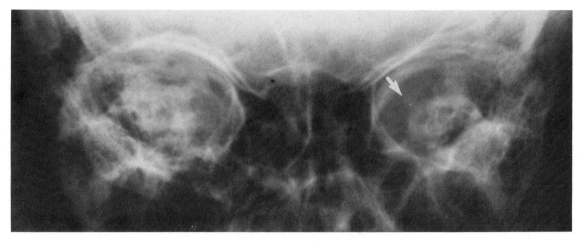

Fig. 250. Metastatic carcinoma in left petrous bone – before treatment.

(2) Preservation of the labyrinth. No matter how extensive the destruction, the bony labyrinth is preserved. Considerable displacement of the labyrinth may occur but invasion does not occur.

Risch (1943) described such a case where a meningioma extensively involved the temporal, sphenoid and occipital bone.

Carcinoma. Secondary involvement of the petrous bone by carcinoma originating in the middle ear is almost inevitable and occurs by contiguous spread. The radiological features are those of destruction of the bony architecture of the mastoid with little or no bony reaction. Cloudiness of the mastoid cells may appear from direct invasion of the cells with tumour tissue or from superadded infection. Blood borne skeletal metastases from distant sites are infrequent and the breast is the commonest site of origin. Figs. 250 and 251 illustrate the typical appearance of an osteolytic

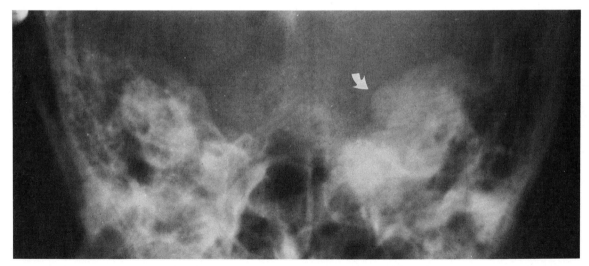

Fig. 251. Metastatic carcinoma – osteosclerotic deposit from breast carcinoma – after treatment with Stilboestrol. Note the extensive reconstruction of bone at the apex of the petrous bone (same case shown in fig. 250).

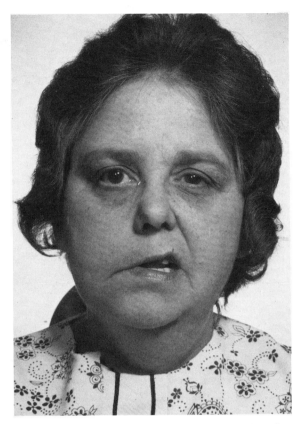

Fig. 252. Patient with breast carcinoma who developed painless facial palsy.

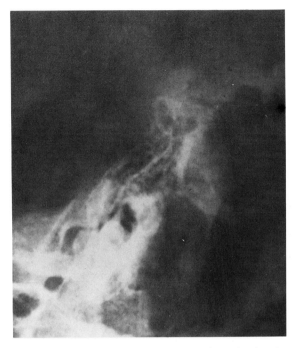

Fig. 253. Lateral mastoid views of patient shown in Fig. 252 showing extensive bone destruction carried by a metastatic deposit from a primary breast cancer involving the facial nerve.

secondary deposit occurring in the temporal bone from a primary growth of the breast. Occasionally a sudden facial palsy may be the first sign of a metastatic deposit (figs 252, 253).

Generalised bony disease involving temporal bone

Generalised skeletal diseases such as Paget's disease or polyostotic fibrous dysplasia may involve the temporal bone and mastoid process.

Paget's disease. It had been accepted until 1950 that the deafness occurring in Paget's disease was the result of direct pressure on the auditory nerve by the new bone produced (Lindsay & Perlman, 1936; Wilson & Anson, 1936). However, work by Newman & Rechtschaffen (1950) showed that changes typical of Paget's disease occur in the bony labyrinth of the internal ear and they consider that deafness is probably secondary to this change rather than due to any pressure effect on the auditory nerve.

The radiological appearances of the bony labyrinth in Paget's disease depend largely on the stage of evolution of the disease. Newman & Rechtschaffen (1950) describe an example of Paget's disease involving the skull where the semicircular canals were unusually visible. They attribute this feature to osteoporosis of the surrounding temporal bone, the osseous labyrinths retaining their normal density.

This undue prominence of the osseous labyrinth in Paget's disease thus only occurs during the stage of osteoporosis circumscripta (fig. 254), and when the diphasic changes of Paget's disease appear, the osseous labyrinth becomes less clearly visualised. When the Paget's changes become advanced the sclerosis may be such as to render the osseous labyrinth completely invisible.

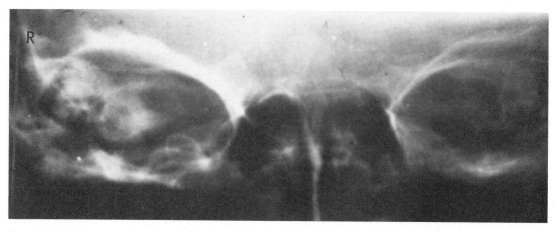

Fig. 254. Osteoporosis circumscripta – decalcification of left petrous bone in Paget's disease mimicking bone loss caused by tumour. The bony labyrinth is not affected and stands out clearly as a consequence of the decalcification of the petrous bone.

Polyostotic fibrous dysplasia. Polyostotic fibrous dysplasia may produce changes in the temporal bone which are identical with change occurring in other bones of the skull. Thickening and loss of texture occur and the bony details of the internal ear are obscured by the dense bone.

REFERENCES

ADAMS, W. S. (1951) The Aetiology of Swimmer's Exostosis of the External Auditory Canals and Associated Changes in Hearing. *J. Lar. Otol.,* **65,** 133.

ADAMS, W. S. & MORRISON, R. (1955) Primary Carcinoma of the Middle Ear and Mastoid. *J. Lar. Otol.,* **69,** 115.

ALEXANDER, E., BRAMER, P. R. & WILLIAMS, J. O. (1951) *J. Neurosurg.,* **8,** 515.

CAPPELL, D. F. & MATHERS, B. P. (1935) Plasmacytoma of the Petrous Temporal Bone and Base of Skull. *J. Lar. Otol.,* **50,** 340.

CINELLI, A. A. (1941) Osteoma Eburneum of the Mastoid. *Archs Otol.,* **33,** 421.

DENNY, W. R. (1955) Diagnosis of Acoustic Nerve Tumours. *J. Lar. Otol.,* **69,** 605.

EAGLETON, W. P. (1936) A New Classification of the Bones Forming the Skull. *Archs Otol.,* **24,** 158.

ELLIOTT, F. A. & McKISSOCK, W. (1954) Acoustic Neuroma. *Lancet,* **ii,** 1185.

ELLIS, M. & BRACY, R. (1954) Carcinoma of the Middle Ear. *Br. med. J.,* **i,** 1413.

FIELD, G. P. (1873) *Manual of the Diseases of the Ear.* 4th Ed. p. 83.

FIGI, F. A. & HEMPSTEAD, B. E. (1943) Malignant Tumours of the Middle Ear and the Mastoid Process. *Archs Otol.,* **37,** 149; *Trans. Am. Acad. Ophthal. Oto-lar.,* **47,** 210.

FISCHER, J. (1923) Hamangiektatischer Tumor des Trommelfells. *Ztschr. f. Hals. Nasen-u. Ohrenh.,* **5,** 221.

FOWLER, E. P. & OSMUN, P. M. (1942) New Bone Growth due to Cold Water in Ears. *Archs Otol.,* **36,** 455.

FRIEDBERG, S. A. (1938) Osteoma of the Mastoid Process. *Archs Otolar.,* **28,** 20.

FURSTENBURG, A. G. (1924) Primary Adenocarcinoma of the Middle Ear and Mastoid. *Ann. Otol. Rhin. Lar.,* **33,** 677.

GARDNER, W. J. & FRAZIER, C. H. (1930) Bilateral Acoustic Neurofibromas. *Archs Neurol Psychiat.,* **23,** 266.

GOEKOOP, C. (1934) Fibro-hamangiom des Felsenbeines und des Mittelohres bei drei Schwestern. *Acta otolar.,* **18,** 153.

GILSE, P. H. G. VAN & BELGRAVER, A. (1938) *Acta otolar.,* **26,** Fasc. 4.

GRAVES, G. O. & EDWARDS, L. F. (1944) *Archs Otolar.,* **39,** 359.

GREIFENSTEIN, A. (1932) Involvement of the Ear, Accessory Nasal Sinuses and Maxilla in Generalised Xanthomatosis. *Arch. Ohr.-, Nas.- u. KehlkHeilk.,* **132,** 337.

GROS, J. C. (1945) Plasmacytoma of Temporal Bone. *Archs Otolar.,* **42,** 188.

HAMPTON, A. O. & SAMPSON, D. A. (1939) Roentgen Diagnosis and Treatment of Angioma of Tympanic Cavity. *Am. J. Roentg.,* **41,** 25.

HARDY, M. & CROWE, S. J. (1936) Early Asymptomatic Acoustic Tumour. *Archs Surg.,* **32,** 292.

HEYMANN, D. (1919) Zur Kenntnis der Knochengeschwulste des Warzenfortsatzes (osteoma eburneum processus mastoidei). *Ztschr. Ohrenh.,* **78,** 23.

HENSCHEN, F. (1915) Zur histologie und pathogenese der Kllin-hirnbrucken-Winkeltumoren. *Arch. Psychiat.,* **56,** 21.

HODES, P. J., PENDERGRASS, E. P. & YOUNG, B. R. (1949) Eighth Nerve Tumours. *Radiology, 53*, 633.

HODES, P. J., PENDERGRASS, E. P. & DENNIS, J. M. (1951) Cerebello-pontine Angle Tumours: their Roentgenologic Manifestations. *Radiology, 57*, 395.

LAPAYOWKER, M. S., CARTER, B. L. & McGANN, M. J. (1962) The Use of Plesiosectional Tomography in the Diagnosis of Eighth Nerve Tumours. *Am. J. Roentg., 88*, 1187.

KIM, B. A. (1971) Malignant External Otitis. *Am. J. Roentg., 112*, 366.

LAWSON, L. J. (1943) Primary Carcinoma of the Eustachian Tube. *Ann. Otol. Rhin. Lar., 52*, 577.

LINDSAY, J. R. & PERLMAN, H. B. (1936) Paget's Disease and Deafness. *Archs Otolar., 23*, 580.

LYSHOLM, E. (1928) Technique of Projection in Roentgenological Examination of Pars Petrosa. *Acta radiol., 9*, 54.

MACONIE, A. C. (1944) Sarcoma of the Middle Ear and Mastoid. *J. Lar. Otol., 59*, 32.

MILLER, M. V. (1949) Haemangioma of Ear and Mastoid Process. *Archs Otolar., 49*, 535.

NEWMAN, E. B. & RECHTSCHAFFEN, J. S. (1950) Surgical Anatomy of Subtentorial Angle, with Special Reference to Acoustic and Trigeminal Nerves. *Lancet, i*, 859.

PROCTOR, P. C. (1912) Two Cases of New Growth involving the Eustachian Tube. *Boston med. surg. J., 166*, 96.

RISCH, O. C. (1943) Meningioma with Unusual Involvement of the Temporal, Sphenoid and Occipital Bones. *Archs Otolar., 37*, 287.

ROSENBERGER, H. C. (1937) Solitary Xanthoma of the External Auditory Canal. *Archs Otolar., 26*, 395.

ROSENWASSER, H. (1940) Neoplasms Involving the Middle Ear. *Archs Otolar., 32*, 38.

ROSENWASSER, H. (1945) Carotid Body Tumours of the Middle Ear and Mastoid. *Archs Otolar., 41*, 64.

SCHALL, L. A. (1935) Neoplasma Involving the Middle Ear. *Archs Otolar., 22*, 548.

SCHUKNECHT, H. F. & PERLMAN, H. B. (1948) Hand-Schuller-Christian Disease: Eosinophilitic Granuloma of the Skull.

SCHUKNECHT, H. G., ALLAN, A. F. & MURAKAMI, Y. (1971) Primary and Metastatic Tumours of the Temporal Bone. *Laryngoscope, 81*, 1273.

SCHUMAKER, P. W. (1940) Primary Carcinoma in the Eustachian Tube. *Ann. Otol. Rhin. Lar., 49*, 1038.

SCOTT, P. & COLLEGE, L. (1939) Discussion on Malignant Disease of the Ear. *Proc. R. Soc. Med., 32*, 1087.

SNAPPER, I. (1946) *Medical Clinics in Bone Diseases.* Chicago: Science Publications.

SPICHT, D. & VOLKER, W. (1929) *Arch. Ohr.-, Nas.- u. KehlkHeilk., 130*, 93.

STIBBE, E. P. (1939) Surgical Anatomy of Subtentorial Angle with Special Reference to Acoustic and Trigeminal Nerves. *Lancet, i*, 859.

STUART, E. A. (1940) Osteoma of the Mastoid. *Archs Otolar., 31*, 838.

SULLIVAN, J. A. (1934) Haemangio-endothelioma of Temporal Bone. *Archs Otolar., 20*, 61.

THANNHAUSER, S. J. & MAGENDANTZ, H. (1938) The Different Clinical Groups of Xanthomatous Diseases; a Clinical Physiological Study of 22 Cases. *Ann. intern. Med., 11*, 1662.

THORELL, I. (1935) Treatment of Malignant Tumours of the Middle Ear. *Acta radiol., 16*, 242.

TOWSON, C. E. (1950) Monostotic Fibrous Dysplasia of the Mastoid and the Temporal Bone. *Archs Otolar., 52*, 709.

VALVASSORI, G. E. (1969) Abnormal Internal Auditory Canal: Acoustic Neuroma. *Radiology, 92*, 449.

VALVASSORI, G. E. (1972) Myelography of the Internal Auditory Meatus. *Am. J. Roentg., 115*, 978.

VALVASSORI, G. E. (1974) Benign Tumours of the Temporal Bone. *Radiologic Clinics of N. America, 12/3*, 533.

WALTNER, J. G. & KARATAY, S. (1947) Cysts of the Mastoid Bone. *Archs Otolar., 46*, 398.

WILSON, J. G. & ANSON, B. J. (1936) Histologic Changes in the Temporal Bone in Osteitis Deformans (Paget's Disease). *Archs Otolar., 23*, 57.

ZIMMERMAN, J. L. (1934) Ewing's Sarcoma of Mastoid. *Penn. med. J., 37*, 654.

ZIZMOR, J. & NOYEK, A. (1969) Tumours and Other Osseous Disorders of the Temporal Bone. *Semin. Roentg., 4*, 151.

CHAPTER 12

Radiology of the post-operative mastoid

Radiological examination is frequently requested to evaluate the post-operative cavity when symptoms develop or persist after operation. A proper understanding of the radiological appearances after the different operations performed is essential before attempting any interpretation of these appearances. Barkhorn (1941) has commended the value of routine post-operative radiography in all cases of mastoid disease to establish a basis for estimation of any pathological change which may subsequently occur in the post-operative mastoid, but this is hardly practical.

From a radiological standpoint the various operations performed on the mastoid process may be grouped as follows (modified from McGuckin, 1949; Mawson, 1972).

Mastoid Operations:

   (i) Cortical mastoidectomy (Heath)
  (ii) Attico-antrostomy
 (iii) Radical mastoidectomy (Schwartz)

End-aural operations:

   (i) Anterior tympanotomy
  (ii) Posterior tympanotomy
 (iii) Combined approach.

Reconstructive operations: Operations primarily directed towards the restoration of hearing:

   (i) Myringoplasty
  (ii) Ossiculoplasty
 (iii) Tympanoplasty

It is well to remember that although there are many variations in surgical approach, *e.g.* in the end-aural operation, the radiological findings may be remarkably similar. In other types of operation the nature of the operation can be more easily deduced from the radiological appearances.

Transmastoid approach. Differentiation of the simple mastoidectomy from the radical or modified radical mastoid operation is based on the presence or absence of the posterior meatal spur (Henle's Spur). Postero-anterior tomographs are essential to assess the extent of bone removal. In the radical mastoid operation the incus and malleus are absent, having been either destroyed by disease or removed by surgical intervention. In the radical mastoid operation an attempt has been made to exteriorise all the mastoid cells although it is seldom that this is successful and pockets of cells usually remain (fig. 255). It is important that, prior to the interpretation of the radiographs, detailed operation notes are available, since an estimate of the degree of bone erosion due to persistent infection can only be made when this information is known.

The post-operation cavity whether from a simple or radical operation, has a clear-cut outline. This feature, however, is not always visible owing to the convex shape of the skull in the mastoid region, the outer table overlapping the operation cavity.

Attico-antrostomy. This operation removes the outer bony wall overlying the antrum. It has limited usefulness and is confined to those patients in whom the cholesteatoma is limited to the attic and who in addition have good hearing.

Radiologically the extent of bone removal in this operation is so limited that unless tomographs are taken the bone defect may not be appreciated.

Radical mastoidectomy

In the radical mastoidectomy the aditus is enlarged by removal of the posterior meatal spur and after

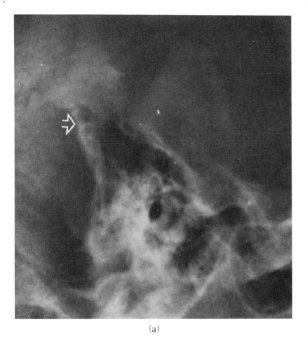

(a)

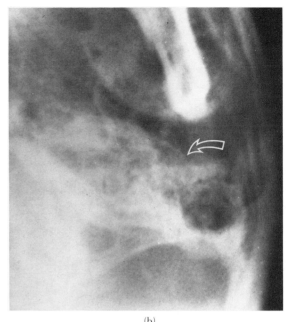

(b)

Fig. 255. A 17-year-old youth who had left cortical mastoid operation at 5 years and had suffered recently from giddiness and otorrhoea.
(a) Lateral oblique view of post-operative cavity. The "cells" remaining (arrow) are probably partly exteriorized into the main cavity.
(b) S.M.V. view of same case. Note that the posterior meatal wall has been removed and the operation cavity drains into the external meatus.

removal of diseased tissue the operation cavity is drained into the meatus. The operative enlargement of the aditus and the removal of the posterior meatal spur can be best seen in tomograms in the postero-anterior plane or in the submentovertical view (fig. 255(b)). In the radical mastoidectomy the malleus and incus may be removed and consequently the shadows of these bones are lost; the stapes is not disturbed.

The number of mastoid cells visible even after an apparently successful radical mastoid operation is always surprising and illustrates the difficulty of their complete removal. Residual cells are most frequently seen in the perisinus region and also near the apex of the petrous bone and tip of the mastoid process. Many of these cells have been exteriorised into the mastoid cavity and although radiographically they appear as unopened cells they are in fact draining into the operation cavity (fig. 255(a)). Errors in interpretation are especially likely if the translucency of these cells remains diminished or if infection persists post-operatively.

End-aural transmeatal approach. The end-aural approach for drainage is fundamentally of a conservative nature, comparatively little bone being removed, consequently only minimal bone loss is seen on the radiograph. The actual surgical approach to the different types of operation varies considerably.

Radiology can provide the following information in all types of post-operative mastoid:

(i) *The type of operation performed.* Reference has already been made to the extent of bone removed in the different types of operation.

(ii) *The extent of the operation cavity.* The extent and outline of the operation cavity can be seen on the plain film. The operation cavity outline is normally clear-cut and sharp. The mastoid antrum usually forms the deepest part of the cavity and the walls slope towards the antrum. In the Stenvers' position the defect usually appears as a triangular radio-lucent area with its apex directed inwards. The roof of the operative bony defect is bounded superiorly by the upper surface of the petrous bone

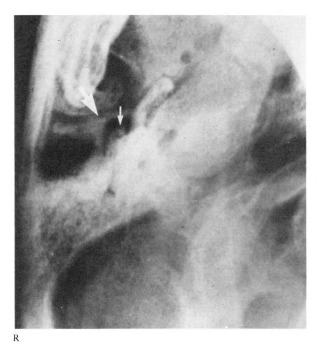 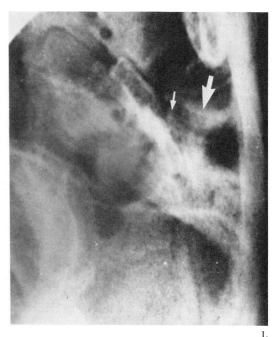

R   L

Fig. 256. Post-operative sequestra. S.M.V. view showing loss of definition of tympanic ring (large arrow) and ossicles (small arrow) on left side. At operation, the tympanic ring and ossicles were found to be sequestrated (see fig. 257).

downwards to the tip of the mastoid process. The base of the triangle is formed by a line connecting these two points.

In the lateral oblique view the operative defect appears as a triangular area bounded above by the tegmen tympani, extending from the middle ear to the junction of the sinus and dural plane, the posterior and anterior borders being formed by lines extending from the mastoid tip to the anterior and posterior ends of the operative defect (Barkhorn, 1941). In the lateral and lateral oblique projections of the mastoid process the posterior walls of the operation cavity do not have the clear-cut outlines seen in the Stenvers' and axial projections owing to the sloping nature of these walls.

(iii) *The extent of the remaining cells.* The basis for the apparent large numbers of mastoid cells remaining after operation has already been considered. If, however, a group of cells or an extension of cells is overlooked such cells may remain the seat of infection and contribute to symptoms persisting after operation.

A forward zygomatic extension of mastoid cells,

an extension deep to the labyrinth, or a perisinus group of cells are the cells most frequently overlooked.

(iv) *The presence of sequestra.* The concomitant bone infection associated with a mastoiditis may be associated with the formation of sequestra. Such sequestra are usually thin and flake-like and may be derived from an intercellular septum or a cell wall. On other occasions they may be derived from the floor of the cavity. Owing to their thinness they are usually best seen when viewed end-on. They are most frequently found on the roof of the operation cavity near the tegmen tympani and can only be clearly demonstrated when the incident beam runs along the long axis of the sequestrum. Stereoscopic films may help in the detection of a sequestrum (Taylor, 1928) (figs. 256, 257) but tomography is a more reliable method.

The cavity wall in the region of the sequestrum also gives an indication of the presence of a sequestrum as this area frequently has a hazy and blurred outline and the smooth, sharply-cut operation cavity is absent. Tomographic films, however, will demonstrate that the bony shadow is

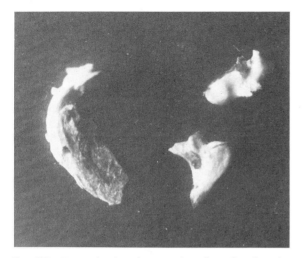

Fig. 257. Tympanic ring, incus and malleus found to be sequestrated at operation (same case as fig. 256).

separate from the wall of the operation cavity, which avoids confusion with a remaining bony intercellular septum.

(v) *The presence of remaining infection.* The detection of persisting infection in the operation cavity radiologically may be extremely difficult. The focus of infection consists of a mass of granulation tissue often admixed with proliferating epithelial cells. Under such conditions decalcification and loss of the sharply-cut outline of the operation cavity may be the only radiographic sign of infection. If sclerosis is present in the mastoid process, a not uncommon finding in these cases, the demonstration of such changes may be impossible.

(vi) *Cholesteatoma formation.* Cholesteatoma formation post-operatively in a mastoid cavity has essentially the same features as that occurring preoperatively. Radiologically, its recognition depends on bone erosion but as this feature may be absent or extremely slight, it may be difficult to recognise cholesteatoma recurring in the operation cavity (fig. 258).

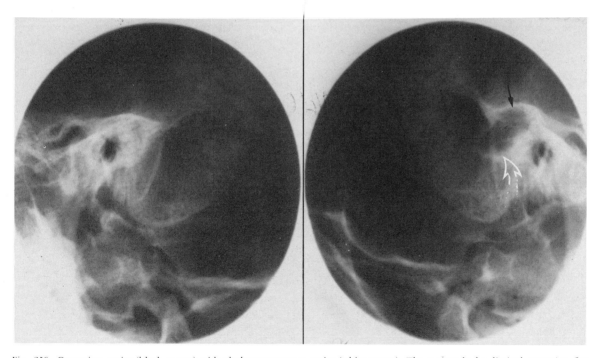

Fig. 258. Operation cavity (black arrow) with cholesteatomatous cavity (white arrow). The patient had a limited operation for mastoiditis six years previously and had recently complained of offensive aural discharge. The rather blurred outline of the operation cavity can be contrasted with the clear definition of the cholesteatoma.

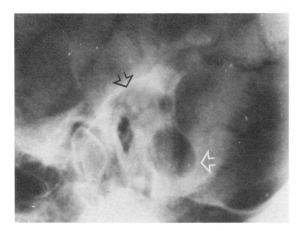

Fig. 259. Post-operative cholesteatoma. Secondary residual cholesteatoma developing near tip of mastoid process.
Operation cavity (black arrow)
Cholesteatoma cavity (white arrow).

Sometimes the cholesteatoma spreads over the surface of the operation cavity, giving rise to practically no bone erosion. Begley & Williams (1951) reported two external cholesteatomatous cysts following incomplete removal and in only one could any signs of the cholesteatomatous cyst be seen on the radiograph (fig. 259).

Localised erosions of bone occurring in a post-operative cavity, and especially if extending outside the limits of the operation cavity, should suggest the diagnosis of a cholesteatoma (fig. 258). Residual cholesteatoma occurring near the tegmen tympani may spread upwards into the cranial cavity eroding this structure.

In other cases the forward spread of a cholesteatoma may be associated with spread into the tympanic tube. This feature can be recognised by widening of the bony margins leading down to the tube (fig. 260).

(vii) *Fistula formation.* A labyrinthine fistula not infrequently occurs as a complication of a radical mastoid operation. The fistula usually occurs into the lateral semicircular canal immediately anterior to its point of maximum convexity. Less frequently the fistula occurs into the vestibule.

Meticulous radiological technique is needed to demonstrate the fistula. The radiological appearances are complicated by the normal thinning of the external bony wall which occurs over the outer aspect of the semicircular canal. Postero-anterior tomographs may conclusively demonstrate the bone loss in this region.

A normal marking caused by the crossing of the posterior semicircular canal over the lateral canal

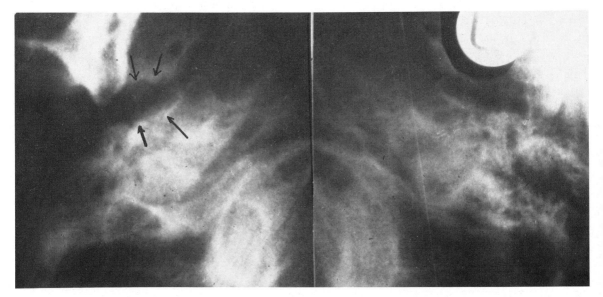

Fig. 260. Post-operative cholesteatoma – near entrance to Eustachian tube. The normal bony outlines are seen on the left side whilst the right side shows expansion of the Eustachian canal. The patient (aged 55 years) had a right radical mastoid operation some years previously and suffered from repeated attacks of discharge and vertigo.

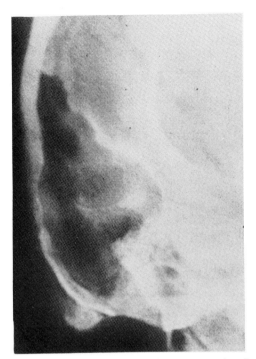

Fig. 261. Post-operative osteomyelitis – extensive bone destruction occurring after a mastoidectomy. A considerable portion of the bone defect is the result of surgical removal.

With other conservative operations where a prosthesis is used, only if it is radio-opaque can it be seen. If a stapedectomy has been performed the larger vestibular window can be demonstrated by tomography. It must be remembered that in some reconstructive operations the malleus is left (Smyth & Kerr, 1969) and can therefore be seen on the radiograph. Repositioning of the incus (Hough, 1970) and the use of cartilage struts can seldom be seen in sufficient clarity to allow radiology to make any contribution to the diagnosis of any malfunctioning of the newly formed chain after operation.

(ix) *Post-operative osteomyelitis*. Extensive spread of infection to surrounding bone is a relic of the pre-antibiotic era but extensive destruction may still occur with specific organisms or with commoner organisms when they are antibiotic resistant (fig. 261).

may be mistakenly interpreted as a fistula. In such instances no decalcification of the surrounding bone can be seen, a feature usually present in the labyrinthine fistula.

(viii) Radiological assistance is frequently required to assess changes when operation for the restoration of hearing has been carried out. Langfeldt (1963) has demonstrated the appearance after the columella operation as shown on tomographs. The alteration in position of the incus or malleus which has been used to form the columella can be seen, but a detailed knowledge of the operative procedure carried out is essential if an accurate assessment of changes is to be made.

REFERENCES

BARKHORN, C. W. (1941) The Acutely Involved Mastoid (Without Complications) Before and After Operation. *Archs Otolar.*, **34,** 69.

BEGLEY, J. W. & WILLIAMS, H. L. (1951) Cholesteatomatous Cysts Secondary to Incomplete Removal of the Cholesteatomatous Matrix. *Archs Otolar.*, **53,** 147.

HOUGH, J. V. D. (1970) Surgical Aspects of Temporal Bone Fractures. *Proc. R. Soc. Med., 63,* 245.

LANGFELDT, B. (1963) Tomography of the Middle Ear in Sound Transmission Disturbances. *Acta radiol.*, **1,** 133.

McGUCKIN, F. (1949) Chronic Otitis Media. *J. Lar. Otol.*, **63,** 328.

MAWSON, S. R. (1972) Management of Chronic Otitis Media. In *Modern Trends in Diseases of the Ear, Nose and Throat*, Series 2, Ed. M. Ellis. London: Butterworths. p. 115.

SMYTH, G. D. & KERR, A. G. (1969) Tympanic Membrane Homografts. *J. Lar. Otol.*, **83,** 1061.

TAYLOR, H. K. (1928) The Roentgenogram in Mastoid Diseases. *Am. J. Roentg.*, **19,** 522.

CHAPTER 13

Radiological examination of the pharynx and larynx

Radiological examination of the pharynx and larynx can provide valuable information without the discomfort and difficulties which may be associated with endoscopic examination. It should be regarded as complementary to rather than a substitute for endoscopy, as final assessment in many cases must come from endoscopy. In children or extremely nervous patients radiography may be the only available method of examination without recourse to endoscopic examination under anaesthesia. In other cases the lower limits of a lesion cannot be determined by endoscopic examination and radiography may be essential to estimate the lower limits of new growths involving the pharynx and larynx.

The radiography of both regions will be considered separately as the technique of examination is different.

PHARYNX

Radiography of the pharynx is either performed by (1) the use of techniques to show the soft tissues, or (2) the use of contrast media to enhance the outlines of these structures.

Two views are used to demonstrate the pharynx, the lateral and submento-vertical. The lateral view is taken with the head in the true lateral position and the incident ray is centred just behind the angle of the mandible (figs. 262, 263). Accurate coning to exclude all but the nasopharynx and pharynx, greatly improves the detail. A Potter Bucky diaphragm is used to improve contrast but it can be dispensed with without significant loss of contrast when examining infants as the shortened exposure time minimises the risk of motional blur.

Whilst the lateral view is extremely valuable in recognising masses arising from the roof or posterior wall of the nasopharynx, it is disappointing in the lack of information supplied about the lateral nasopharyngeal wall where quite large tumours may exist without any evidence of their presence (figs. 263, 264). The lobe of the ear, according to its size, may overlap the nasopharynx and may cause a confusing soft tissue shadow (fig. 286).

The submento-vertical view provides invaluable information by demonstrating the lateral nasopharyngeal walls and encroachment on the air space by masses arising from the lateral wall. In addition, infiltration of those structures can be recognised by erosion of the base of the skull (Jönsson, 1941) (fig. 264). The technique to obtain a submento-vertical view of the nasopharynx is identical to that described under the examination of the sphenoid sinuses (see Chapter 1). There is no doubt that a fine focus tube greatly improves detail in all the examinations of the nasopharynx.

In the newborn and in small infants radiography of the nasopharynx is frequently requested to determine the cause of respiratory obstruction. Radiography of these structures in infants presents a technical challenge but the use of high output generators and short exposure times enables satisfactory radiographs to be obtained. In infants and babies some form of restraining device may be necessary. In older infants the child should be seated on the mother's lap and a film held against the child's shoulder with a second assistant firmly holding the child's head in a true lateral position. Needless to say, the child and mother should be adequately protected with lead aprons to avoid scattered radiation. Care should be taken to see that the tongue is pushed forwards between the incisor teeth so that the soft tissue shadow of the base of the tongue can be clearly seen.

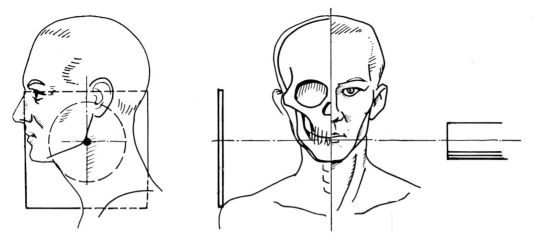

Fig. 262. Position for lateral radiograph of pharynx. The centering point is just behind the angle of the jaw.

Supplementary lateral views with the mouth and nose held closed during forcible expiration allow distension of the nasopharyngeal air space and assist in the detection of early growths. Lateral radiographs during the performance of the foregoing test should be regarded as complementary to the lateral film taken at rest. In infants blowing a balloon or whistle is generally the easiest way of obtaining a film in forced expiration.

Lateral tomography or zonography (thick-section tomography) in the midline plane and with serial sections on either side of the midline is a valuable addition to the soft tissue radiography of the nasopharynx. In a relatively small series of nasopharyngeal tumours investigated by Epstein (1951) it was found that midline tomographs (fig. 265) were superior to routine lateral views in demonstrating soft tissues, but that tomograms of the base of the skull were not superior to stereoscopic films in demonstrating bony involvement. Zonograms in the lateral position using the Polytome however, have proved a most successful method of demonstrating bone erosion of the base of the skull.

Another frequent request for radiological examination of the nasopharynx is for the estimation of the function of the soft palate, especially before and after cleft palate operation. The lateral film is taken with the patient phonating "aa" and "ee" and the closure of the nasopharynx by the palate can be assessed. Cinefluorography

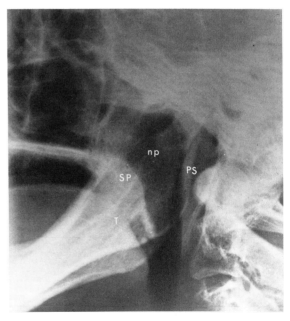

Fig. 263. Lateral radiograph of pharynx showing the normal markings and an apparently normal nasopharynx. Fig. 264 shows how a large tumour arising on the lateral wall of the nasopharynx may not be visible in this view.

SP   soft palate
np   —nasopharynx
T   —tongue
PS   —post-nasal soft tissues.

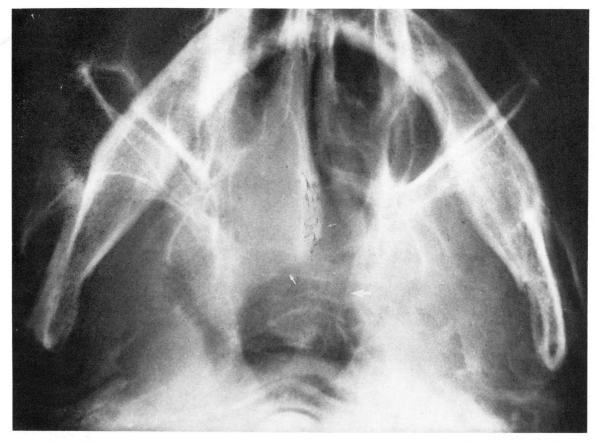

Fig. 264. Large arrow indicates normal left lateral wall of nasopharynx. A large soft tissue tumour arising from the right lateral wall is seen (small arrows) in this view and is unrecognizable in the lateral view (fig. 263).

(Blackfield *et al.,* 1963) and videotape examination have been used in the investigation of cleft palate speech problems. 100 mm film with an exposure rate of 6 films/second is a very convenient method of estimating and recording palatal function.

Nasopharyngeal escape is recognised by the failure of the palate to adequately close off the nasopharynx during speech. During phonation the palate initially angulates in its mid part, its free edge hanging downwards inert, and in a second movement the whole bent palate moves upwards towards the posterior pharyngeal wall to effect closure of the nasopharynx.

Contrast examination (Nasopharyngograms). The nasopharynx can also be investigated by the instillation of contrast medium into the nasopharynx. With the patient's head extended in the submento-vertical position and lying below the body level, 10–20 ml of oily Dionosil are instilled through a polythene catheter into one nostril and the patient instructed not to swallow (figs. 266–268).

Lateral and submento-vertical films are taken without moving the head. The lateral film demonstrates any forward displacement of the contrast medium but the submento-vertical film is more useful in demonstrating masses involving the lateral wall of the nasopharynx. Whilst lateral soft tissue views readily demonstrate masses involving the mid-line, quite large masses may be present on the lateral wall of the nasopharynx without any apparent alteration in the lateral film. These laterally placed tumours become obvious in the contrast studies by the inward displacement of the contrast medium.

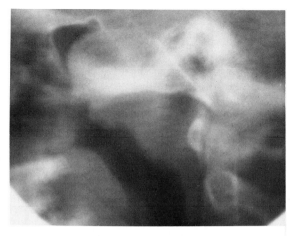

Fig. 265. Zonogram of nasopharynx (6° Polytome, 125 kV, 3 mm brass filtration). Soft tissue mass invading the sphenoid sinus and extending into the nasopharynx can be readily appreciated. This is an extremely valuable method for determining the extent of nasopharyngeal tumours.

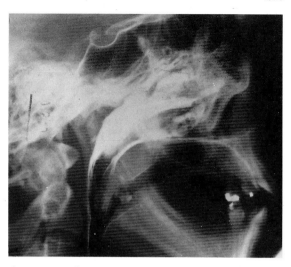

Fig. 267. Nasopharyngogram. Lateral view showing Dionosil in nasopharynx. The head is in the inverted position so that the Dionosil remains in the nasopharynx.

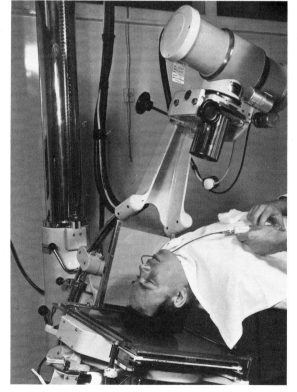

Fig. 266. Nasopharyngogram showing position of patient and operator for instillation of contrast medium. The head is hyperextended to keep the Dionosil located in the nasopharynx.

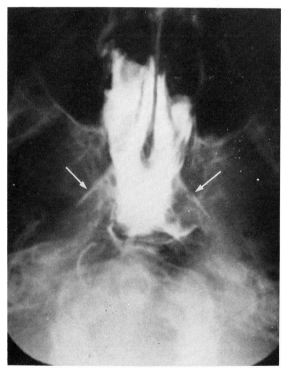

Fig. 268. Nasopharyngogram. Submentovertical view showing the nasopharynx outlined with contrast medium and the Eustachian tubes filled on both sides.

Adenoids appear as relatively symmetrical smooth masses indenting the contrast filled nasopharynx. Malignant tumours tend to give unilateral irregular deformities of the contrast filled nasopharynx.

If the Valsalva manoeuvre is performed after the nasopharynx has been filled and the contrast medium swallowed, filling of the cartilaginous Eustachian tube will occur (fig. 268).

Oily contrast media such as Lipiodol, Neohydriol or Dionosil instilled through a nasal catheter are generally used. Water solutions of contrast medium have also been used for this purpose (Rüedi & Zuppinger, 1934). Apart from its spectacular success demonstrating choanal atresia and narrowing, this method of investigation adds considerably to the information obtained from plain films. Some observers have attempted to outline the soft tissues of the nasopharynx by the insufflation of tantalum powder. This method would appear to have no advantage over endoscopy which can supply more reliable information without any greater discomfort to the patient. A contrast medium capable of outlining the lateral walls of the nasopharynx and which could be administered through an aerosol spray, would make a significant improvement in radiological diagnosis but still awaits development. Computerised axial tomography has yet to be fully explored in the diagnosis of early, and particularly lateral, spread of lesions in the nasopharynx, but holds out great promise for the future.

In the oropharynx and hypopharynx contrast examination by barium swallow is essential and the use of cineradiography has enabled the rapid swallowing motion of this area to be recorded and analysed. Cineradiographic examination of the swallowing of a thick bolus of barium will enable motor dysfunctions to be appreciated, whilst cineradiography in the antero-posterior and lateral positions swallowing air after the ingestion of barium enables the mucosal lining to be demonstrated by a double contrast method. Barium swallow in the recumbent position will assist in recognising small lesions but the advent of cineradiography enable the act of swallowing to be recorded and later analysed in slow motion (Kemp & Ardran, 1951; Ardran & Kemp, 1975).

Lateral soft tissue films of the nasopharynx are an invaluable record in planning the fields of x-ray therapy, in control of the effects of treatment, and in the evaluation of results (Fletcher & Matzinger, 1951).

The functional anatomy of the oropharynx and hypopharynx during deglutition can be studied by means of a barium swallow examination. In the antero-posterior view the various phases of deglutition are demonstrated. During the act of swallowing the barium first fills and coats the tongue and the lateral recesses of the tonsillar fossa; immediately before swallowing the larynx is elevated.

The larynx itself impresses into the barium filled pharynx producing a round half-shadow appearance which is especially well seen if the head is extended during swallowing. During swallowing the larynx is elevated and the appearances alter, the normal air filled shadows of the larynx disappear, the lateral recesses of the valleculae are filled out and the barium passes through a smooth tube into the hypopharynx. The mucosal relief which is demonstrated after the bolus of barium has been swallowed is of utmost value in demonstrating the normal transverse mucosal folds which occur at this point. Lateral views of the pharynx demonstrate the shallowness of the smooth laryngeal impression which is hardly appreciated in the lateral view. On the anterior wall of the cervical portion of the oesophagus a small linear defect is frequently seen which has to be differentiated from a web. This has been ascribed to a venous plexus lying behind the larynx (Pitman & Fraser, 1965).

LARYNX

(i) **Lateral radiograph.** The larynx is best examined in the lateral position, as in the antero-posterior position the cervical spine largely obliterates the outlines of the air structures of the larynx. The lateral radiograph is obtained by centering the incident ray at a point just behind the prominence of the thyroid cartilage. The film is placed against the shoulder and the anode film distance is increased to 6 ft (2 m) to minimise geometric distortion. The film is taken with the breath held and the neck in the neutral position – it is important to avoid over-extension as the soft tissues anterior to the larynx are thinned out and consequently over-exposed. Accurate coning helps to improve contrast and no grid is used. Lateral films should be taken at rest and when phonating "ee" as this helps to visualise the anterior ends of the cords and the anterior commissure – a feature of importance as malignant growths of the cord and their relationship to the thyroepiglottic ligament (conus elasticus) can be assessed (Powers, Holtz & Ogura, 1964).

Valvassori & Goldstein (1970) have suggested that lateral films should include:

(i) with quick breathing, with mouth closed and producing maximal abduction of cords
(ii) expirating phonation with "ee" producing adduction of cords. If the patient is unable to "ee", a sound which can be produced without effort should be made (Ardran & Kemp, 1975)
(iii) modified Valsalva manoeuvre with patient puffing out of his cheeks, with his lips closed producing distension of the supraglottic larynx and hypopharynx
(iv) reverse or inspiratory phonation often delineates the laryngeal ventricle.

Antero-posterior radiographs of the larynx using kilovoltages of 125–150 kV and a 2 mm brass or combination filter (Thoreus) have the effect of obliterating the obtruding shadows of the cervical vertebrae and allowing the larynx to be seen (bone free) more clearly.

(ii) **Displacement method.** By utilising the mobility of the larynx this structure can be displaced from midline by a lucite rod and oblique films will reveal the details of the larynx free from the overlapping cervical spine. The displacement can be controlled under fluoroscopy and serial films taken at the appropriate degree of displacement. Unfortunately when growths affect the larynx the sensitivity of the structures is such that the free displacement of the larynx, such as occurs normally, is seldom possible and the method consequently loses much of its effectiveness.

(iii) **Tomography.** Radiographic examination of the larynx is incomplete without tomography (Young, 1940; Leborgne, 1940; Ardran & Kemp, 1967). The value of tomography in examination of the larynx may be summarised as follows:

(a) The method is free from discomfort and only demands the co-operation of the patient to the

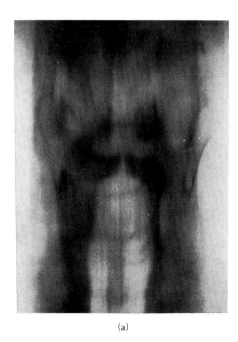

(a)

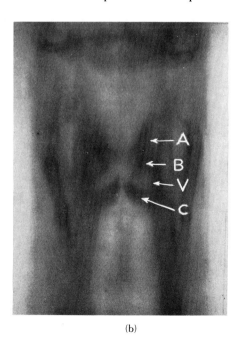

(b)

Fig. 269. Tomographs of the larynx in the antero-posterior position showing the normal markings in two different planes of depth. (a) anterior plane of section through larynx in the antero-posterior position. (b) posterior plane of section showing the relationship of the arytenoid cartilages to the vocal cords.

A—arytenoid fold   V—ventricle
B—false vocal cord   C—true vocal cord.

extent of suspending respiration during the examination.

(b) Tomography enables the outline of the laryngeal soft tissues to be clearly seen without overlap of the bony shadows of the cervical spine.

(c) It enables the lower limits of tumours and extensions into the subglottic space to be defined.

(d) Tomography enables lesions in the subglottic space, frequently invisible to endoscopic methods, to be demonstrated.

The tomographic movement usually used in the larynx has been a linear movement with the patient supine but hypocycloidal movement may be useful in avoiding the summation of shadows which frequently cause disturbing shadows in the linear tomographs.

Accurate coning and the use of small fields are essential in producing films of high quality necessary for diagnosis. An angle of swing of 35°–40° is necessary to obtain a section of sufficient thinness and films are taken at 0·5 cm levels through the larynx; in this manner the whole of the length of the vocal cords and ventricular bands can be seen. The extent of separation of the tomographic sections is nearer 1·0 cm than the 1–2 mm often claimed (Ardran & Emrys Roberts, 1965) (fig. 269).

The examination is carried out with the patient sitting or lying and the neck is straightened so as to bring the larynx as far as possible parallel with the plane of section. The exposure is made with the patient phonating "ee" as this enables approximation of the vocal cords and their outlines can be more clearly seen in relation to the surrounding air.

Tomographs taken at a slightly lower level are invaluable in determining the tracheal relationship at the thoracic inlet. Retrosternal extensions of thyroid enlargements can be well assessed by this method.

Tomographic views of the larynx in the lateral plane are disappointing as the relation of the contained air and soft tissues does not allow the anatomical planes to be clearly differentiated.

The relative values of tomography and laryngography have been admirably summed up by Valvassori & Goldstein (1970) as follows.

(i) Tomography is the study of choice in ascertaining the true extent of glottic and subglottic

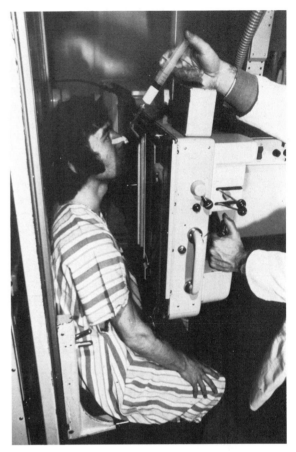

Fig. 270. Laryngogram. The patient sits on an erect screening stand with the catheter in position and the contrast medium is injected under fluoroscopic control.

disease.

(ii) Laryngography is more helpful in ascertaining the precise location and involvement of supraglottic and extrinsic lesions.

(iii) Linear tomography is especially valuable for supraglottic, true cord, laryngeal ventricle and false cord lesions. Linear tomography has the disadvantage of unreliable visualisation of the laryngeal vestibule and pyriform sinus.

(iv) **Contrast examination (laryngograms).** Contrast studies of the larynx and pharynx using oily Dionosil are invaluable in outlining the laryngeal structures.

The technique (Powers, McGee & Seaman, 1957) consists in premedicating the patient with Nembutal and atropine and using a topical spray of

1% lignocaine or cocaine to produce local anaesthesia. 10–20 ml of oily Dionosil are then dripped slowly over the tongue during quiet inspiration. Frontal and lateral films with a spot filming device are then taken during nasal inspiration, phonation and Valsalva and reverse Valsalva manoeuvres (fig. 270). Recently tantalum powder has been used by insufflation as a contrast medium. It may have some advantage in outlining the subglottic region.

Contrast studies have the advantage that the whole of the larynx and hypopharynx are visualised at the one examination. The mucosal coating with contrast medium allows early changes in these structure to be seen and establishes the superiority of this method over all other radiological methods. Antero-posterior, oblique and lateral views of the larynx must be taken to see that the whole length of the ventricle and ventricular bands is shown.

Certain interesting anatomical features are noted in this method, namely:

(i) In nasal inspiration the cords are retracted and not seen.
(ii) The ventricular bands, the vocal cords and the ventricles are symmetrical.
(iii) The cords form a right angle with the trachea.
(iv) The lateral wall of the pyriform fossa may be asymmetrical; the medial wall is uniformly constant on both sides.
(v) The upper surface of the vocal cord may show a normal corrugated appearance (Hemmingson, 1973).

Comparison of the value of the methods used for the investigation of the larynx is shown in the following Table.

TABLE I

COMPARISON OF THE DIAGNOSTIC VALUE OF THE THREE COMMONLY USED ROENTGEN EXAMINATIONS (AFTER JING, 1975)

		Lateral soft tissue Roentgenogram of the neck	Frontal tomogram	Contrast laryngogram
A.	Projections	Lateral	Frontal	Frontal and lateral
B.	Characteristics	Static	Static	Dynamic
C.	Anatomical abnormalities:			
	1. Tumour mass			
	a. small lesion	−	?	+
	b. infiltrative lesion	+	+	+ +
	c. exophytic lesion	+	+	+ +
	2. Mucosal irregularity	−	−	+
D.	Functional abnormalities:			
	a. Change in mobility of mobile structures	−	−	+
	b. Change in distensibility of distensible structures	−	−	+
E.	Specific areas:			
	a. Anterior commissure	−	−	+
	b. Inferior margin of true cord	−	?	+
	c. Subglottic space	+ (anterior)	+ (lateral)	+ (anterior and lateral)
	d. Base of epiglottis	?	−	+
	e. Area distal to supraglottic tumour	?	−	+
	f. Pre-epiglottic space	+	−	?
	g. Thyroid cartilage	+	?	?

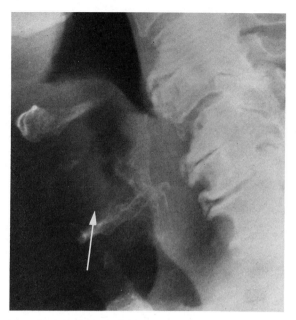

Fig. 271. Carcinoma of larynx. Conventional lateral view showing invasion of thyroid cartilage by an advanced carcinoma of larynx.

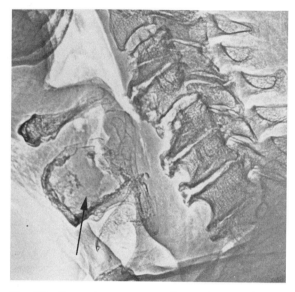

Fig. 272. Comparison xerogram of case shown in fig. 271, showing the bone detail of the larynx and cervical spine more clearly.

Cleft palate. The radiographic investigation of a cleft palate is designed to show the effectiveness of pharyngeal closure during speech and the extent of nasopharyngeal escape.

Cineradiography will clearly show the movements of the palate but serial films of the nasopharynx taken during the phonation of the consonants will indicate the degree of nasopharyngeal closure (Owsley, 1962).

Cineradiography. Considerable information with regard to vocal cord movements, as well as to the mechanism of swallowing, can be obtained by cineradiography of the larynx during speech and of the pharynx during a barium swallow. Kemp & Ardran (1951) have shown the cineradiographic movements of a paralysed vocal cord during speech.

Xerography of the larynx. The use of xerography using the specially charged selenium plates has been made to produce lateral "radiographs". The detail of the laryngeal cartilages and soft tissue produced is remarkable. Unfortunately the radiation dose needed to produce radiographs is high and comparison of xerograms in contrast to routine radiographs reveals that although

aesthetically they are more pleasing, the information obtained is not greater (Samuel, 1975) (figs. 271, 272).

References

ARDRAN, G. M. & EMRYS ROBERTS, E. (1965) Tomography of the Larynx. *Clin. Radiol.,* **16,** 369.

ARDRAN, G. M. & KEMP, F. H. (1967) The Mechanism of the Larynx, Parts I and II. *Br. J. Radiol.,* **39,** 341; **40,** 372.

ARDRAN, G. M. & KEMP, F. H. (1975) The Larynx. In *Modern Trends in Radiology.* Edinburgh: Churchill Livingstone. Chap. 5.

BLACKFIELD, H., OWSLEY, J. O., JR., MULLER, E. L. & LAWSON, L. E. (1963) Cinefluorographic Analysis of the Surgical Treatment of Cleft Palate Speech. *Plastic reconstr. Surg.,* **31,** 542.

EPSTEIN, B. S. (1951) Laminography in the Diagnosis of Nasopharyngeal Tumours. *Radiology,* **56,** 355.

FLETCHER, G. H. & MATZINGER, K. E. (1951) Value of Soft Tissue Technique in the Diagnosis and Treatment of Head and Neck Tumours. *Radiology,* **57,** 305.

HEMMINGSON, A. (1973) Corrugated Vocal Cords. *Acta radiol. Diag.,* **14,** 289.

JING, B.-S. (1975) Roentgen Examination of Laryngeal Cancer: a Critical Evaluation. *Can. J. Otolar.,* **4,** 64.

JÖNSSON, G. (1941) The Roentgenographic Diagnosis of Pathological Conditions in the Nasopharynx. *Acta radiol.,* **22,** 651.

KEMP, F. H. & ARDRAN, G. M. (1951) The Mechanism of Swallowing. *Proc. R. Soc. Med.,* **44,** 1038.

LEBORGNE, F. (1940) Tomographic Study of Cancer of the Larynx. *Am. J. Roentg.,* **43,** 493.

OWSLEY, W. C., JR. (1962) Palate and Pharynx: Roentgenographic Evaluation in the Management of Cleft Palate and Related Deformities. *Am. J. Roentg.,* **87,** 811.

PITMAN, R. G. & FRASER, G. M. (1965) The Post-cricoid Impression on the Oesophagus. *Clin. Radiol.,* **16,** 34.

POWERS, W. E., McGEE, H. H., JR. & SEAMAN, W. B. (1957) Contrast Examination of Larynx and Pharynx. *Radiology,* **68,** 169.

POWERS, W. E., HOLTZ, S. & OGURA, J. (1964) Contrast Examination of Larynx and Pharynx: Inspiratory Phonation. *Am. J. Roentg.,* **92,** 685.

RÜEDI, L. & ZUPPINGER, A. (1934) Zur rontgen-kontrastuntersuchung des Nasopharynx. *Z. Hals-Nasen-Ohrenheilk.,* **35,** 500.

SAMUEL, E. (1975) Xerography or Conventional Radiography for Laryngeal Examination? *Can. J. Otolar.,* **4,** 59.

VALVASSORI, G. E. & GOLDSTEIN, C. (1970) Radiographic Evaluation of the Larynx. *Otol. Clin. N. America,* **3**/3.

YOUNG, B. R. (1940) Recent Advances in Roentgen Examination of the Neck. *Am. J. Roentg.,* **44,** 519.

CHAPTER 14

Development and anatomy of the pharynx and larynx

Embryology. The larynx is developed as an intrinsic part of the respiratory system. It first appears as a groove on the ventral wall of the pharynx. The groove deepens and becomes a tube, the laryngotracheal tube, the cephalic part forms the larynx, the intermediate part the trachea and the terminal portion the lung buds.

On each side of the rudimentary groove which forms the larynx two arytenoid swellings appear and they become approximated to each other and to the furcula (the posterior part of the hypobranchial eminence). The furcula forms the epiglottis and the upper aperture of the larynx forms a vertical slit which later forms the glottis (Frazer, 1940). The upper aperture of the larynx is closed by the adherence of the two arytenoid swellings to each other and this remains closed until the third month when it re-opens (Gray, 1973).

The arytenoid swellings differentiate to form the arytenoid and corniculate cartilages and the folds joining the arytenoid swellings to the posterior end of the hypobranchial arch form the aryepiglottic folds.

The cartilaginous development is as follows:- the arytenoid and corniculate cartilages arise from the arytenoid swellings. The cuneiform cartilage is derived from the epiglottis whilst the thyroid cartilage is derived as two plates from the ventral ends of the fourth and fifth branchial arches. These plates fuse ventrally in the midline by membrane which later chondrifies (Fawcett, 1916).

PHARYNX

The common channel between the mouth, and oesophagus, nose and the larynx is the pharynx. Anatomically (fig. 273) it is subdivided into:

(a) **Nasopharynx,** which represents that portion of the pharynx between the posterior choanae and an arbitrary line drawn at the lower limits of the soft palate.
(b) **Oropharynx,** representing that portion of the pharynx between the level of the soft palate and the level of the hyoid bone.
(c) **Hypopharynx,** connecting the oropharynx and the oesophagus.

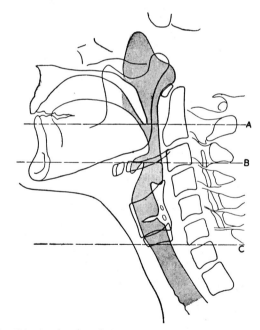

Fig. 273. Line drawing of pharynx.
Plane A: represents the lower border of the nasopharynx drawn through the tip of the palate.
Plane B: The lower border of the oropharynx drawn through the tip of the epiglottis.
Plane C: At the level of the cricoid cartilage representing the lower border of the hypopharynx.

212

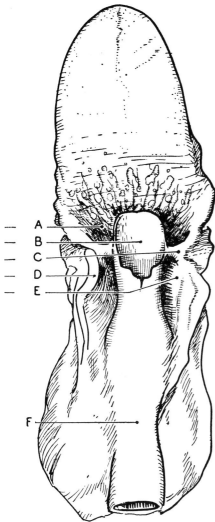

Fig. 274. Line drawing of pharynx and larynx.

A—base of tongue   D—thyroid cartilage
B—epiglottis   E—pyriform fossa
C—aryepiglottic folds   F—trachea

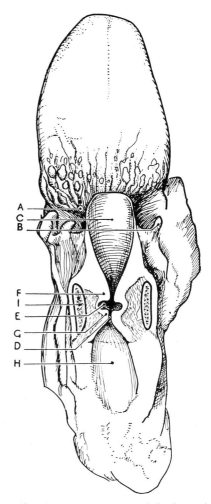

Fig. 275. After the posterior aspect of the larynx has been removed.

A—base of tongue   F—false vocal cord
B—hyoid bone   G—true vocal cord
C—epiglottis   H—subglottic space
D—rima glottidis   I —thyroid cartilage.
E —ventricle of larynx

This subdivision of the pharynx is not only of anatomical interest as pathological conditions arising in each subdivision tend to have specific features (figs. 274, 275).

(a) **Nasopharynx.** On the lateral wall of the nasopharynx lies the slit-like opening of the Eustachian tube and posteriorly is the prominence formed by an aggregation of lymphoid tissue, the Eustachian tubercle.

(b) **Oropharynx.** Anteriorly the oropharynx is bounded by the sloping posterior aspect of the base of the tongue. This is formed by the continuation of the soft tissues downwards from the nasopharynx and inferiorly by an arbitrary line drawn through the hyoid cartilage representing the lower level.

(c) **Hypopharynx.** The hypopharynx extends from the lower edge of the hyoid bone to the mouth of the oesophagus (located at the upper level

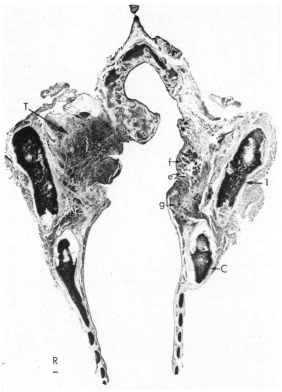

Fig. 276. Thin longitudinal section of larynx showing the normal anatomical markings on the left side corresponding to fig. 275. The cut surfaces of the thyroid and cricoid cartilages are shown. On the right side a laryngeal carcinoma (T) arising from the false vocal cord is seen, and its lateral extension towards the pyriform fossa can be well appreciated.

T—tumour   g —true vocal cord
f —false vocal cord   I —thyroid cartilage (see fig. 275)
e —ventricle   C—cricoid cartilage.
(*Courtesy of Professor D. N. Harrison.*)

of the cricoid cartilage). The upper portion of the hypopharynx is wide, tapering funnel-like into the lower narrower portion. Anteriorly, it is bounded by the aryepiglottic folds whilst posteriorly, the soft tissue shadow covering the vertebral column forms the posterior wall. Lower down the mucosa covering the posterior surface of the cricoid cartilage forms the anterior wall of the hypopharynx (figs. 274, 275, 276).

LARYNX

The larynx representing the uppermost part of the air passage into the lungs, is largely concerned with

speech. It lies in the neck opposite the anterior surfaces of the third to the sixth cervical vertebrae projecting forwards between the great vessels of the neck, and being covered by the depressor muscles of the hyoid bone.

In children and females the larynx lies at a higher level than in the male and until puberty there is no difference between the appearances of the male and female larynx. After puberty considerable differences occur in both sexes, the male larynx shows a considerable increase in size of the cartilage and the rima glottidis is nearly doubled in size.

The larynx is composed of a fibro-muscular organ supported by a cartilaginous skeleton. This supporting cartilage skeleton is composed of nine cartilages, three single and three paired. The unpaired cartilages are the epiglottis, thyroid and cricoid cartilage. The paired cartilages are, two arytenoid, two corniculate, and two cuneiform cartilages. The details of the anatomical features are well seen in laryngograms (figs. 277–279).

The Epiglottis. The epiglottic cartilage is thin, leaf-like and is composed of yellow fibro-cartilage. It projects upwards from beneath the root of the tongue and forms a guard over the entrance to the larynx. The free end of the epiglottis is blunt and rounded – the attached end is long and narrow and is connected by an elastic ligament, the thyro-epiglottic ligament to the superior angle formed by the junction of the lateral plates of the thyroid cartilage. This membrane has an important influence on the spread of laryngeal carcinoma.

The sides of the epiglottis are attached to the laminae of the thyroid cartilage by folds of mucous membrane – the aryepiglottic folds. The mucous membrane is also reflected from the anterior surface of the epiglottis on to the base of the tongue as the glosso-epiglottic folds (a single median fold divides this space into two compartments known as the valleculae).

The radiographic appearances of the epiglottis can best be seen in lateral views of the larynx. The delicate curved appearance can be clearly seen and the aryepiglottic folds running from the lateral walls of the larynx to the epiglottis can be recognised. The valleculae can be seen lying anterior to the epiglottis. During deglutition these vallecular fossae may fill with swallowed material. In the postero-anterior plane the epiglottis seldom casts a sufficiently dense shadow to be visualised and even with special techniques such as

ANATOMIC- MARKINGS – LARYNGOGRAM

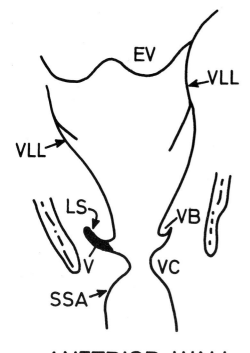

ANTERIOR WALL

Fig. 277. (a) Anterior wall:
V   —ventricle
VC —vocal cord
VB —ventricular band
VLL —lateral wall of larynx
EV —pyriform fossa
LS —laryngeal saccule
SSA —subglottic area.

POSTERIOR WALL

(b) Posterior wall:
SP   —pyriform sinus
A   —arytenoid
HA   —medial raphe
MW/SP—mucosal pattern over posterior wall
TC   —thyroid cartilage.

(after Landman)

tomography it is seldom possible to visualise the epiglottis in this plane.

The thyroid cartilage. The thyroid cartilage is composed of two laminae which are fused anteriorly to form the laryngeal prominence.

Above the laryngeal prominence there is a notch – the suprathyroid notch. The laminae of the thyroid are quadrilateral in shape and their posterior angles are prolonged into superior and inferior cornua. The laminae of the thyroid form protection for the vocal cords and an attachment for the intrinsic muscles of the larynx.

The angle formed by the fusion of both laminae of the thyroid cartilage has a sex difference. In males the angle is approximately 90° and in the female 120°. To the superior cornu of the thyroid cartilage is attached the lateral thyrohyoid ligament whilst on the inferior cornu there is an oval facet for articulation with the cricoid cartilage.

The radiographic visualisation of the thyroid cartilage is largely dependent on the degree of ossification present within the cartilage (fig. 280). Ossification commences in early adult life and involves the posterior free edge of the thyroid cartilage. Ossification then spreads forward into the main lamina of the cartilage (fig. 280). In the

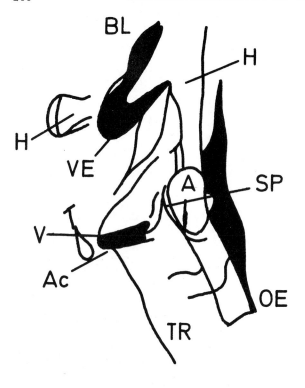

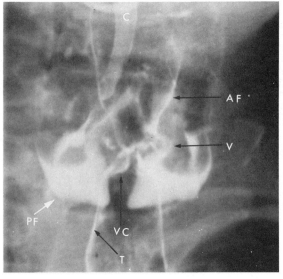

Fig. 279. Laryngogram in antero-posterior projection.

V	—ventricle	AF	—aryepiglottic fold
VC	—vocal cord	PF	—pyriform fossa
T	—lateral wall of trachea	C	—catheter.

LAT. RADIOGRAPHY

Fig. 278. Lateral radiography.

H	—hyoid	OE	—oesophagus
HY	—hypopharynx	SP	—pyriform fossa
VE	—vallecula	V	—ventricle
A	—arytenoid	Ac	—anterior commissure.

(after Landman)

lateral view the posterior margins of the thyroid cartilage, which may be the only part ossified, may lie across the cervical soft tissues and may be mistaken for a swallowed fish bone. The ossification in the lamina of the thyroid is extremely irregular, a feature which must be evaluated when estimating malignant invasion or in the diagnosis of fractures of thyroid cartilage. Keen & Wainwright (1957) have shown that ossification in the thyroid cartilage is genetically determined and not a simple degenerative process associated with advancing age. Vastine & Vastine (1952) have reported that ossification of all the laryngeal cartilages was similar in identical twins and this would appear to

confirm the importance of genetic factors in determining the pattern of ossification.

The cricoid cartilage. The cricoid cartilage is shaped like a signet ring, and is most inferior of the laryngeal cartilages. It consists of a posterior quadrate lamina and a narrow anterior arch. Anteriorly, the arch is attached to the thyroid cartilage by the crico-thyroid ligament whilst below it is joined to the first ring of the trachea by the crico-tracheal ligament.

Ossification of the cartilage of the cricoid occurs in early life and again, as in the thyroid cartilage, the ossification process commences in the posterior quadrate lamina of the cartilage.

Arytenoid cartilages. The arytenoid cartilages are paired and are situated at the upper border of the lamina of the cricoid cartilage at the back of the larynx. Each is pyramidal in shape and has three surfaces, a base and an apex. The base has a smooth surface for articulation with the cricoid cartilage. **The anterior angle (vocal process) is sharp and** projects forward to give attachment to the vocal cords.

The arytenoids can be readily demonstrated on the radiograph owing to the frequency with which they ossify. It is claimed that the vocal process of

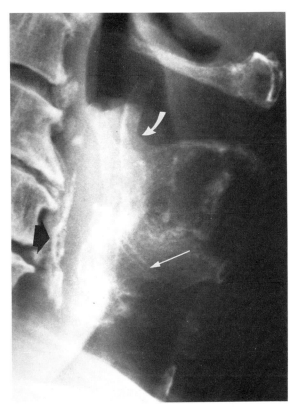

Fig. 280. Extensive ossification in the thyroid (superior cornua indicated by curved arrow) and cricoid cartilages (thin arrow). Note the extensive calcification posteriorly which lies in the carotid artery (black arrow).

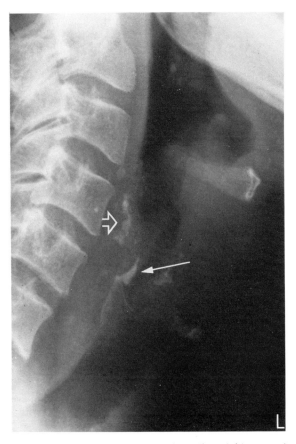

Fig. 281. Ossification in arytenoid cartilage (white arrow) appearing as dense shadows due to superimposition of both arytenoids. Hollow arrow indicates calcification in carotid artery overlying thyroid cartilage and triangular calcified appearance of cricoid cartilage posteriorly is clearly seen.

the arytenoid cartilage does not ossify. The paired nature of the cartilages enables them to be easily recognised but in the lateral position they may be superimposed and the single dense shadow thrown has been mistaken for a foreign body (fig. 281).

The two other paired cartilages, the corniculate (Santorini) and cuneiform (Wrisberg) cartilages cannot be demonstrated on the radiograph unless they are ossified.

The corniculate cartilages. The corniculate cartilages are two small conical nodules of yellow elastic cartilage which articulate with the summits of the arytenoid cartilages and serve to prolong them backwards and medially.

The cuneiform cartilages. The cuneiform cartilages are two small nodules of yellow elastic cartilage placed one on each side in the

aryepiglottic fold. Another small cartilage which may ossify and become demonstrable on the radiograph is the Cartilago Triticea which lies in the thyrohyoid ligament halfway between the thyroid cartilage and the hyoid bone.

All the intrinsic cartilages of the larynx are joined together by the ligaments and the presence of diarthrodial joints between the cartilages allows rotary and gliding movements to take place. Rarely a false joint forms between the greater cornua of the hyoid and thyroid cartilages (fig. 282).

Ossification may occur in the ligaments of the larynx. The commonest ligament to ossify is the stylohyoid ligament. Ossification in the stylohyoid

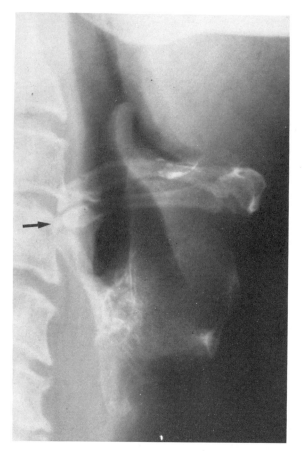

Fig. 282. Abnormal articulation between greater cornua of the hyoid bone and superior horns of thyroid cartilage.

The portion of the larynx above the false vocal cords is the vestibule of the larynx. It is wide above and narrow below, and the anterior wall is considerably longer than the posterior wall. The anterior wall is formed by the inner surfaces of the aryepiglottic folds. The vestibule of the larynx can be clearly visualised in the lateral radiograph.

The ventricle of the larynx is a fusiform recess which arises from the middle part of the larynx and lies between the true and false vocal cords. From its upper surface arises the appendix of the ventricle which ascends between the ventricular fold and the inner surface of the thyroid cartilage.

The ventricle of the larynx can be clearly seen in the lateral radiograph and the true and false vocal cords are easily identifiable. The appendix of the ventricle unless it is enlarged cannot be visualised.

The ventricular folds (false vocal cords) are two thick folds of mucous membrane enclosing the ventricular ligament. The vocal folds (true vocal cords) consist of a band of yellow elastic tissue attached in front to the angle of the thyroid cartilage, and behind to the vocal process of the arytenoid cartilage. The vocalis muscle lies lateral to and parallel to the vocal ligament.

The ventricular and vocal folds can be clearly seen in the lateral films of the larynx. In the antero-posterior tomograms the vocal folds are readily recognised and the rima glottidis stands out clearly. The mucosal surfaces of the soft tissues of the larynx can however be best visualised by contrast laryngography. Normal mucosal irregularity on the upper surface of the vocal cords (corrugated vocal cords) Hemmingson (1973) must not be mistaken for early malignancy.

During the performance of a barium swallow the normal larynx produces an impression on the swallow which may be mistaken for a tumour mass (fig 283).

ligament may appear as an anomalous hyoid bone (Klinefelter, 1952). The crico-thyroid membrane is the next commonest ligament in the larynx to show ossification.

The cavity of the larynx (cavum laryngis) extends from the laryngo-pharyngeal entrance to the level of the upper ring of the trachea where it is continuous with the cavity of the trachea.

Two pairs of folds of mucous membrane project into the laryngeal cavity and divide it into three compartments. The upper pair of folds are known as the ventricular folds (false vocal cords) and the fissure between them is called the rima vestibuli. The lower pair of folds are called the vocal folds (true vocal cords) and the fissure between them is known as the rima glottidis.

REFERENCES

FAWCETT, E. (1916) *Proceedings of the Anatomical Society of Great Britain and Ireland.*

FRAZER, J.E. (1940) *Manual of Embryology,* 2nd Ed. Baltimore: Williams and Wilkins. p. 242.

GRAY, H. (1973) *Gray's Anatomy,* 35th Ed. Ed. R. Warwick. London: Longmans.

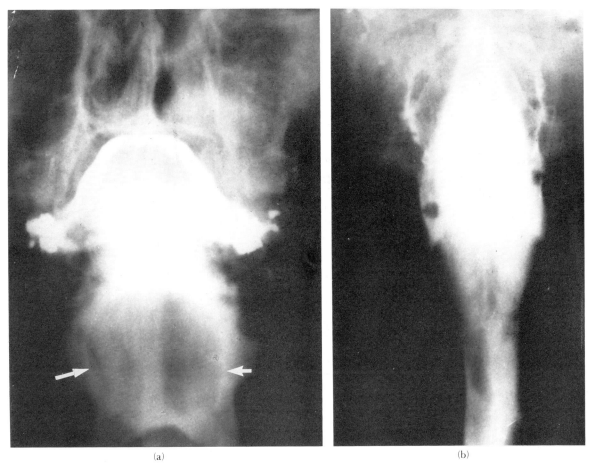

(a)   (b)

Fig. 283. Laryngeal impression on barium swallow. Barium swallow showing normal laryngeal impression on the barium-filled oesophagus. Note that the impression of a soft tissue tumour is transient.
(a) During initial phase as the barium bolus passes over the tongue.
(b) During a later phase of deglutition.

HEMMINGSON, A. (1973) Corrugated Vocal Cords. *Acta radiol.*, **14,** 289.

KEEN, J.A. & WAINWRIGHT, J. (1957) Ossification of the Thyroid, Cricoid and Arytenoid Cartilages. *S. Afr. J. Lab. clin. Med.*, **58,** 83.

KLINEFELTER, F.W. (1952) The Anomalous Hyoid. *Radiology*, **58,** 221.

LANDMAN, G. H. M. (1970) *Laryngography and Cinelaryngography.* Excerpta Medica Foundation.

VASTINE, J.H. & VASTINE, M.F. (1952) Calcification in the Laryngeal Cartilages. *Archs Otol.*, **55,** 1.

CHAPTER 15

Non-malignant lesions of the pharynx and larynx

FOREIGN BODIES

Foreign bodies lodging in the upper respiratory passages usually draw attention to themselves by violent symptoms of choking and coughing. In some instances, however, the foreign body may cause relatively minor or even no symptoms and thus may remain undetected for a considerable time. This is especially so in infants where a comparatively large foreign body lodged in the pharynx or larynx may remain apparently asymptomatic for a long period. In such cases the foreign body is usually lodged in the vallecula, less commonly between the false vocal cords.

Radiological appearances. If the foreign body is radio-opaque it can be seen in the lateral and postero-anterior views. The widespread use of plastic materials of low radio opacity constitutes a new hazard in the detection of foreign bodies aspirated into the air passages.

Fragments of animal or fish bone of comparatively low density may be mistaken for calcification in the thyroid or cricoid cartilages, and likewise the arytenoid cartilage when ossified may be mistaken for a foreign body (fig. 281). The paired nature of the ossified arytenoid may not be apparent as in lateral films the shadows of both arytenoids may be superimposed. The resemblance of an ossified arytenoid to a foreign body may be heightened by the fact that the arytenoid may be well ossified when no other laryngeal cartilage may show such change.

Calcification occurring in the wall of the common carotid artery near its bifurcation may be also projected (in the lateral view) over the post-cricoid space and cause confusion with a swallowed foreign body (fig. 280).

Air in the post-cricoid portion of the oesophagus may signify a non-opaque foreign body lodged at a slightly lower level in the oesophagus. This is not invariably so as air may be normally present in this region of the oesophagus in elderly subjects.

TRAUMA

Injuries to the pharynx generally result from direct blows or gunshot wounds. In such cases radiographic examination is mainly of value to determine the extent of damage to the hyoid bone. In evaluating fractures of the hyoid bone it must be remembered that the hyoid bone develops from several ossific centres and non-fusion of these should not be mistaken for fractures. Radiographic examination of the hyoid bone may have medico-legal implications in cases of suspected strangulation and radiographic examination of the cadaver before the larynx is removed may be an important factor in assessing damage in such cases. Indirect injury to the pharynx may result in damage to the muscular wall with the formation of a traumatic hernia.

Hankins (1944) records a case of traumatic hernia of the lateral pharyngeal walls occurring in a trumpet player. Radiological examination during forced expiration showed that the pyriform sinuses were dilated and bulged on both sides above the level of the larynx. The symmetrical nature and sites of the bulges enabled them to be differentiated from true laryngoceles.

A sequel of penetrating traumatic lesions of the pharynx is the development of palato- and glosso-pharyngeal stenosis. The radiological features of traumatic and other forms of pharyngeal stenosis are discussed by Dohlman & Thulin (1949) who report eight cases of stenosis due to diverse causes.

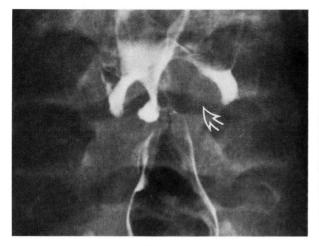

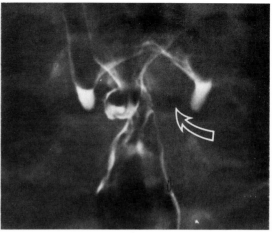

Fig. 284. Dislocated arytenoid cartilage. A young Mormon preacher who had been attacked by a bull and butted in the throat. Subsequently he had noticed voice weakness and hoarseness.

Fig. 285. Same case as fig. 284 during phonation, showing the abnormal movement of the cord on the affected side and the soft tissue swelling.

Radiology can demonstrate the extent and degree of stenosis during voluntary distension of the pharynx with air after the swallowing of thick barium to coat the pharyngeal wall, when a double contrast picture is obtained.

Injuries to the larynx may result from injuries to the neck caused by closed or penetrating wounds. Kicks and blows to the larynx may cause dislocation of the arytenoid cartilage without any fracture of the thyroid cartilage. The presenting symptom is usually a voice change and the dislocated arytenoid can be demonstrated by contrast laryngography (figs. 284, 285). Endoscopic examination reveals a bulge in the mucosa in the site of the normal arytenoid cartilage.

In closed injuries of the larynx three clinical stages present. In Stage I – the acute reactive stage, oedema and haematoma formation distort the laryngeal soft tissues. At this stage only conventional radiographic views are possible.

Stage II occurs from three days to several weeks after injury when the acute swelling has subsided. Tomography is usually possible at this stage and provides a better analysis of the extent of the lesion.

Stage III is the sequel of laryngeal trauma when cicatricial stenosis or web formation may occur. Examination by laryngography is essential to evaluate such lesions and in cases when a laryngo-oesophageal fistula is suspected a Gastrografin

swallow may demonstrate the fistulous track (Valvassori & Goldstein, 1970).

Penetrating injuries due to missiles, e.g. gunshot wounds and stab wounds, form a high percentage of laryngeal injuries. Lederer & Howard (1946) record 43 wartime injuries affecting the larynx. In this latter series radiology was used mainly to determine the site and size of the foreign body.

Surgical fulguration of laryngeal papilloma if excessive may result in a perichondritis of a laryngeal cartilage with the development of a stricture.

Radiation treatment of cervical adenopathy or post-cricoid carcinoma may result in stricture formation in the pharynx and in the cervical oesophagus.

In the nasopharynx post-operative fibrosis of the palate after repair of a cleft palate may be referred for investigation. Fibrosis of the palate results in a failure of the palate to close off the nasopharynx during speech with "nasopharyngeal escape" of air. Voice production is affected by this nasopharyngeal escape and examination of the soft palate in the lateral view or during phonation of various consonants will demonstrate the degree of effective closure of the nasopharynx. Cineradiographic studies and 70 mm film taken at even slower rates of 3 frames/second will help in the evaluation of palatal movement (Owsley, 1962).

LYMPHOID TISSUE

The orifice of the oropharynx is surrounded by a ring of lymphoid tissue, the tonsil, adenoid and lingual tonsil. Infection, reticulo-endotheliosis and other conditions may cause general enlargement of one member or all this group. An enlargement, especially of the adenoid pad, may occur to such a degree as to completely obliterate the nasopharynx. Obstruction to the nasal air space may result in mouth breathing and the clinical features of the "adenoid facies".

Clinical examination of the pharynx is generally sufficient to obtain all the necessary information relevant to the pharyngeal and lingual tonsils.

With adenoid enlargement, however, inspection by a nasopharyngeal mirror, necessary to obtain

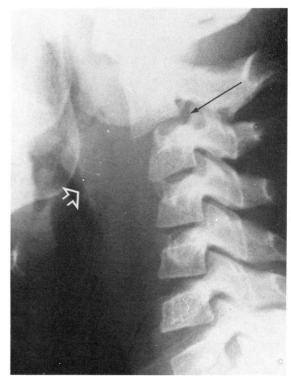

Fig. 287. Dislocation of axis on 3rd cervical vertebra after adenoidectomy. The child complained of stiffness and pain in the neck. The forward slip of the 2nd on the 3rd cervical vertebra (black arrow) is seen, and the swelling of the prevertebral soft tissues is visible (hollow arrow).

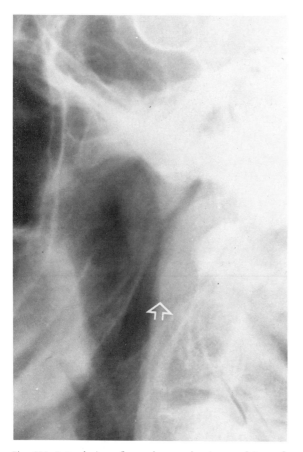

Fig. 286. Lateral view of nasopharynx showing overlying soft tissue shadow of lobule of ear mimicking a soft tissue polyp in the nasopharynx.

the requisite information may sometimes be difficult or impossible in children. In such cases lateral views of the nasopharynx will reveal the size of the adenoid pad (Groth, 1933). Care should be taken not to confuse the lobule of the ear with the shadow caused by an enlarged adenoid pad (fig. 286). Injuries to the cervical spine may occur after adenoidectomy (figs 287, 288).

Enlarged and hypertrophied tonsillar shadows can also be revealed (fig. 289). The demonstration of the soft tissue structures projecting into the nasopharynx is aided if the air content, and consequently the contrast, is increased by the performance of Valsalva's manoeuvre during the exposure. Calcification in the tonsil probably represents calcification in epithelial debris within the crypts of the tonsil. Such calcified opacities (tonsilloliths) may cause confusion in lateral views

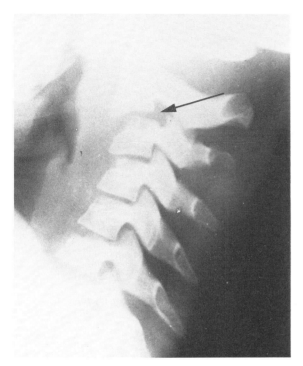

Fig. 288. Same case as fig. 287, in flexion showing an increase in the degree of subluxation.

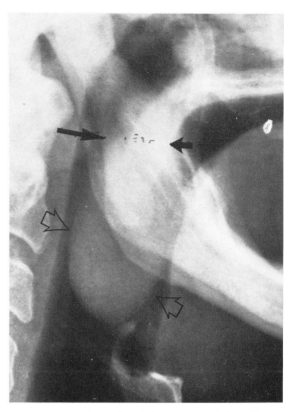

Fig. 289. Enlarged tonsillar shadows – particularly well seen. Soft palate indicated (dense arrows) and tonsillar shadow (hollow arrows). Histological section showed simply hypertrophied tonsillar tissue.

of the neck. They are most frequently mistaken for calcified tuberculous glands.

The soft tissue shadow of the adenoid pad can be seen projecting from the posterior and superior wall of the nasopharynx into the nasopharyngeal air space towards the shadow cast by the soft palate. The enlargement of this adenoid pad may be to such a degree as to completely obliterate the nasopharyngeal air space.

Clifford, Neuhauser & Ferguson (1944) and Calthrop (1940) advocate radiology as an accurate means of defining the exact size of the mass of the adenoid pad. The radiographic technique advocated by these authors for a child aged two years is a lateral projection taken at a focal film distance of 1 m with 1/60th second exposure at 200 milliamperes and 65 kilovolts. Films should be exposed when there is most air present in the nasopharynx, i.e. at the beginning of the cry in an infant, and on exhalation through the nose in older children.

Weitz (1946) has measured the soft tissue mass projecting from the nasopharynx and has attempted to classify adenoid hyperplasia according to these measurements. He considers that a soft tissue shadow of more than 6–7 mm projecting from the roof of the nasopharynx is pathological, and that 7–9 mm represents slight adenoid enlargement, 1–1·5 cm moderate hyperplasia, and more than 1·5 cm marked hyperplasia, usually with complete occlusion of the nasopharynx.

Widening of the retro-pharyngeal soft tissue space may also present a problem in radiological diagnosis. Usually widening of this space is due to enlargement of the retro-pharyngeal lymph glands. Rathbone (1940) has attempted to formulate actual radiographic measurements of this space. In this author's experience in infants and children the width should not exceed 11 mm. Table I shows the average measurements and Table II the commonest causes of widening of this space.

TABLE I

NORMAL MEASUREMENTS

	Exposure during Insp.		28–48 inch target distance			
Age	Under 1 year		1–2 years		2–3 years	
No. of cases	40		19		21	
	Retro-pharyngeal	Retro-tracheal	Retro-pharyngeal	Retro-tracheal	Retro-pharyngeal	Retro-tracheal
Extremes	11–3 mm	18–8 mm	11–4 mm	16–8 mm	11–3 mm	14–8 mm
Average	7 mm	10 mm	8 mm	11 mm	8 mm	10 mm

TABLE II

CLINICAL DIAGNOSIS IN TWENTY CASES WHICH RADIOLOGICALLY SHOWED RETROPHARYNGEAL WIDENING

Diagnosis	No. of cases	Age
Nasopharyngitis or sinus disease . .	6	18/12, 19/12, 24/12, 8/12, 16/12, 18/12
Enlarged thymus	5	4/52, 5/52, 6/52, 3/12, 12/12
Otitis media	4	7/12, 9/12, 10/12, 20/12
Foreign body	2	14/12, 19/12
Unexplained fever	1	19/12
Cervical adenitis	2	2½ years, 3 years

LARYNX

Infections

Infections involving the nasopharynx or larynx, unless a local abscess forms, seldom give rise to a soft tissue enlargement to a degree that needs radiographic examination.

Acute infections of the epiglottis. Infection or abscess formation in the epiglottis (epiglottitis) is relatively uncommon but when it occurs it is associated with huge swelling of the epiglottis and the symptoms of acute upper respiratory tract obstruction. Oedema of the glottis may develop as a complication of an acute infection of the epiglottis.

As direct or indirect laryngoscopy may be impossible radiography may be the only means of visualisation. The lateral radiograph of the nasopharynx will reveal an enormous swelling of the epiglottis bulging into the oropharyngeal air space and associated with loss of the normally sharp soft tissue contours of the epiglottis (fig. 290).

Acute infections of the larynx. The features of acute infections are blurring of the soft tissue outlines with an encroachment on the air space. The ventricle of the larynx disappears and the margins of the mucosal folds of the larynx, *i.e.* the aryepiglottic folds, normally sharp, become blurred.

In diphtheria with membrane formation the membrane is usually located in the vicinity of the vocal cords and in the area immediately below them. Radiological investigation is seldom required. Post-diphtheritic strictures are usually in the subglottic region and in the trachea immediately below.

Radiological investigation of post-diphtheritic strictures may be of inestimable value as the extent, especially the length of the stricture, can be estimated by this method (figs. 291, 292). Endoscopic methods of examination can only show the upper limit of the stricture and contrast laryngography is the easiest means of determining the length of the stricture (fig. 295).

The roentgen findings are those of a funnel-shaped column of air with its base directed towards the larynx, ending in a stricture in the cricoid region. The lower limit of the stricture can be

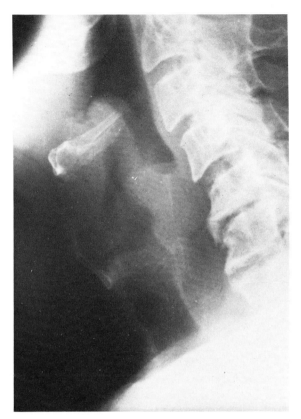

Fig. 290. Acute epiglottitis – general swelling of epiglottis and to a lesser extent of the aryepiglottic folds. The cavity of the larynx is not involved.

Rhinoscleroma. Another granulomatous lesion which affects the upper respiratory passages and which may give rise to granulomatous masses is rhinoscleroma. Hoover & King (1953) reported a male, aged 56 years, who presented with a mass in the nose. In other cases the lesion progresses downwards along the larynx and may give rise to stricture formation in the larynx or subglottic region.

Laryngeal obstruction in infancy

Laryngeal or tracheal stridor in infancy is an ever recurring problem. It has become generally accepted that stridor in infants tends to disappear as the child grows and the larynx enlarges quicker than general body growth. The paediatric opinion is that unless there is failure of the infant to thrive the stridor need not be regarded too seriously (Franklin, 1952). Birrell (1952) feels that at the end of one year in most instances the stridor has disappeared without any apparent cause being found. According to Pracy (1965) this type of congenital stridor does not account for more than 25% of cases.

Radiographic examination is a relatively simple but extremely useful means of investigating causes of stridor, but an appreciation of the variability of tracheal size is an important consideration in assessing stridor. Kinking of the trachea readily occurs with alterations in position of the infant's head, and these variations must not be mistaken as the cause of stridor.

The causes of stridor have been classified as follows:

(a) *Intrinsic*
    (i) Laryngomalacia (congenital laryngeal stridor)
    (ii) Unilateral vocal cord paralysis
    (iii) Laryngeal cysts
    (iv) Subglottic stenosis
    (v) Laryngeal webs and atresias
    (vi) Acute or subacute laryngitis
    (vii) Multiple papillomas

(b) *Extrinsic*
    (i) Vascular rings
    (ii) Retropharyngeal abscess
    (iii) Paralaryngeal cyst

determined by the extent of interruption of the air column. Occasionally, the strictures may be multiple.

Tuberculosis. Tuberculosis may involve the vocal cords and arytenoids. A generalised swelling of all the soft tissues with an obliteration of the ventricle of the larynx may be present. The radiograph shows obliteration of the shadow of the ventricle and of the vocal cords. The radiographic appearances in the larynx in themselves are not diagnostic but any generalised swelling of the laryngeal soft tissues should suggest the necessity of a radiograph of the chest (figs. 293, 294).

Syphilis. Syphilitic chondritis and perichondritis do not give any specific radiological appearances and the investigation and radiological appearances of syphilitic strictures do not differ from other laryngeal strictures.

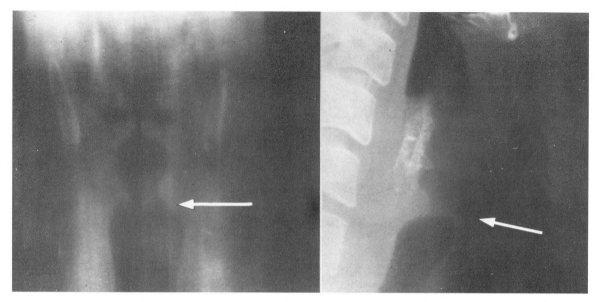

Fig. 291. Larynx showing stricture following misplaced tracheostomy. A.P. tomogram showing stricture in subglottic region.

Fig. 292. Lateral view of same case as fig. 291 showing stricture.

(iv) Congenital goitre
(v) Undiagnosed.

The majority of extrinsic causes result in tracheal as opposed to laryngeal stridor and apart from congenital goitre, which can be readily recognised clinically, the stridor is usually the result of constricting lesions surrounding the trachea in the upper mediastinum.

The commonest cause is a vascular ring and the commonest anomaly is a double aortic arch but an anomalous right or left subclavian artery may also give rise to considerable tracheal compression (Neuhauser, 1946). These vascular abnormalities may be detected by their impressions on the barium filled oesophagus but arteriography is usually necessary to confirm the diagnosis.

Congenital laryngeal stridor (laryngomalacia). Congenital laryngeal stridor tends to disappear spontaneously between the first and third years (Birrell, 1952) and unless it is associated with failure of the infant to thrive need not be the cause of serious concern (Franklin, 1952).

The value of radiographic examination is mainly to exclude other causes of stridor.

Unilateral vocal cord paralysis. Unilateral paralysis, like cysts, laryngomalacia and vascular rings, gives rise to stridor at birth; bilateral adductor paralysis does not produce symptoms until a month or so after birth. In adult life **unilateral paralysis does not produce stridor.**

Radiological examination, especially cineradiography, demonstrates the "cadaveric" position of the affected cord with the characteristic bulge in the subglottic region (Ardran & Kemp, 1975).

In functional paralysis of the cord the following features may be seen:

(1) The involved cord is partly abducted at rest.
(2) The laryngeal ventricle is more obvious and appears larger.
(3) The cord is immobile during phonation.
(4) The false cord is more prominent on the opposite side to the lesion.
(5) The pyriform sinus is more prominent on the affected side (Valvassori & Goldstein, 1970).
(6) A subglottic bulge is invariably present on the affected side (Ardran & Kemp, 1975).

Laryngeal cysts. Laryngeal cysts may be suspected clinically when the stridor is more pronounced, when the infant is completely relaxed and asleep.

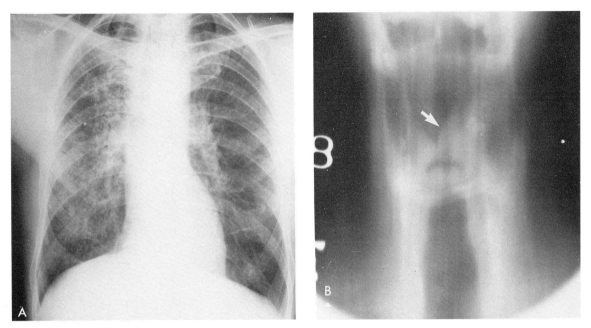

Fig. 293. Tuberculosis of larynx. Male aged 61 years who had complained of dryness and sticking in the left side of his pharynx. A teleradiogram of the chest shows extensive tuberculous infiltration of the right upper lobe (fig. 293A). Tomographs of the larynx (fig. 293B) showed a swollen and thickened left false vocal cord. No mucosal ulceration could be seen.

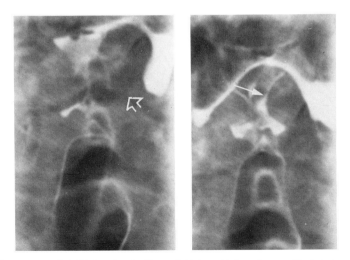

Fig. 294. Laryngogram of same case as fig. 293 showing swollen and thickened left cord covered by intact mucosa. Histological examination of a biopsy specimen showed typical tuberculous granulation tissue.
(Courtesy of Dr. A. G. Maran and Dr. A. J. A. Wightman.)

Feeding difficulties are uncommon (Pracy, 1965).

Lateral radiographs of the neck may show a soft tissue swelling with a smooth outline. Laryngeal cysts have to be differentiated from laryngeal papillomas, which may be difficult if the papilloma has a smooth outline and does not show any of the characteristic pitting of the surface of the papilloma. Antero-posterior tomography may give further details of the site, size and extent of the cyst (fig. 319).

Subglottic stenosis. This may be associated with laryngeal webs and cartilaginous masses may develop around the cricoid cartilage (figs. 295–297). Holinger, Johnson & Schiller (1954) found 34 cases of subglottic stenosis out of 379 congenital abnormalities of the larynx of all types.

Cavanagh (1965) reporting on the value of lateral radiography in the demonstration of subglottic stenosis described two cases of laryngeal web who had additional subglottic stenosis. Histological examination in one of these cases which ended fatally showed a dense fibrous mass intimately blending with the cricoid. The lateral radiograph in this case demonstrated a soft tissue mass with an inward projection from the tracheal walls in the subglottic region (figs. 295, 296, 297).

Laryngeal webs and atresias. Zurhelle (1869) reported the first case of congenital laryngeal web diagnosed by indirect laryngoscopy although they had been noted at post-morten examination previously. McHugh and Loch (1942) found 133 such cases reported in the literature, 100 at cord level, 10 subglottic and 7 complete atresia. Holinger et al. (1954) found 19 laryngeal webs in a total of 379 congenital abnormalities. Over 11% of cases of laryngeal webs are associated with other congenital abnormalities (McHugh and Loch, 1942); the majority of associated congenital lesions affect the palate, lips, eyes, toes, feet and anus.

The web may affect the whole or part of the laryngeal space between the vocal cords. Lateral films do not usually reveal any abnormality if simple web formation is present and are mainly of value in excluding associated subglottic stenosis. Contrast laryngography will be helpful in outlining the web and is of especial value in excluding more than one stricture.

Acute or subacute laryngitis. Stridor in these conditions is a sequel of inflammatory oedema (laryngitis stridulosa). There are no specific radiological features in these conditions.

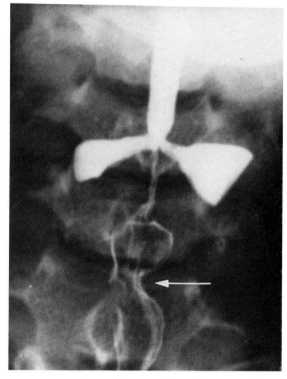

Fig. 295. Laryngeal stricture subglottic. Laryngogram demonstrating the clear outline of the stricture and the normal mucosa covering the stricture.

Laryngeal papilloma occurs in young infants when the vocal cords become the site of papillomatous formation. The frequency of laryngeal papilloma varies between 1 in 6,000 (Clark, 1905) and 1 in 14,000 (Ferguson & Scott, 1944). The infantile type of laryngeal papilloma resembles the adult type in the frequency of its recurrence after removal but differs in the absence of any tendency towards malignant change. According to Ferguson & Scott (1944) these laryngeal papillomas tend to recur although they finally disappear at puberty.

The symptoms of laryngeal papilloma are mainly produced by mechanical obstruction to speech and respiration. The diagnosis of laryngeal papilloma is best made by direct laryngoscopy but lateral radiographs and tomographs in the antero-posterior position will equally well show the exact site and extent of the papillomatosis. Serial radiography particularly with contrast laryn-

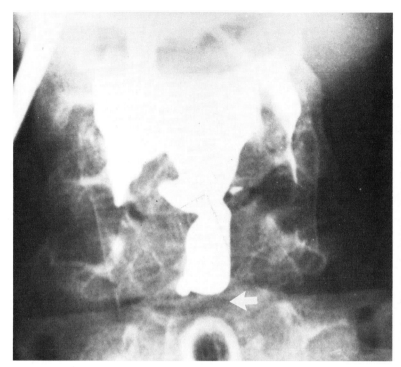

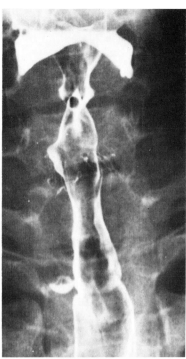

Fig. 296. Laryngeal stricture, post-diphtheritic, showing complete obstruction above the tracheostomy opening. No contrast media extends beyond the stricture. The tracheostomy is seen at the lower end of the film.

Fig. 297. Laryngeal stricture – same case as fig. 296, after surgical repair of stricture. Note that a small diverticulum has occurred in the tracheal wall below the site of stricture.

gography is the best means of keeping a record of the progress and the response to therapy.

Radiological appearances. (i) In the lateral radiograph the papilloma can be seen arising as a soft tissue swelling from the vocal cords. It has a smooth outline but often has a mottled appearance due to air lying in the interstices of the papilloma (a radiological feature which when present, enables it to be distinguished from a congenital laryngeal cyst) (fig. 298).

(ii) In the antero-posterior tomograms a soft tissue mass arising from the vocal cords can be seen.

(iii) Contrast laryngograms will coat the papilloma and often allow its exact site of origin to be ascertained.

Displacements of the larynx and trachea

Extrinsic masses in the neck may cause marked compression or displacement of the larynx or trachea. Radiological investigation enables the exact site of the larynx and cervical portion of the trachea involved to be determined and the extent of compression ascertained.

The conditions which displace and compress the cervical trachea may be divided into:

(a) Thyroid swellings.
(b) Other cervical masses.

The subdivision into these two groups is a result of the intimate relationship borne by the thyroid to the trachea. The thyroid swellings envelop the trachea and cause side to side compression as well as displacement of the trachea. In the large goitres the displacement of the cervical portion of the trachea is considerably more than the degree of lateral compression. In other conditions of the thyroid gland, *e.g.* Riedel's thyroiditis, marked lateral compression may not be associated with any displacement of the trachea. Antero-posterior compression of the trachea usually implies

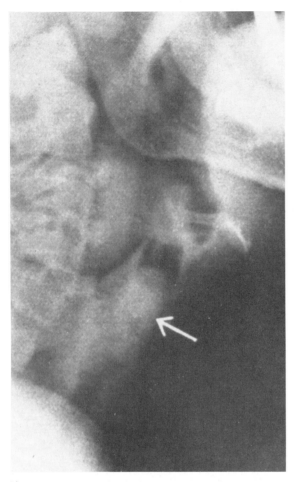

Fig. 298. Papilloma of larynx. A 3-year-old girl who had suffered from choking attacks and a weak voice. Cyanosis of the lips was present and dyspnoea was exaggerated in the recumbent position. The lateral radiograph shows a soft tissue shadow occupying the larynx with distension of the hypopharynx. Endoscopy showed a papillomatous tumour involving the larynx. The thin streaks of air in the body of the mass are a radiological feature indicating its papillomatous nature.

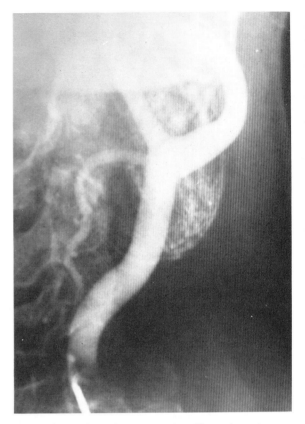

Fig. 299. Carotid body tumour. Carotid arteriography may enable soft tissue masses displacing the trachea, *e.g.* carotid body tumour, to be recognized. The arteriogram shows the typical appearances of the carotid body tumour in the arterial phase showing tumour staining and splaying of the internal and external carotid vessels.

involvement of the thyroid isthmus and is most frequently seen in malignant tumours of the thyroid gland. The separation of the trachea from the oesophagus by extension of the retro-laryngeal portion of the thyroid is another diagnostic feature of thyroid enlargement. Other cervical masses which displace the larynx and trachea do so without any radiological feature to indicate the nature of the mass. Branchial cysts, glandular masses either malignant or benign, and carotid body tumours (fig. 299) all may cause displacement of the larynx and cervical portion of the trachea.

Laryngocele (pneumocele)

This is an air-filled sac arising from the lateral aspect of the larynx and probably represents a dilated sacculus of the larynx. Horowitz (1951) classified laryngoceles into internal, when they lie within the larynx proper, and external when they present outside the larynx. The first type he regards as **primary (congenital)** and it is usually **asymptomatic**, while the **secondary (extrinsic)** usually causes symptoms. Simpson (1938) regards the majority of laryngoceles as congenital in origin. In some of the higher primates, *e.g.* the gorilla, the sacculus arising from the ventricle of the larynx is enormously developed and the laryngocele in the human probably represents a similar developmental structure.

Clinically, laryngoceles present as soft cyst-like tumours on the lateral aspect of the larynx which are soft and doughy to the touch (Blewett, 1939). In other instances voice changes or shortness of breath may be the predominant feature (Harrison, 1950). They can be made to vary in size by Valsalva's experiment. They show an impulse on coughing and have to be differentiated from cystic hygromas and branchial cysts.

Radiological appearances. Radiographic examination is diagnostic as the large air-filled space communicating with the larynx is readily recognisable and the increase in size with Valsalva's test is diagnostic. Tomograms in the antero posterior plane are necessary to outline the intrinsic type of laryngocele (fig. 300).

Jackson (1945) recommends tomography as a useful means of determining the size and shape of the laryngocele (fig. 301). Lindsay (1940) prefers radiography whilst the patient forcibly expires against a closed nose and mouth. In children the easiest means, although the noisiest, is to obtain a radiograph whilst blowing a whistle.

Differential diagnosis. Cystic hygromas and branchial cysts cast shadows which are of the same density as the other soft tissue structures in the neck. Lipomas cast a shadow of somewhat less density than normal structures but their radiolucency is not as great as a laryngocele and they do not show the same alteration in size with Valsalva's test. Furthermore, their outline is seldom as clearly defined as a laryngocele.

The development of speech after laryngectomy

Radiographic investigation of the development of the speech mechanism in laryngectomised patients forms an interesting study (Kallen, 1934; Bangs, 1947).

Three types of speech appear to develop after total laryngectomy.

(a) *Buccal speech.* A whispered sound produced from air displaced from the buccal cavity. This is an extremely poor form of speech and only a few words can be formed. This probably represents the

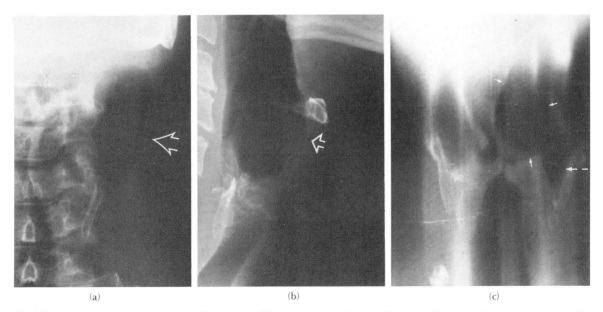

(a) (b) (c)

Fig. 300. Laryngocele. Showing an internal and external laryngocele (a) A.P. view. The external laryngocele is clearly seen but the internal laryngocele less well so. The A.P. tomogram (c) shows the internal laryngocele clearly displacing the false cord. The lateral view (b) does not show the laryngocele clearly due to superimposition on the air filled pharynx. The pyriform fossa on the left side is distended with air (broken arrow).

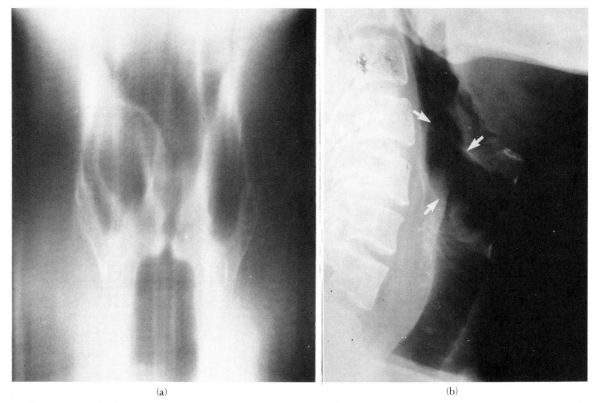

(a)   (b)

Fig. 301. Laryngocele. (a) P.A. tomogram. Internal laryngocele showing no external component. The whole sac lying within the thyroid cartilage. (b) Lateral view. Small laryngoceles may be easily overlooked in the lateral view even when the sac is distended.

first stage in the development of speech after laryngectomy.

(b) *Pharyngeal speech.* This represents a later stage and the air reservoir is the pharynx. Prior to phonation the pharynx is seen to balloon to a considerable degree but no air passes the crico-pharyngeus muscle, into the oesophagus. A considerable quantity of air is present in the buccal sulci of the cheek. Probably in these cases the pharyngeal pillars form the resonating mechanism. Pharyngeal speech forms the second stage in the evolution of post-laryngectomy speech.

(c) *Oesophageal speech.* This type of speech represents the highest degree of developed speech in laryngectomised patients. The oesophagus acts as a reservoir for the air column and the cricopharyngeus as the pseudo-glottis to resonate the air column. This type of speech allows formation of complete sentences. The air is aspirated into the oesophagus during and between phonation. The gastric air bubble may act as a reservoir for the air column in the oesophagus (Brighton & Boone, 1937; Morrison, 1931). Froeschels (1951) and Bateman (1953) hold that the gastric air bubble plays no part in oesophageal speech, the latter basing his arguments on the relations of kymographic pressure recordings and the radiographs.

PHARYNX

Inflammatory lesions

Simple or specific inflammations of the pharynx do not call for radiological examination as they are easily accessible to direct inspection.

Abscess. Abscess formation in the tissues around

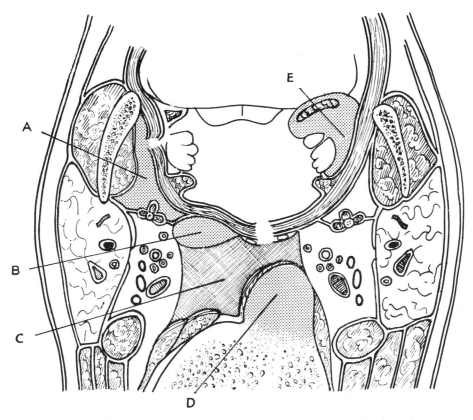

Fig. 302. Line drawing illustrating the anatomical spaces around the pharynx. The commonest sites of abscess are:

A. Parapharyngeal   C. Postvisceral   E. Peritonsillar.
B. Peripharyngeal   D. Prevertebral

the pharynx more frequently demands radiographic examination to determine the extent and possible cause of the abscess rather than for actual diagnosis of abscess formation.

The anatomical spaces around the pharynx are 15 in number (Tschiassny, 1945) and any of these may be involved (fig. 302) although significant abscess formation from a radiological standpoint is usually para-pharyngeal or retro-pharyngeal. The causes of abscess around the pharynx are many. The para-pharyngeal abscess is almost invariably of tonsillar origin. Perforation by foreign bodies, *e.g.* fish bones, may also give rise to para-pharyngeal abscess.

Retro-pharyngeal abscess may lie anterior or posterior to the prevertebral fascia. These retro-pharyngeal abscesses which lie posterior to the prevertebral fascia generally arise from the cervical vertebrae. Those abscesses which lie anteriorly are rather derived from perforations of the pharynx or from suppuration in lymphatic glands. The increasing number of endoscopic procedures performed has increased the number of instrumental injuries although the early use of antibiotics has prevented the development of an excessive number of retro-pharyngeal abscesses.

Very rarely these retro-pharyngeal abscesses are tuberculous in origin and the primary tuberculous focus may be either in the cervical spine or in the lymphatic glands. Healing with calcification in the retro-pharyngeal abscess may occur when the abscess is tuberculous.

Radiological appearances. The radiological appearances of the retro-pharyngeal abscess are:

(a) A large soft tissue swelling lying behind the pharyngeal air space, displacing the air space forwards and narrowing it in its antero-posterior diameter (fig. 303).

(b) Infrequently a radio-opaque foreign body may be visible within the abscess.

(c) In the erect position a small gas cap and a fluid level may be visible.

(d) Calcification may be visible within the abscess if tuberculous in origin or if calcification is not visible within the abscess it may be visible in other cervical lymphatic glands.

(e) Erosion and destruction of cervical vertebrae may occur if the abscess is secondary to tuberculous disease of the cervical spine (fig. 304). Other infections of the cervical spine such as staphylococcal osteomyelitis seldom produce abscess formation although they may cause considerable new bone formation and are probably more frequent today than tuberculous disease.

Congenital lesions

Pharyngeal pouches form one of the commonest congenital lesions in the pharynx. Although the

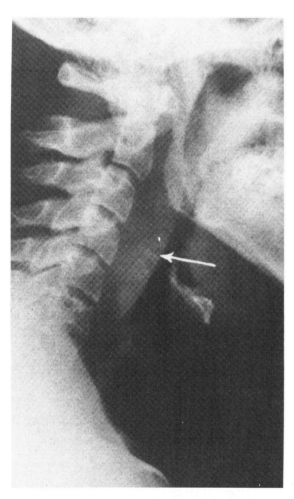

Fig. 303. Retropharyngeal abscess – following perforation of the posterior pharyngeal wall by a foreign body – the widened prevertebral space with the forward displacement of the air filled trachea can be seen.

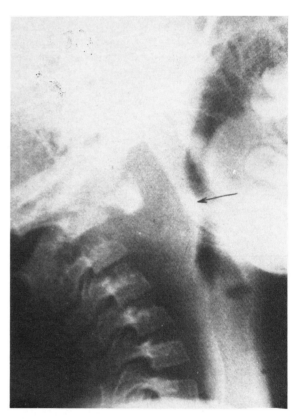

Fig. 304. Prevertebral retropharyngeal abscess associated with tuberculous destruction of the 2nd cervical vertebra. The large soft tissue shadow of the abscess is seen displacing the air filled pharynx forwards.

underlying defect is congenital these pouches only develop during growth and seldom cause symptoms until adult life. Pharyngeal pouches may be of two types.

(a) Lateral, arising from the second branchial cleft, and
(b) Posterior.

The lateral pharyngeal pouches do not grow to a large size and may only be recognised when the barium swallow is carried out in the supine position. Cine studies of the barium swallow allow them to be more easily recognised as they seldom remain filled with barium for any length of time.

The posterior pharyngeal pouch arises at the junction of the posterior pharyngeal and oesophageal wall. The mucosa in this area herniates through an unsupported muscular portion of the posterior pharyngeal wall. This lies between the oblique and circular fibres of the crico-pharyngeus muscle (Killian's dehiscence).

An increased pharyngeal pressure results in bulging of the pharynx and the continual pressure associated with swallowing results in a progressive enlargement of the pouch. This enlargement is further hastened by the change in the alignment of the oesophagus which is displaced by the pouch out of the direct path of the swallowed bolus. Consequently this results in a filling of the pouch with each swallow and only when it is filled out does food regurgitate into the oesophagus.

The pouch enlarges generally towards the left side of the neck and may present in the supraclavicular fossa. In other cases the pouch enlarges down into the superior mediastinum and may simulate a mediastinal tumour.

Radiological appearances. (i) In the erect film the fluid contents and gas in the pouch separate and a fluid level may be seen in the lower part of the neck. The well demarcated outline of the gas bubble enables the fluid level to be differentiated from that occurring in an abscess.

(ii) In the early stages, the barium swallow reveals a small dimple in the posterior pharyngeal wall often only seen in cineradiographic studies of the barium swallow. As the pouch enlarges, the barium-filled pouch can be seen and the oesophagus is displaced forwards and to the right side (fig. 305).

(iii) The neck of the pouch remains narrow and the weight of the contents serves to keep the neck

narrow. The sac may enlarge and spread down to the superior mediastinum.

(iv) The barium may show a mottling in the pouch due to the food remaining in the pouch. Care must be taken not to confuse the filling defects produced by growths in the pouch with filling defects produced by residual food remnants. These conditions can be differentiated by the fact that the filling defects of malignant change are usually eccentric and occur near the neck, whereas filling defects due to debris occur in the fundus of the sac (fig. 306).

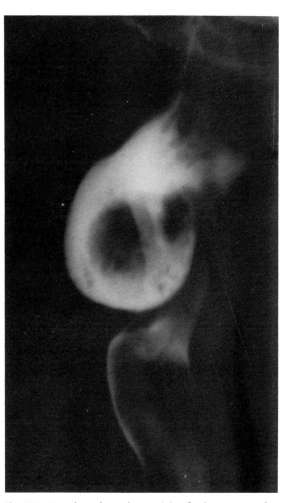

Fig. 305. Oesophageal pouch containing food remnants, often mistaken for tumour. Note that the outline of the pouch is not destroyed as with carcinomatous change (see fig. 306).

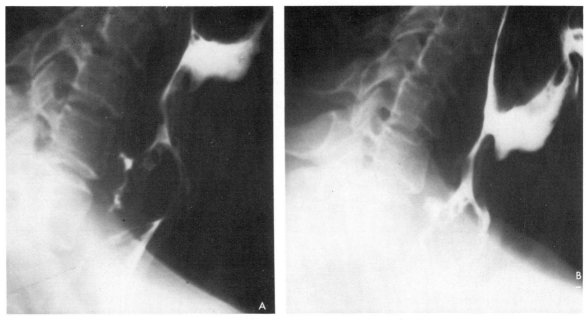

Fig. 306. Pharyngeal pouch – with malignant change in pouch. The lumen of the pouch is obliterated and the oesophagus is displaced forwards by the tumour mass.

Strictures of the pharynx

Congenital. Congenital strictures of the pharynx are infrequent. Complete strictures are not compatible with life but partial degrees of stricture may be present without causing any marked symptoms. Web formation in the post-cricoid portion of the pharynx and upper part of the oesophagus is frequently associated with Plummer-Vinson syndrome (sideropenic dysphagia) (Walstrom & Kjellberg) 1939. These webs can be recognised with a barium swallow and usually project backwards into the barium-filled column from the anterior wall. Templeton (1944) describes web formation in five patients in whom there was no evidence of iron deficiency anaemia.

Radiologically, demonstration of these webs is best made by examination of the barium swallow with the patient lying or standing in the lateral position. Cineradiographic studies at 16 frames/second are invaluable in detecting the presence of a web. A normal filling defect on the anterior wall of the oesophagus considered to be due to defects produced by the post-cricoid venous plexus (Pitman & Fraser, 1965) must not be confused with

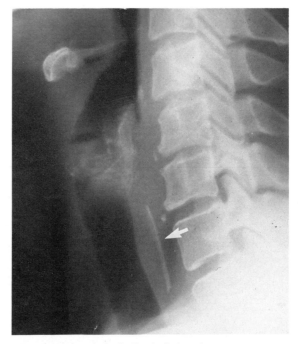

Fig. 307. Fishbone lodged at level of crico-pharyngeus.
(Reproduced by permission from Sutton's Textbook of Radiology. Edinburgh: E & S. Livingstone.)

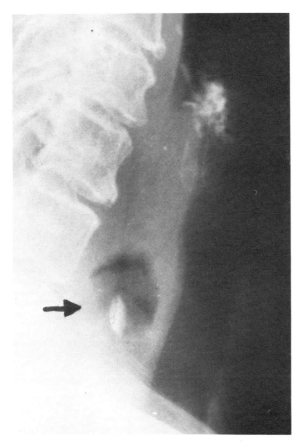

Fig. 308. Fragment of food lodged at level of cricopharyngeus muscle. An "air cap" outlines the soft tissues attached to the swallowed bone. Rarely such an appearance without a central bony fragment may be seen.

web formation. These venous defects vary with swallowing and are partly covered with redundant mucosa (Stiennon, 1963).

Acquired. Acquired strictures of the pharynx are relatively uncommon. They usually occur in one of two sites:

(a) At the level of the pillars of the fauces (glossopharyngeal strictures);
(b) at the junction of pharynx and oesophagus.

The majority of glossopharyngeal strictures are inflammatory (post-diphtheritic) or post-surgical, e.g. (cleft palate operation). Strictures may also follow guillotine tonsillectomy, a sequel which has fortunately largely disappeared with the more universal adoption of dissection tonsillectomy.

Post-irradiation stricture of the lower end of the pharynx may follow irradiation treatment of carcinoma of the larynx. The increased survival following modern irradiation treatment is unfortunately liable to increase the potential number of such strictures.

Radiological appearances. The post-irradiation stricture is situated at the pharyngo-oesophageal junction in the lowermost part of the pharynx and the upper part of the pharynx is usually dilated above the stricture. The outline of the strictures is smooth and well defined.

Foreign bodies

Foreign bodies lodged in the pharynx and oesophagus are an ever-recurring problem (fig. 307). The most frequent sites of lodgement are:

(a) In the tonsillar fossae;
(b) in the valleculae;
(c) at the level of the crico-pharyngeus;
(d) in the mid-oesophagus;
(e) at the lower end of the oesophagus.

The commonest type of foreign body is a meat or fish bone. The smaller, thinner hair-like fish bones tend to lodge in the tonsillar fossae or valleculae.

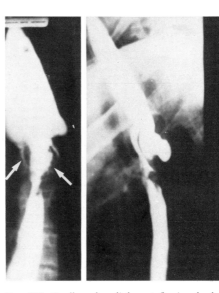

Fig. 309. Swallowed radiolucent foreign body (fragment of dental plate) which had been *in situ* for three weeks with intermittent dysphagia. Note the filling defect in the barium column and the localized perforation.

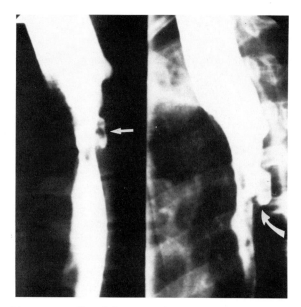

Fig. 310. Swallowed foreign body (same case as fig. 309), showing formation of traumatic diverticulum three weeks later at the site of local perforation.

Radiography in such cases is of little value as the shadow cast is too ill-defined to be appreciated. If perforation and a retro-pharyngeal abscess develop then the soft tissue swelling of the abscess can be clearly demonstrated (fig. 303).

Fish bones which lodge at lower levels in the oesophagus or pharynx tend to be of the larger variety and can be seen with direct radiography. Administration of barium-soaked pledglets of cotton wool will also show a hold-up at the site of the foreign body. If the foreign body has been lodged for any length of time the consequent oedema of the surrounding structures enhances the ease with which the foreign body can be seen (figs. 309, 310). Epstein (1955) advises radiography in the lateral projection during deglutition when low placed foreign bodies lying below the level of the clavicle may rise above the clavicle and become visible.

REFERENCES

ARDRAN, G. M. & KEMP, F. (1975) The Larynx. In *Recent Advances in Radiology*. Edinburgh: Churchill Livingstone: chap. 5.

BANGS, J. L. (1947) Oesophageal Speech. *J. Speech Hear. Disorders*, **12**, 339.

BATEMAN, G. H. (1953) Oesophageal Speech after Laryngectomy. *Acta Otolar.*, **43**, 133.

BIRRELL, J. F. (1952) Discussion of Stridor in Infants. *Proc. R. Soc. Med.*, **45**, 360.

BLEWETT, J. (1939) Laryngocele. *Br. J. Radiol.*, **12**, 163.

BRIGHTON, G. R. & BOONE, W. A. (1937) Roentgenographic Demonstration of Method of Speech in Cases of Complete Laryngectomy. *Am. J. Roentg.*, **38**, 571.

CALTHROP, G. T. (1940) Radiological Demonstration of Adenoids. *Lancet*, **i**, 1005.

CAVANAGH, F. (1965). Congenital Laryngeal Web. *Proc. R. Soc. Med.*, **58**, 272.

CLARK, J. P. (1905). Papilloma of the Larynx in Children. *Trans. Am. Lar. Ass.*, **27**, 185.

CLIFFORD, S. H., NEUHAUSER, E. B. D. & FERGUSON, C. F. (1944) Adenoid Bronchosinusitis in Infants and Children. *Med. Clins N. Am.*, **28**, 1091.

DOHLMAN, G. & THULIN, A. (1949) Stenosis of Pharynx. *Acta otolar.*, **37**, 361.

EPSTEIN, B. S. (1955) A Roentgenographic Aid to the Diagnosis of Radio-opaque Foreign Bodies in the Upper Intrathoracic Oesophagus. *Am. J. Roentg.*, **73**, 115.

FERGUSON, C. F. & SCOTT, H. W. (1944) Papillomatosis of Larynx in Childhood. *New Engl. J. Med.*, **230**, 477.

FRANKLIN, A. E. (1952) Discussion of Stridor in Infants. *Proc. R. Soc. Med.*, **45**, 358.

FROESCHELS, E. (1951) Therapy of the Laryngeal Voice Following Laryngectomy. *Archs Otolar.*, **53**, 77.

GROTH, K. E. (1933). The Roentgen Picture of the Epipharynx of Children under Normal Conditions and by Adenoid Vegetations. *Acta radiol.*, **14**, 463.

HANKINS, W. D. (1944) Traumatic Hernia of Lateral Pharyngeal Walls. *Radiology*, **42**, 499.

HARRISON, K. (1950) Laryngoceles in the Human. *J. Lar. Otol.*, **64**, 777.

HOLINGER, P. H., JOHNSON, K. C. & SCHILLER, F. (1954) *Ann. Otol. Rhinol. Lar.*, **63**, 581.

HOOVER, W. B. & KING, G. D. (1953) Rhinoscleroma. *Archs Otolar.*, **57**, 79.

HOROWITZ, S. (1951) Laryngoceles. *J. Lar. Otol.*, **65**, 724.

JACKSON, C. L. (1945) Laryngocele. *Archs Otolar.*, **41**, 93.

KALLEN, L. A. (1934) Vicarious Vocal Mechanisms. Anatomy, Physiology and Development of Speech in Laryngectomised Persons. *Archs Otolar.*, **20**, 460.

LEDERER, F. L. & HOWARD, J. C. (1946). Wartime Laryngeal Injuries. *Archs Otolar.*, **43**, 331.

LINDSAY, J. R. (1940) Laryngocele Ventricularis. *Ann. Otol. Rhinol. Lar.*, **49**, 661.

McHUGH, J. & LOCH, W. E. (1942) *Laryngoscope, St. Louis*, **52**, 43.

MORRISON, W. W. (1931) The Production of Voice and Speech Following Total Laryngectomy. *Archs Otolar.*, **14**, 413.

NEUHAUSER, E. B. D. (1946) The Roentgen Diagnosis of Double Aortic Arch and Other Anomalies of the Great Vessels. *Am. J. Roentg.,* **56,** .

OWSLEY, W. C. Jr. (1962) Palate and Pharynx: Roentgenographic Evaluation in the Management of Cleft Palate and Related Deformities. *Am. J. Roentg.,* **87,** 811.

PITMAN, R. G. & FRASER, G. M. (1965) The Post-Cricoid Impression on the Oesophagus. *Clin. Radiol.,* **16,** 34.

PRACY, R. (1965) An Assessment of Stridor in Infants and Young Children. *Proc. R. Soc. Med.,* **68,** 267.

RATHBONE, R. R. (1940) Roentgen Diagnosis of Therapy of Retroperitoneal Adenitis. *Am. J. Roentg.,* **43,** 25.

SIMPSON, W. L. (1938) Laryngocele. *Ann. Otol. Rhinol. Lar.,* **47,** 1054.

STIENNON, O. A. (1963) The Anatomic Basis for the Lower Esophageal Contraction Ring. *Am. J. Roentg.,* **90,** 811.

TEMPLETON, F. (1944) *Radiology of the Stomach and Duodenum.* Chicago: University of Chicago Press.

TSCHIASSNY, K. (1945) "Juxtapharyngeal" Spaces as Carriers and Barriers of Suppurations. *Cincinn. J. Med.,* **26,** 337.

VALVASSORI, G. & GOLDSTEIN, C. T. (1970) Radiographic Evaluation of the Larynx. *Otol. Clins N. Am.,* 3/3.

WALSTROM, J. & KJELLBERG, S. R. (1939) The Roentgenologic Diagnosis of Sideropenic Dysphagia. *Acta Radiol.,* **20,** 618.

WEITZ, H. L. (1946) Roentgenography of Adenoids. *Radiology,* **47,** 66.

ZURHELLE, F. (1869) *Berl. klin. Wschr.,* **50,** 544.

CHAPTER 16

Tumours of the pharynx and larynx

PHARYNX

The pharynx is subdivisible into three main areas – the nasopharynx, the oropharynx and the hypopharynx. This subdivision is not only of anatomical merit but also has clinical value as growths occurring in each of these areas have to some extent specific features.

Nasopharynx

Benign tumours. The commonest benign tumour of the nasopharynx is the FIBROMA (ANGIOFIBROMA) OF PUBERTY (fig. 311). It almost invariably occurs in the male. It is generally a sessile, globular, relatively hard tumour arising from mucosa over the body of the sphenoid or from the roof of the posterior nares.

Histologically the tumour is composed of dense fibrous tissue intermixed with numerous cavernous blood spaces (Friedberg, 1940). Although it is said to disappear spontaneously after adolescence (Martin, Ehrlich & Abels, 1948) few authenticated records of this phenomenon exist. Clinically there may be nasal obstruction, epistaxis, facial deformity and sometimes proptosis (Steinberg, 1954). The tumour has a tendency to occupy the pterygo-maxillary groove and to extend into the sphenoid sinus. Radiologically the tumour presents as a soft tissue mass in the nasopharynx, or when it occupies the pterygo-maxillary groove the rounded soft tissue tumour may be superimposed on the maxillary antrum and resemble an antral polyp. Holman & Miller (1965) describe a characteristic feature of this tumour, which depends upon its typical location in the pterygo-maxillary groove. This is the so-called antral sign, and consists of an anterior bowing of the posterior wall of the maxillary antrum, best seen on a lateral projection (figs 312, 313). Other characteristic features are optimally demonstrated by tomography, for example the involvement of the sphenoid sinus, which shows a total opacity continuous with the soft tissue mass in the nasopharynx and a defect in the floor of the sinus. The sphenoid is often expanded. Carotid angiography may be diagnostic but is not always necessary in management of these

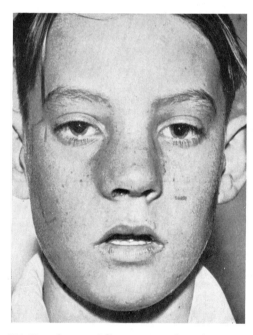

Fig. 311 Nasopharyngeal fibroma. A youth aged 12 years who had noticed nasal obstruction for several years. Some nasal bleeding had occurred from the right nostril. Section of the tissue from the nasopharynx and the right nostril showed a fibroma.

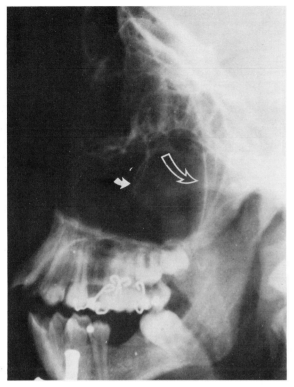

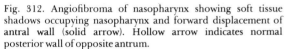

Fig. 312. Angiofibroma of nasopharynx showing soft tissue shadows occupying nasopharynx and forward displacement of antral wall (solid arrow). Hollow arrow indicates normal posterior wall of opposite antrum.

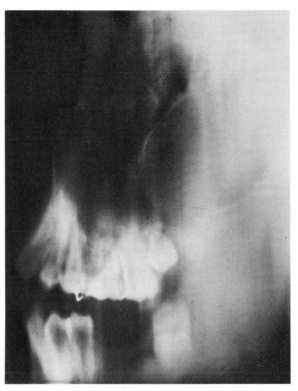

Fig. 313. Tomogram of case shown in fig. 312. The mass in the nasopharynx and the "antral wall sign" are more easily seen.

tumours. They are exceptionally rich in vessels and draw their main blood supply from the external carotid. They usually give a strong tumour blush on arteriography, a feature which can best be appreciated in subtraction films.

Other types of fibroma such as NEUROFIBROMA may also occur. Such tumours usually occur in adults (Freundlich & Hodes, 1963). Neurofibromas occurring in later life may produce bone erosion and optic atrophy by local pressure. They are exceedingly rare but Albanese (1945) has recorded a case of neurofibroma arising in the retro-pharyngeal space and displacing the trachea and pharynx forwards. Turchik (1946) reports a schwannoma of the vocal cords associated with paralysis of the vocal cords. These tumours do not give any specific radiological appearances and can merely be demonstrated as soft tissue tumours. Computerised axial tomography is a valuable

method of detecting bone change and the extent of spread of the tumour.

ODONTOMES may also occur in the nasopharynx and in such cases (McClure, 1946) radiological detection of fragments of teeth in the mass enables the correct diagnosis to be made.

SARCOIDOSIS. Larsson (1951) has reported 10 cases of histologically proven sarcoid lesions involving the nasopharynx which caused difficulties in differential diagnosis. The lesions presented as small soft tissue swellings resembling adenoid pads, while some larger lesions resembled malignant tumours. They were associated with signs of sarcoidosis in the lungs or bones.

Malignant tumours. Malignant tumours of the nasopharynx may be subdivided into:

(a) Sarcoma, (either chondro-, fibro-, myxo- or lymphosarcoma).

(b) Lymphoepithelioma.
(c) Epithelioma.
(d) Chordoma.

This classification is based on the histological nature of the tumour but apart from chondrosarcoma which may show speckled calcification it is impossible to differentiate these individual types radiologically.

In a series of 34 cases of all types of nasopharyngeal tumours reported by Davis (1948) the frequency of the various tumours was as follows:

19 carcinoma,
 4 lymphosarcoma
10 angiofibroma, and
 1 myxosarcoma of doubtful origin.

Sarcoma. FIBROSARCOMA. This tumour has to be differentiated from the recurrent angiofibroma.

This may be extremely difficult even on histological examination, and it is likely that many recurrent nasopharyngeal fibromas are probably fibrosarcomas.

The presenting symptoms are those of nasal obstruction, post-nasal discharge and bleeding.

Radiological appearances. Fibrosarcomas are best demonstrated in the lateral projection of the nasopharynx and the features are:

(1) A soft tissue mass with a smooth outline projecting into the nasopharynx from the roof or posterior wall. The mass is generally sessile and broad based.
(2) The edges of the mass are ill-defined and blend with the soft tissue shadow of the nasopharynx.
(3) Destruction of the bony roof of the nasopharynx is unusual and generally only occurs late in the course of the disease.

MYXOSARCOMA. Myxosarcoma and myofibrosarcoma are indistinguishable from fibrosarcoma and the diagnosis can only be made on histological examination.

LYMPHOSARCOMA. Baclesse (1949) has classified lymphosarcomas in the nasopharynx into three groups depending on their site of origin.

In order of frequency the sites of origin are:

(a) From the pharyngeal tonsil and the pharyngeal recess of Rosenmuller.
(b) From the adenoid tissue around the orifice of the Eustachian tube.
(c) Rarely from the posterior surface of the palate.

Radiographically these varieties can be classified as:

(a) A posterior superior variety (pharyngeal tonsil).
(b) Lateral variety (tube).
(c) Anterior variety (palate).

In many cases the disease is so advanced when first seen that determination of the real site of origin is not possible. In such cases it is generally possible at some time during radiation therapy, when the growth has partially shrunk, to identify the exact site of origin.

Lymphoepithelioma. Lymphoepitheliomas arise from mucosa covering lymphoid tissue and to some extent in their clinical course resemble sarcomas. They tend to cast a massive soft tissue shadow with smooth contours.

Epithelioma. Malignant change may occur in any part of the epithelium of the nasopharynx. In the cauliflower type of growth the soft tissue shadow shown can be readily seen on the radiograph against the air-filled nasopharynx. With infiltrative and ulcerative growths the radiographic changes are negligible. Baclesse (1949) advises the use of Lipiodol contrast medium to outline the nasopharynx in such cases but careful endoscopy and biopsy under anaesthesia is a far surer method of detection of early malignant change in this region. Nasopharyngograms using oily Dionosil as a contrast medium, may demonstrate tumours on the lateral wall of the nasopharynx when they are submucosal and direct inspection reveals no abnormality (Hartley *et al.,* 1965).

Nasopharyngeal carcinoma may be associated with hypertrophic pulmonary arthropathy usually when pulmonary metastases are present. However, a single instance without pulmonary involvement has been reported (Zornova *et al.,* 1977).

Radiological appearances. The radiological signs of epithelioma may be subdivided into three groups:

(a) *Soft tissue masses*
    (i) Nasopharyngeal masses projecting into the air space of the nasopharynx are best seen in the lateral projection (figs. 314, 315). Sarcomatous masses tend to give larger soft tissue swellings than epithelioma and the ulcerative form of epithelioma may not produce any appreciable soft tissue shadow.
    (ii) Soft tissue mass in the sphenoid sinus. An opacity in the sphenoid sinus may follow tumour invasion or superadded infection.

(b) *Bone invasion*

The sites of bone destruction in the skull base correspond to the routes of invasion of the tumour, and erosion of bone when it occurs is the result rather than the cause of intracranial extension (Martin & Blady, 1940): in other words it is usual for invasion to occur through the foramina prior to the demonstration of bone destruction by radiology. This is substantiated by venographic studies, which may reveal the presence of cavernous sinus obstruction before demonstrable bone erosion. Since the fossa of Rosenmuller lies directly under the medial part of the foramen lacerum, the neoplasm may extend by direct continuity from the nasopharynx *via* the foramen lacerum and carotid canal into the cranium. Invasion of the parapharyngeal space (Lederman, 1961) permits destruction of the greater wing of the sphenoid near the foramen ovale without obvious destruction of the petrous temporal bone. The floor of the sphenoid sinus forms the

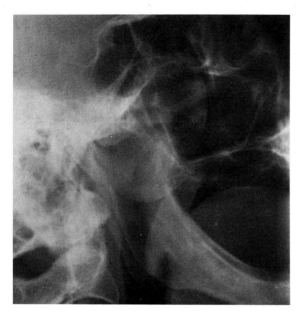

Fig. 314. Carcinoma of nasopharynx. Lateral view showing soft tissue mass projecting into nasopharynx.

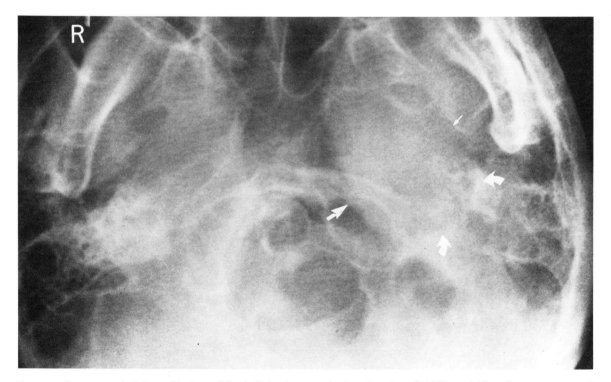

Fig. 315. Submento-vertical views of the base of the skull showing extensive bony invasion of middle cranial fossa from a carcinoma of the nasopharynx.

roof of the nasopharynx and can be invaded very early by tumour affecting the roof and posterior wall with expansion and destruction of the sinus walls and destruction of the floor of the pituitary fossa. Extension forward from this central position may produce bone destruction in the maxillo-ethmoidal region, and extension posteriorly may result in invasion of the retropharyngeal space and involvement of the lateral mass of the atlas. These changes are best demonstrated by hypocycloidal tomography and coronal, lateral and axial studies are necessary for full assessment. Computerised axial tomography is also useful in outlining the full extent of the tumour.

In addition to osteolytic changes, neoplastic invasion may provoke a sclerotic reaction in the basi-sphenoid or floor of the sphenoid sinus and in the adjacent pterygoid laminae.

(c) *Opacity in the paranasal sinuses*
This may be the result of actual invasion of the sinuses by the growth, or of associated infection (Belanger & Dyke, 1943).

Oropharynx

The upper level of the oropharynx is an arbitrary line passing through the soft palate, and its lower level the hyoid bone. Its posterior boundaries are the posterior pharyngeal wall covering the second and third cervical vertebrae, and anteriorly the posterior aspect of the tongue leading to the vallecula and anterior portion of the epiglottis.

Abnormal radiological features in this region are most easily seen in the lateral radiograph. In this position an accurate determination of the extent of tumour development is often better as clinical methods of examination may completely fail to reveal the lower limits of the tumour.

Diamond & Perkins (1948) have described an unusual calcified mass occurring in the oropharynx. This mass which was densely calcified with well-defined boundaries, proved to be a calcified haematoma secondary to a gunshot wound. Such a calcification has to be differentiated from calcified lymphatic glands in the neck or prevertebral retropharyngeal space.

Tumours. Tumours arising from this portion of the pharynx are almost invariably malignant and the anterior wall (including the root of the tongue)

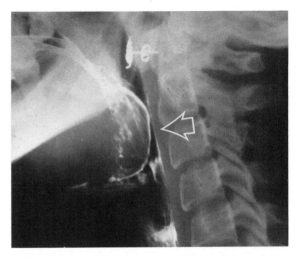

Fig. 316. Carcinoma of the base of the tongue projecting into the oropharynx. The barium swallow has coated the tumour and shows its limits clearly.

is a frequent site for the development of carcinoma. Epithelioma arising from the root of the tongue can be classified into the following types (Baclesse, 1949):

PROLIFERATIVE VARIETY. In this variety there is a soft tissue mass arising from the base of the tongue. Its outline is clear-cut and the soft tissue tumour can be seen projecting backwards into the oropharyngeal air space (fig. 316). This type of tumour is associated with a relatively good prognosis. It should be confirmed that the tongue has been protruded during the exposure of the lateral film as a retracted tongue may cause prominence of the palmate folds normally present over the posterior portion of the tongue and mimic a soft tissue swelling in this region.

The second type of tumour is the ULCERO-PROLIFERATIVE VARIETY which does not cause any appreciable loss of substance of the tongue. The ulcerative lesion is caused by necrosis in the centre of the growth. According to Baclesse (1949) the prognosis in this type of case is less favourable. In the lateral radiograph the soft tissue swelling due to the growth can be easily recognised and the ulcer crater in the centre of the growth may also be seen (fig. 317).

The third type of epithelioma arising from the root of the tongue is the INFILTRATIVE variety which produces little or no change in radiological

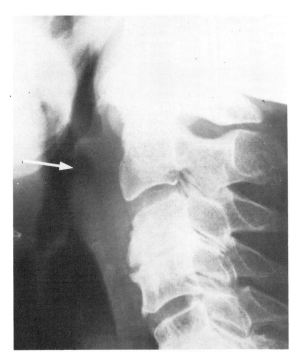

Fig. 317. Carcinoma of the posterior pharyngeal wall. A soft tissue mass with superficial ulceration (arrow) can be seen. The changes in the intervertebral disc between the 3rd and 4th cervical vertebrae are probably spondylitic in nature.

appearances. This type is the most frequently overlooked on the radiograph.

The ULCERATIVE variety is the fourth type and the loss of substance involves the whole thickness of the base of the tongue. Radiographically the lesion presents as a deep ulcer in the root of the tongue appearing on the anterior wall of the nasopharynx. The prognosis of this type of growth, according to Baclesse is extremely poor. The assistance of radiographic examination in determining the loss of substance in the root of the tongue is extremely valuable in planning therapy.

Other tumours of the oropharynx, apart from the malignant growths, are extremely rare. The commonest type is a chordoma and its radiological features have already been described (see Chapter 5).

Hypopharynx

The hypopharynx extends from the hyoid bone to the lower edge of the cricoid cartilage and anteriorly it is subdivided into a right and left pharyngo-laryngeal channel. On either side of the midline the valleculae, fossae subdivided by a median raphe, can be identified.

The hypopharynx can be subdivided into two parts – an upper air containing section lying between the cornua of the hyoid bones above and the upper edge of the thyroid cartilage below, and a lower non-air containing opaque part which is formed anteriorly by the posterior pharyngo-laryngeal shadow. There is a notch corresponding to the crico-arytenoid space. The lower portion is composed of the posterior plate of the cricoid cartilage covered by the soft tissues.

This subdivision of the hypopharynx into two portions is not only of anatomical interest as tumours arising in the upper part of the hypopharynx have a far better prognosis than tumours arising in the lower portion.

Radiological appearances. Growths arising in the upper part of the hypopharynx most commonly arise from the aryepiglottic folds. Their radiological features are (Coutard, 1932):

(a) The hypopharynx lying between the hyoid and the upper border of the thyroid cartilage which generally can be well seen, becomes filled with tumour tissue with obliteration of the normal air space.

(b) The upper portion of the thyroid cartilage becomes displaced forwards.

(c) The distensibility of the pharynx is normal when Valsalva's test is applied.

Growths arising from the lower portion of the hypopharynx (post-cricoid growths) give the following radiological signs (fig. 318):

(a) There is generalised thickening of the soft tissue shadow in the post-cricoid space. The width of this space varies with the degree of extension of the cervical spine. Normally the width of the soft tissue space is about the same as that of a cervical vertebral body and widening beyond this should be regarded with suspicion.

(b) The thyroid cartilage becomes displaced forwards.

(c) The barium swallow shows a marked irregularity of the mucosal pattern at the site of growth. Contrast studies with barium are necessary to outline the size and extent of growth.

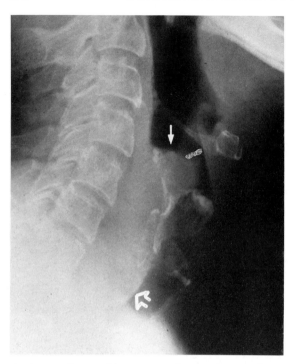

Fig. 318. Carcinoma of the post-cricoid region showing upward extension into the pyriform fossa (white arrow) and marked forward displacement of the trachea (hollow arrow).

LARYNX

Benign cysts and tumours

Laryngeal cysts. Cysts involving the larynx are not uncommon in adults. New & Erich (1938) found 35 examples in a series of 722 cases of benign laryngeal tumours at the Mayo Clinic. Cysts of the larynx may be classified into retention and congenital cysts. Retention cysts comprise more than 50% of the total of laryngeal cysts and the vast majority of retention cysts occur in the epiglottis.

Congenital cysts are usually responsible for symptoms dating from birth or early infancy. Only 20 cases have so far been described in the literature. Such cysts present within the first weeks of life and the symptoms may be grouped under:

(a) Respiratory obstruction.
(b) Cyanosis.
(c) Voice changes.
(d) Disturbances of feeding (Ahlén & Ranström, 1944).

Dyspnoea is usually the outstanding symptom but cyanosis only develops later in the course of the disease. Position of the head profoundly affects the degree of dyspnoea. Congenital cysts of the larynx carry a poor prognosis.

Radiological appearances. The radiological findings in congenital laryngeal cysts are vitally important as endoscopic examination of the larynx in young infants is often a formidable undertaking. The appearances noted are as follows (fig. 319):

(i) *Absence of air from the larynx (cavum laryngis).* In many cases the laryngeal cyst completely fills the cavity of the larynx obscuring the soft tissue landmarks of the larynx.

(ii) *Ballooning of the pharynx and oropharynx.* As a consequence of the respiratory obstruction the pharyngeal air space above the larynx becomes over distended.

(iii) *Visualisation of the soft tissue shadow.* The upper outline of the cyst may frequently be visible against the air-filled hypopharynx. In rare cases the whole soft tissue outline of the cyst may be visualised (Marx, 1928; Kleinfeld, 1934). In infants the soft tissue shadow produced by the laryngeal cyst must be differentiated from laryngeal papillomas which may occur in young infants. Laryngeal papillomas tend to have more irregular soft tissue shadows and often tend to have a mottled appearance due to air trapped between the individual papillomas. The importance of lateral radiography in the diagnosis of laryngeal cysts cannot be overestimated as direct laryngoscopy may not reveal the cyst as in Ahlén & Ranström's case (1944).

Radiography has further value in excluding cardiac, thymic or pulmonary pathology as other causes of the dyspnoea.

Chondroma of the larynx. McCall, Dupertius & Gardiner (1944) presented two cases of chondroma occurring in the larynx. These authors were only able to find a total of 85 cases in the literature. The majority of cases occur between the ages of 40 and 60 years and the symptoms are due to mechanical pressure on the surrounding structures. Speech is interfered with and the airway may be obstructed by the growth of the tumour into the air space. Chondroma show a special tendency to grow upwards (Gay, Wilkins & Sagels, 1958).

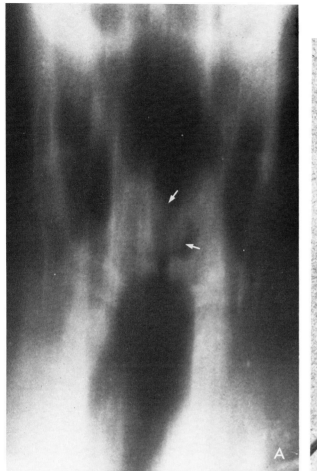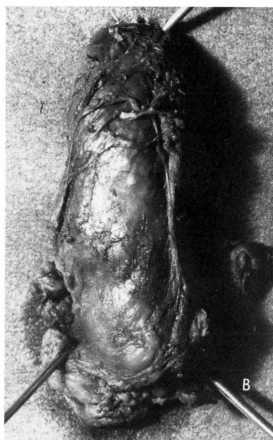

Fig. 319. Laryngeal cysts. A. P.A. tomographic film showing soft tissue shadow with well-defined outlines arising from the right ventricular band – projecting into larynx. The vocal cords are not involved. B. Laryngeal cyst showing specimen of cyst removed at operation.

The commonest sites of origin of these tumours are from the posterior part of the cricoid cartilage, the thyroid cartilage and, less frequently, from the epiglottis, arytenoids and vocal cords (Kelly, 1950).

Radiography with anteroposterior, lateral views and tomography will demonstrate a soft tissue swelling with clearly defined outlines projecting into the laryngeal air space (fig. 320). Unless the tumour contains calcium, differentiation by radiological means from other soft tissue tumours cannot be made (Ryan & Zizmor, 1949).

If the chondroma arises from the lateral surface of the thyroid cartilage the differential diagnosis from a calcified adenoma of the thyroid must be considered (fig. 321). Malignant change with the development of a chondrosarcoma can only be recognised by a rapid increase in growth and the extent of infiltration (fig. 322).

Haemangioma of the larynx. Haemangioma of the larynx is an extremely rare condition, only 123 cases having been described (Ferguson, 1944). Two types occur – an adult and an infantile type. Lateral radiography of the larynx is valuable in determining the exact extent of the tumour.

The tumour is not malignant but its haemorrhagic nature makes surgical removal a formidable undertaking.

Cystadenoma of the larynx. This tumour may be

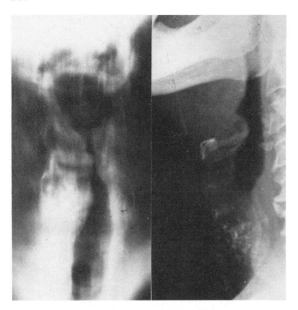

Fig. 320. Chondroma of larynx showing calcification best seen in the lateral view (b) but forming an intrinsic part of the larynx.

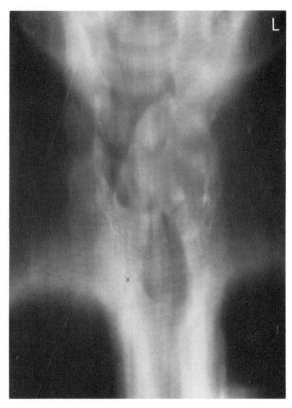

Fig. 322. Chondrosarcoma of larynx – showing soft tissue tumour invasion of the air space. The appearances are similar to a chondroma and it is only the rate of spread which may be the differentiating feature.

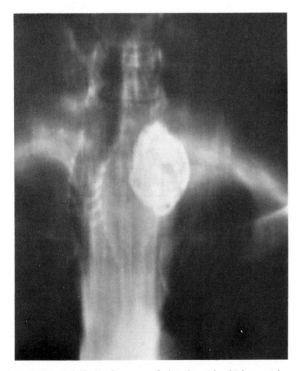

Fig. 321. Calcified adenoma of the thyroid which may be mistaken for a chondroma of larynx seen in an anteroposterior tomogram to be separate from the larynx.

regarded as an adenoma which has undergone cystic degeneration (Figi, Rowland & New, 1944). It may be analogous to that occurring in the breast. Only a few cases of this type have been reported in the literature but the above-named authors describe four such cases.

Fibromyxoma and neurofibroma. Fibromyxomas are practically confined to adult males. Little is known about their origin but they appear to be associated with chronic laryngitis. Chronic irritation may be an aetiological factor and the singer's nodule may be considered as an example of this condition. Histologically they are composed of fibrous tissue although myxomatous degeneration may occur.

The symptoms produced by these fibromas are determined by their shape and size. They can readily be seen by direct or indirect laryngoscopy and usually they do not attain sufficient size to be demonstrated on the radiograph.

Neurofibromas may involve the larynx. They are excessively rare, only three cases having been described in the literature (Oliver, Diab & Abu-Jaudeh, 1948). These authors added a further case of their own where the tumour arose from the lateral wall of the larynx above the vocal cords.

Extramedullary plasmacytoma of the larynx. The first recorded case of plasmacytoma of the larynx was by Boit in 1907. This is a rare type of tumour most commonly met with in males between the fifth, sixth and seventh decades. Figi, Broders & Havens (1945) found that 82% of these tumours occurred between these ages.

Stout & Kenney (1949) found that 104 cases of the extramedullary plasmacytoma originated in the air passages or the oral cavity. Ewing & Foote (1952) found that the single local deposit was ultimately followed by the appearance of multiple scattered deposits (multiple myeloma). The tumour, however, has a relatively slow course and conversion into the diffuse disease, multiple myeloma, may not occur for many years.

Macroscopically, plasmacytoma of the larynx may be single or multiple, polypoid, sessile or infiltrating. The polypoid tumours tend to be benign and the infiltrative form relatively malignant. These tumours have a predilection to occur in sites where lymphatic tissue occurs. To the naked eye these tumours appear grey or yellowish grey and vary considerably in size. Multiple benign plasmacytoma tend to occur as polypoid tumours situated in the larynx, trachea or nasopharynx and they show a marked tendency to recur after removal. About 45% of extra-osseous plasmacytoma occurring in the nasopharynx may remain solitary but the remaining 55% are more or less malignant from inception, metastases first occurring in lymph nodes although bone metastases may occur after many years (Jackson, Parker & Bethea, 1931).

Histologically, respiratory tract plasmacytomas show the same features as those occurring in the bone marrow. The main cellular component is the plasma cell with its characteristic "clock-faced" nucleus. Multi-nucleated giant cells are also found in the tumour. The stroma of the tumour is generally a fine spindle-celled one. The tumour mass tends to invade the surrounding soft tissues. With laryngeal plasmacytoma, death may occur

from respiratory obstruction but more commonly from the development of multiple myelomatosis.

Radiologically, plasmacytoma occurring in the larynx appears as a soft tissue tumour either with a smooth outline in the benign groups or with an ill-defined outline and radiologically indistinguishable from a carcinoma or a papilloma in the more malignant varieties.

Granuloma of the larynx. Clausen (1932) first recorded bilateral polypoid granuloma of the larynx following endotracheal anaesthesia. Epstein & Winston (1957) reviewed the literature and added their own personal experience. These granulomas are not sufficiently large to show any radiological features.

Amyloid disease. Tumour-like deposits are most often found in or near tissues containing cartilage and are more frequently found in the upper part of the respiratory tract than in any other part of the body. In New & Erich's (1938) series of 722 cases, 18 cases of amyloid were found; 4 of these were localised tumours and 9 inflammatory tumours which had undergone amyloid deterioration.

Laryngeal papilloma. Laryngeal papillomas occur at two distinct age groups. There is the first type which occurs in infants and young children, and the second in adults, which has a marked tendency to malignant change.

PAPILLOMA IN INFANTS. This type of growth, which histologically is benign with no tendency to malignant change, is nevertheless of great importance owing to the dangerous respiratory symptoms which may occur.

Histologically, papilloma is composed of columnar epithelium of variable height.

Clinically, papillomas present with hoarseness, loss of voice and dyspnoea. An interesting feature is the manner in which posture affects the dyspnoea, the child often adopting a semi-erect crouching position for relief.

Radiological appearances. Owing to the difficulties of laryngoscopy in small infants, radiological examination of suspected infantile papilloma is extremely valuable. Conventional films should be taken in the lateral position and, if the child is sufficiently cooperative, should be supplemented by tomographs in the antero-posterior plane. In the lateral films an irregular soft tissue mass can be seen projecting into the air space of the larynx. Tomographs will reveal the extent of the mass. Subglottic extensions should be carefully looked for as knowledge of such extensions is invaluable in planning the operation. Tomographs in the lateral position seldom provide additional information.

PAPILLOMA IN ADULTS. This tumour has the same histological characters as papilloma arising from the same type of epithelium in other parts of the body. Differentiation from an early carcinoma is not possible by radiological methods alone. Tomography and contrast laryngography in the antero-posterior position may be especially valuable in demonstrating the exact size and site of the papilloma.

Malignant tumours

Laryngeal growths are classified into glottic (arising from the vocal cords or commissure) and supraglottic and subglottic. Baclesse (1946) classified laryngeal tumours into intrinsic and extrinsic groups and the extrinsic group further into the supraglottic growths, growths arising from the false vocal cords, and subglottic growths. Tucker (1962) impressed by the way in which laryngeal cancers spread deep into the mucosa has proposed the concept of a paraglottic space (bounded above by the mucosa of the pyriform sinus, laterally by the ala of the thyroid cartilage, medially by the quadrangular membrane above and the conus elasticus below). The paraglottic spaces include the paired structures of the larynx. The other areas comprise the supra-glottic region (epiglottic and pre-epiglottic space), the glottic (anterior commissure tendon and inter-arytenoid muscle) and the subglottic (cricothyroid ligament).

Definition of these boundaries is important as the submucosal spread of laryngeal tumours tends in part to be bounded by these fibrous septa and the escape routes of laryngeal carcinoma can be predicted by reference to them.

The value of radiographic examination in the management of laryngeal carcinoma has always been in dispute. Jorgensen and others (1975) have attempted to quantify the indications and evaluate the significance of radiography in the management of laryngeal carcinoma. In an analysis of 64 cases of primary laryngeal carcinoma, routine radiography did not contribute to the extent of the sub- or supraglottic extension of small tumours and is not recommended in the primary laryngeal carcinomas in T_1 and T_2 (1972) stage U.I.C.C. Classification. It is indicated if direct laryngoscopy is not feasible.

Only extensive supra- or subglottic extension can be detected. It has great importance in classifying T_3 and T_4 tumours. Demonstration of invasion of cartilage may convert a T_3 to a T_4 classification.

Radiography is of particular value in detecting the extent of recurrence and is indicated in such a case to determine the extent of the recurrence. Jorgensen and others did not use contrast laryngography in this study which must limit the value of their findings.

The differentiation of post-radiation oedema from recurrent tumour is another problem which may cause considerable difficulty and even with laryngography the differentiation of tumour recurrence from post-radiation oedema may be impossible.

Intrinsic (glottic) carcinoma of the larynx. The true vocal cord is a relatively frequent site for the development of a primary carcinoma (214 cases out of a series of 340 laryngeal growths, Baclesse, 1946). Initially the growth is limited to the vocal cord proper but some extension of the growth outside the cord soon occurs (Baclesse & Henry, 1950). Baclesse distinguishes three sites of origin of carcinoma of the vocal cord:

(a) Arising from the membranous part of the cord.
(b) Arising in the anterior commissure.
(c) Involving the cartilaginous part of the cord.

Growths arising on the vocal cords are generally easily available for inspection by direct and indirect laryngoscopy and the particular value of radiography is to determine the lower limits and deeper extensions of the growth (Tucker, 1961) (figs. 323, 324).

Growths arising in the anterior portion of the vocal cords (anterior commissure growths) (Baclesse & Henry, 1950) tend to be less accessible to laryngoscopic examination as they are obscured by the epiglottis. Widespread infiltration may occur without any clinical symptoms or signs. They are of two types:

(a) the PROLIFERATIVE, which invades slowly but which gives rise early to a soft tissue tumour projecting from the larynx, and
(b) the INFILTRATIVE or ULCERO-EROSIVE TYPE, which spreads forward anteriorly and rapidly invades the thyroid cartilage.

Early invasion of the anterior commissure either by growths arising in this site or extending from the

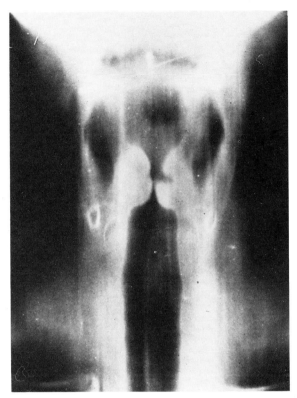

Fig. 323. Carcinoma of right vocal cord – obliterating ventricle but showing no downward or lateral extension.

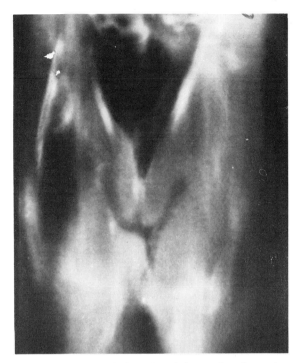

Fig. 324. Carcinoma of left vocal cord showing lateral spread to pyriform fossa. The air-filled pyriform fossa on the right side is clearly seen. Some subglottic extension is seen anteriorly.

cord are best seen in the laryngogram, particularly in the oblique views. Irregularity of the mucosa, increased tissue thickness in this region, or failure of this part to fill indicate invasion of this site. When the growth is extensive plain lateral radiographs show the growth clearly (Jing, 1975) (fig. 326).

Extension into the ala of the thyroid cartilage is a grave sequel of laryngeal growths. There may be no clinical signs to indicate this extension. The radiological interpretation of cartilage invasion is difficult owing to the irregular nature in which the laryngeal cartilage ossifies. Baclesse (1946) gives the following radiological signs as being indicative of involvement of the laryngeal cartilages.

(a) The anterior part of the ala of the thyroid cartilage becomes mottled due to patchy infiltration and rarefaction. This site is most frequently involved in supraglottic tumours.

(b) With laryngeal growths involving the true and false vocal cords the central portion of the thyroid cartilage is most frequently involved and the edges of the areas of destruction are serrated. This destruction has to be distinguished from irregular ossification (fig. 272). An increase in the width of the soft tissue space between the air-filled ventricle and the inner surface of the thyroid cartilage is an indication of spread of laryngeal growth across the anterior commissure. In the lateral radiograph the extent of this invasive process can be clearly assessed and the growth can spread into the base of the epiglottis and even the pre-thyro-cricoid tissues.

(c) The inferior and anterior part of the ala of the thyroid cartilage becomes involved by growths which spread from the anterior commissure. This portion of the cartilage is always ossified in males but seldom in females.

Extrinsic tumours. Extrinsic growths of the larynx are those which arise outside the true vocal

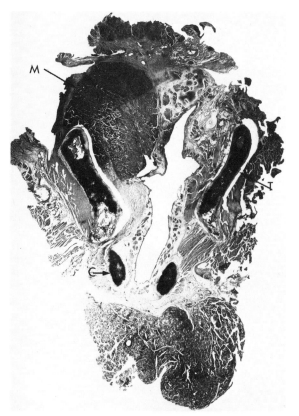

Fig. 325. Thin section showing spread of an extrinsic tumour of the larynx upwards and above the thyroid cartilage. Note the almost complete lack of spread of the growth inferiorly.
M. Tumour mass. T. Cut ala of thyroid cartilage. C. Cricoid cartilage.
(*Courtesy of Professor D. N. Harrison.*)

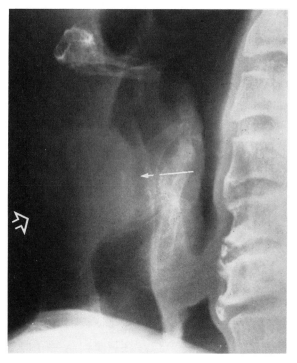

Fig. 326. Anterior spread of carcinoma of larynx. Shows soft tissue mass anteriorly.

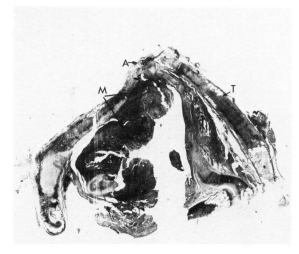

Fig. 327. Horizontal thin section through larynx showing anterior spread of growth across the anterior commissure.
M—growth arising from right vocal cord
A —anterior commissure
T —cut section of thyroid lamina.
(*Courtesy of Professor D. N. Harrison.*)

cord. They can be subdivided into two main groups:

(a) Supraglottic growths.
(b) Subglottic growths.

SUPRAGLOTTIC GROWTHS (carcinoma of the vestibule). The original researches of Coutard (1932) and Baclesse & Henry (1950) greatly clarified our radiographic knowledge of supraglottic carcinoma. These authors emphasised the importance of serial radiography during treatment in assessing the actual size and site of origin of the growth. In many cases when examined initially the growth is so extensive as to make the determination of the actual site of origin impossible; under treatment, as the growth regresses it does so centripetally so that the last remaining mass represents the actual site of origin. The determination of the actual site of origin of growth is of considerable importance in prognosis as Baclesse & Henry (1950) have shown that the incidence of glandular metastases in growths arising in the posterior half of the larynx is considerably less than those arising in the anterior part.

The are five common sites of origin of carcinomas arising in the supraglottic portion of the larynx (Baclesse and Henry, 1950).

1. *Cancer of the epiglottis* (fig. 328). May be supra-hyoid or infra-hyoid. Both sites may show proliferative or invasive types. The proliferative supra-hyoid growth may attain a formidable size before it is recognised. The infiltrative supra-hyoid epiglottic cancer spreads anteriorly to the vallecula, base of tongue and pre-epiglottic space. The lateral soft tissue film is particularly valuable in outlining the extent of the growth and tomography adds little to the diagnosis.

Cancer of the infra-hyoid portion of the epiglottis equally is of the proliferative and invasive types and lateral films and contrast laryngography are the radiological examinations which best demonstrate the lesion. Examination of the mobility of the epiglottis on contrast laryngography helps to assess the degree of spread to the pre-epiglottic soft tissues.

2. *Anterior half of the false vocal cords.* These carcinomas arise from the anterior part of the false vocal cord and tend to spread into the base of the epiglottis and across to the opposite side of the larynx. These growths do not infiltrate the true cords by submucous spread. Coutard (1932) and Hautant (1939) believe that this type of growth is more radiosensitive than any other type of extrinsic growth of the larynx.

3. *Posterior part of the false vocal cords.* These growths tend to infiltrate deeply and involve the arytenoid cartilages early and spread upwards into the aryepiglottic fold. Whilst tomography can demonstrate thickening of the cord with obliteration of normal structures, *e.g.* the ventricle, differentiation from oedema may only be possible by contrast laryngography. This may show destruction of the mucosa and impaired mobility of the cord, indicating cancer to be recognised. Involvement of the epiglottis or laryngeal cartilages may be evident in the lateral soft tissue views.

4. *Arising in the supero-lateral part of the vestibule* (aryepiglottic fold), fig. 329. Growths may arise in the

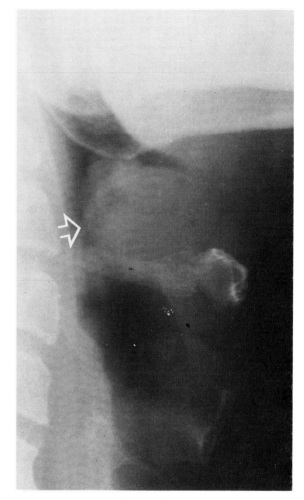

Fig. 328. Carcinoma of the epiglottis. An extensive tumour involving and destroying the bulk of the epiglottis. The destruction of the epiglottic cartilage can be seen.

superior part of the vestibule just below the level of the hyoid bone near the junction of the aryepiglottic fold with the pharynx. Advanced lesions involve the laryngeal surface of the epiglottis, the pyriform sinus, the posterior surface of the arytenoid and the posterior cricoid region. Extension into the ventricle of the larynx is unusual although the false vocal cord may be involved.

5. *Arising from the ventricle of the larynx.* These growths arise from between the true and false vocal cords. They spread rapidly upwards and downwards to involve both the true and false vocal

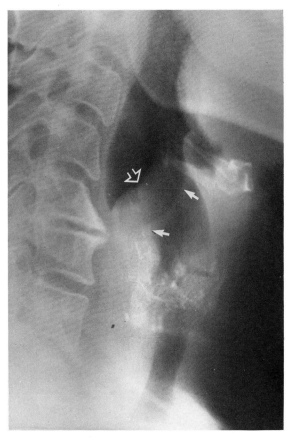

Fig. 329. Carcinoma of aryepiglottic folds. Solid white arrows indicate normal fold, hollow arrow shows upper limits of infiltrated aryepiglottic fold.

cords. They can be differentiated from growths arising in other parts of the true vestibule as these growths do not involve the true vocal cord.

Intrinsic growths arising in the vocal cord which have extended widely before treatment may be impossible to distinguish from growths of the ventricle.

SUBGLOTTIC GROWTHS. These growths arise in the true subglottic space and usually arise on the lateral walls. They invade the vocal cords only when the growth is advanced.

Radiological appearances. It has already been emphasised that when the growth is advanced to any degree it may not be possible to determine the actual site of origin until the growth has begun to recede under treatment. Basically, however, there is a general radiological pattern for these growths.

They are best examined in the lateral and in the postero-anterior tomograms. The features of these growths are:

(a) *Soft tissue tumour.* This feature is naturally more marked in the proliferative type of tumour. Early infiltrative lesions may be overlooked unless considerable care is taken in examining the films. With the infiltrative lesions thickening of a normal soft tissue marking may be the only radiological feature detectable and contrast laryngography is needed to show this change.

(b) *Distortion of the normal soft tissue markings.* The normal soft tissue markings may be obliterated or distorted. Diffuse thickening of the soft tissues usually implies infection or non-inflammatory swelling whilst localised thickening generally implies an infiltrative growth.

(c) *Mucosal changes.* Growths may also distort the normal markings by increasing the size and density of the soft tissue markings and replacement of the normal smooth mucosa by an irregular appearance may occur.

(d) *Fixity of the normal laryngeal structures.* Loss of density and loss of mobility of the laryngeal structures usually implies malignant infiltration.

(e) *Invasion of the laryngeal cartilages.* Upwards invasion of the root of the epiglottis can be mainly appreciated by the soft tissue enlargement of this structure. If the epiglottis is calcified then invasion and destruction of the ossified cartilage may be seen.

Invasion of the ala of the thyroid cartilage is more difficult to appreciate radiographically owing to the irregular manner in which the cartilage ossifies. Comparison with the ala of the opposite side is also valueless, but occasionally in the postero-anterior tomogram it may be possible to detect alterations in the structure of the thyroid cartilage indicating malignant invasion.

(f) *Recurrent laryngeal tumours.* Assessment of the recurrence of growth after radiotherapeutic treatment is one of the most difficult radiological problems. After radiotherapeutic treatment the soft tissues of the larynx show a generalised oedema maximal in about five weeks after treatment and gradually returning to normal.

Reliance on tomography with dynamic studies, *i.e.* films taken in (a) phonation, (b) blowing against resistance, and (c) at rest, are invaluable in assessing the signs described below.

Laryngography is not as successful in the treated case as adequate mucosal coating with contrast medium is more difficult to achieve under these conditions.

Of 21 cases in which radiographic examination was requested for the diagnosis of recurrent growth, nine cases showed recurrent tumour, four cases were reported x-ray positive, two suggestive and three recurrences were not detected. Twelve cases showed no recurrence and 10 cases were reported negative, and two more were incorrectly reported as showing recurrence (Rideout, 1975).

The radiological criteria for the diagnosis of recurrent tumour were:

(i) *Progressive localised swelling.* Persistent localised oedema following radiotherapy almost invariably means that some tumour remains, particularly so if the local swelling increases.

(ii) *Ulceration.* The development of ulceration almost invariably indicates recurrent growth.

(iii) *Decalcification* of the mineralised laryngeal cartilages also indicates spread of growth but it must be remembered that post-irradiation necrosis may develop. Xerography is useful in detecting fractures in the latter condition.

(iv) *Fixation and asymmetry* of the soft tissue shadows usually indicates progressive growth.

Sarcoma of the larynx. Havens & Parkhills (1941) observed that at the Mayo Clinic over a period of 30 years the ratio of sarcoma to carcinoma was 1:100. Although many types of sarcoma may involve the larynx, the fibrosarcoma (Clerf, 1946) is the commonest. Fibrosarcoma grows slowly and does not metastasise early but local recurrence may grow considerably faster than the original growth.

Figi (1933) maintained that as fibrosarcomas tend to infiltrate the laryngeal tissues less than carcinomas they remain operable for a considerably longer period. Chondrosarcoma may arise from laryngeal cartilage and may represent a malignant change in a chondroma (fig. 322).

Tracheal tumours

Tumours of the trachea are relatively uncommon. Cylindroma occurs most frequently in the cervical portion of the trachea (Clagett, Moersch & Grindlay, 1953), but carcinoma involving the lower third is by far the commonest tumour (Tinney, Moersch & McDonald, 1945).

These tumours present with wheezing or tickling in the throat, dyspnoea too is a prominent symptom. Routine x-ray studies are of no great value but tomography and Lipiodol contrast studies (tracheograms) may be diagnostic.

Histologically these tumours may be cylindroma, haemangio-endothelioma, squamous or adeno-carcinoma. Radiologically all four types appear as soft tissue tumours. Metastatic tumours may occur in the tracheal wall particularly arising from primary thyroid carcinomas (fig. 330).

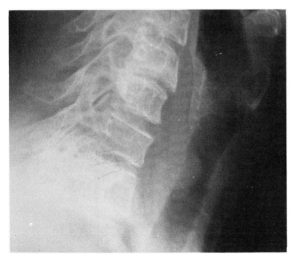

Fig. 330. Secondary deposit in trachea seen in lateral view. Primary growth in thyroid gland.

REFERENCES

AHLEN, G. & RANSTRÖM, S. (1944) Congenital Cysts in Early Infancy. *Acta otolar.,* **32,** 483.

ALBANESE, A. R. (1945) Duello: Tumor del Espacio Retrofaringoes: Neurofibroms. *Prensa méd. argent.,* **32,** 1763.

BACLESSE, F. (1946) Radiotherapie des cancers du larynx. *J. Radiol. Électrol.,* **27,** 63.

BACLESSE, F. (1949) Roentgentherapy in Cancer of Hypopharynx. *J. Am. med. Assoc.,* **140,** 525.

BACLESSE, F. & HENRY, R. (1950) Anterior Glottic Cancers, Radiographic and Radiotherapeutic Considerations. *J. Radiol. Électrol.,* **31,** 1.

BELANGER, W. G. & DYKE, C. G. (1943) Roentgen Diagnosis of Malignant Tumours. *Am. J. Roentg.,* **50,** 9.

CLAGETT, O. T., MOERSCH, H. J. & GRINDLAY, J. H. (1953) Intrathoracic tracheal tumours: Development of Surgical Technics for their Removal. *Trans. Am. surg. Ass., 70,* 224.

CLAUSEN (1932) Unusual Sequela of Tracheal Intubation. *Proc. R. Soc. Med., 25,* 1507.

CLERF, L. H. (1946) Sarcoma of Larynx: Report of 8 Cases. *Archs Otolar., 44,* 517.

COUTARD, H. (1932) Roentgen Diagnosis During Course of Roentgen Therapy of Epitheliomas of Larynx and Hypopharynx. *Am. J. Radiol., 28,* 293.

DAVIS, E. D. D. (1948) The Diagnosis and Treatment of Tumours of the Nasopharynx. *J. Lar. Otol., 62,* 192.

DIAMOND, E. H. & PERKINS, C. W. (1948) Calcified Haematoma of the Oropharynx Secondary to a Gunshot Wound. *Archs Otolar., 47,* 64.

EPSTEIN, B. S. & WINSTON, P. (1957) Intubation Granuloma. *J. Lar. Otol., 71,* 37.

EWING, M. R. & FOOTE, F. W. Jr. (1952) Plasma Cell Tumours of the Mouth and Upper Air Passages. *Cancer, N.Y., 5,* 499.

FERGUSON, G. B. (1944) Haemangioma of the Adult and of the Infant Larynx. *Archs Otolar., 40,* 189.

FIGI, F. A. (1933). Sarcoma of the Larynx. *Archs Otolar., 18,* 21.

FIGI, F. A., BRODERS, A. C. & HAVENS, F. Z. (1945) Plasma Cell Tumours of the Upper Part of the Respiratory Tract. *Ann. Otol. Rhinol. Lar., 54,* 283.

FIGI, F. A., ROWLAND, W. D. & NEW, G. B. (1944) Cystadenoma of the Larynx. *Archs Otolar., 40,* 445.

FREUNDLICH, I. M. & HODES, P. J. (1963) A Nasopharyngeal Fibroma Presenting with Pituitary and Optic Nerve Symptomatology. *Am. J. Roentg., 89,* 41.

FRIEDBERG, S. A. (1940) *Archs Otolar., 31,* 313.

GAY, B. B., WILKINS, S. A. & SAGELS, E. P. (1958) The Roentgen Characteristics of Chondroma of the Larynx. *Am. J. Roentg., 80,* 987.

HARTLEY, W., EVISON, G. & SAMUEL, E. (1965) The Pattern of Ossification in the Laryngeal Cartilages: a Radiological Study. *Br. J. Radiol., 38,* 585.

HAUTANT, A. (1939) *Ann. Otolar., 3,* 296.

HAVENS, F. Z. & PARKHILLS, M. (1941) Tumours of the Larynx Other than Squamous Cell Epithelioma. *Archs Otolar., 34,* 1113.

HOLMAN, C. B. & MILLER, W. E. (1965) Juvenile Nasopharyngeal Fibroma. *Am. J. Roentg., 94,* 292.

JACKSON, H., PARKER, F. & BETHEA, J. M. (1931) Plasmacytomata and their Relation to Multiple Myelomata. *Am. J. med. Sci., 181,* 169.

JING, B.-S. (1975) Roentgen Examination of Laryngeal Cancer: a Critical Evaluation. *Can. J. Otolar., 4,* 64.

JORGENSEN, J. et al. (1975) Radiography of Laryngeal Carcinoma. Assessment of Value. *Acta radiol. (Diag.), 16,* 367.

KELLY, D. B. (1950) Chondroma of Vocal Cord. *J. Lar. Otol., 64,* 195.

KLEINFELD, L. (1934) Laryngeal Cyst in Newborn. *Archs Otolar., 19,* 590.

LARSSON, L. G. (1951) Nasopharyngeal Lesions in Sarcoidosis. *Acta radiol., 36,* 361.

LEDERMAN, M. (1961) *Cancer of the Nasopharynx. Its Natural History and Treatment.* Springfield, Illinois: C. C. Thomas.

MARTIN, H. & BLADY, J. V. (1940) Cancer of Nasopharynx. *Archs Otolar., 32,* 692.

MARTIN, H., EHRLICH, H. F. & ABELS, J. C. (1948) Juvenile Nasopharyngeal Angiofibroma. *Ann. Surg., 127,* 513.

MARX, H. (1928) *Z. Hals-Nasen-u. Ohrenheilk., 21,* 376.

McCALL, J. W., DUPERTIUS, S. W. & GARDINER, F. S. (1944) Chondroma of the Larynx. *Laryngoscope, 54,* 1.

McCLURE, G. (1946) Odontoma of Nasopharynx. *Archs Otolar., 44,* 51.

NEW, G. B. & ERICH, J. B. (1938) Benign Tumours of the Larynx. *Archs Otolar., 28,* 841.

OLIVER, K. S., DIAB, A. E. & ABU-JAUDEH, C. N. (1948) Solitary Neurofibroma of the Larynx. *Archs Otolar., 47,* 177.

RIDEOUT, D. F. (1975) Appearances of the Larynx after Radiation Therapy. *Can. J. Otolar., 4,* 98.

RYAN, M. D. & ZIZMOR, J. (1949) Chondroma of Larynx. *Am. J. Roentg., 62,* 715.

STEINBERG, S. S. (1954) Pathology of Juvenile Angiofibroma, Lesion of Adolescent Males. *Cancer, N.Y., 7,* 15.

STOUT, A. P. & KENNEY, F. R. (1949) Primary Plasma Cell Tumours of the Upper Air Passages and Oral Cavity. *Cancer, N.Y., 2,* 261.

TINNEY, W. S., MOERSCH, H. J. & McDONALD, J. R. (1945) Tumours of the Trachea. *Archs Otolar., 41,* 284.

TUCKER, G. F. (1961) A Histological Method for the Study of Spread of Cancer Within the Larynx. *Ann. Otolar., 70,* 910.

TUCKER, G. F. (1962) A Histological Demonstration of the Development of Laryngeal Connective Tissue Compartments. *Trans. Am. Acad. Ophthal. Oto-Lar., 66,* 308.

TURCHIK, F. (1946) Schwannoma of Pharynx with Paralysis of Vocal Cord. *Archs Otolar., 44,* 568.

ZORNOVA, J., CANGIR, A. & GREEN, B. (1977) Hypertrophic Osteoarthropathy Associated with Nasopharyngeal Carcinoma. *Am. J. Roentg., 128,* 679.

Index

257